Nocturne

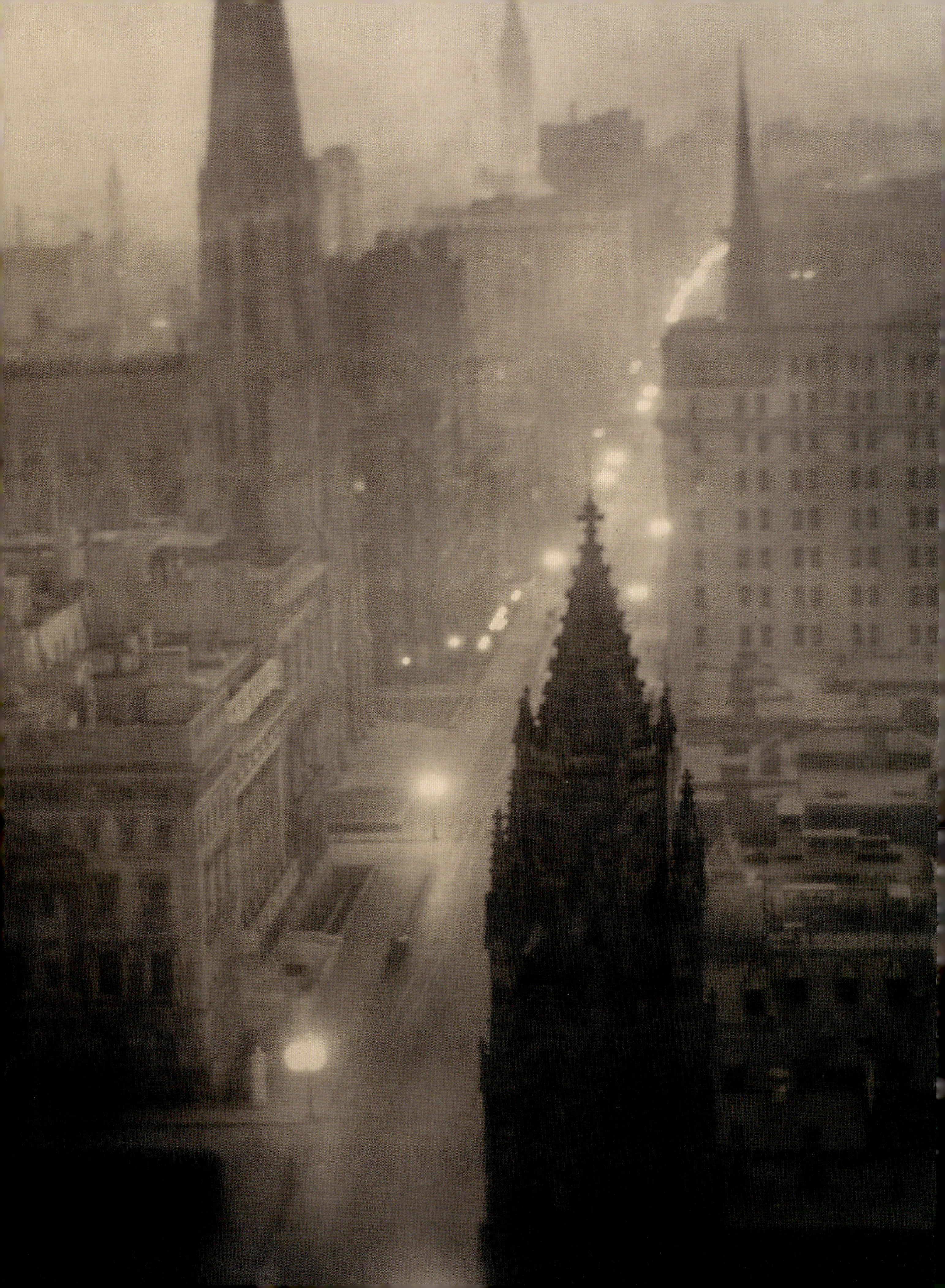

Nocturne

Night in American Art, 1890–1917

Hélène Valance

Translated by Jane Marie Todd

Yale University Press New Haven and London

This publication has been made possible through support from the Terra Foundation for American Art.

TERRA
FOUNDATION FOR AMERICAN ART

yalebooks.com/art

Designed by Leslie Fitch and Julie Allred
Set in Crimson and Source Sans Pro type by BW&A Books, Inc.
Printed in China by Regent Publishing Services Limited

Library of Congress Control Number: 2017961776
ISBN 978-0-300-22399-6

A catalogue record for this book is available from the British Library.

This paper meets the requirements of ANSI/NISO Z39.48-1992 (Permanence of Paper).

10 9 8 7 6 5 4 3 2

Jacket illustrations: (front) Childe Hassam, *Nocturne, Railway Crossing, Chicago,* 1893 (fig. 125, detail); (back) Winslow Homer, *Summer Night,* 1890 (fig. 9, destail).
Frontispiece: Alvin Langdon Coburn, *Fifth Avenue from the St. Regis,* c. 1905 (fig. 146).

For Elisabeth and Suzanne

Contents

Acknowledgments

Writing this book has been far from a solitary venture, and over the long course of its maturation I have received the help of many more people than I would be able to list here. I am grateful, first, to François Brunet and Michael Leja for their solid and constant support from the very first months of my doctoral research.

I have been time and again surprised by the generosity of American art scholars; from eminent professors to young scholars, many have taken the time to read and offer insightful criticisms on various stages of this manuscript. I owe much to Cynthia Mills and Bill Truettner, with whom I broached the topic of nocturne paintings more than ten years ago. I enjoyed discussing night and artificial lighting with Hollis Clayson, Sandy Isenstadt, and William Sharpe, and I hope to continue our conversations beyond this book. Sarah Burns, Martin Berger, Alan Braddock, and Alexander Nemerov provided great suggestions, as did my co-fellows at the Smithsonian American Art Museum: Anna Aranbindan-Kesson, Lacey Baradel, Sarah Beetham, Maggie Cao, Liam Considine, Seth Feman, Mazie Harris, Sara Levavy, Emily Liebert, Erin Pauwels, Alex Taylor, and Tatsiana Zhurauliova. Our weekly writing workshops remain among the most exciting and satisfying intellectual exchanges I ever experienced. The Terra Foundation for American Art summer residency in Giverny was the occasion of lively discussions with a community of young colleagues, among whom I particularly thank Ellery Foutch and Alison J. Carr for their astute reading of important passages of this book. I am tremendously thankful for Sophie Cras's admirable way of being at once so kind and so smart in her suggestions on vast parts of the manuscript.

I was impressed by the availability and warmth of the many museum curators I met during my research, and I am grateful for the conversations I had with Nancy Anderson at the National Gallery of Art in Washington, Anna Marley at the Pennsylvania Academy for the Fine Arts, Kathleen Foster at the Philadelphia Museum of Art, Joyce Schiller at the Delaware Art Museum, Kenneth Myers at the Detroit Institute of Art, Scott Shields at the Crocker Art Museum, and Harvey Jones at the Oakland Museum of California. The Terra Foundation for American Art has provided several generous grants and fellowships which, rather than simply make my research possible, turned it into an exceptionally comfortable venture. Above all, though, I am grateful to Veerle Thielemans, Francesca Rose, and Ewa Bobrowska at the Terra Foundation's offices in Paris. They have always offered helpful and benevolent advice as they watched this project grow through the years.

I feel very lucky for the friends I have made in the American art community, but I am just as thankful for the support of friends and family for whom this project could appear a bit exotic. I owe special thanks to my parents for patiently letting me wander so far away from them, and to Rémi Gauthier, who has followed me long enough to become an American art connoisseur malgré lui.

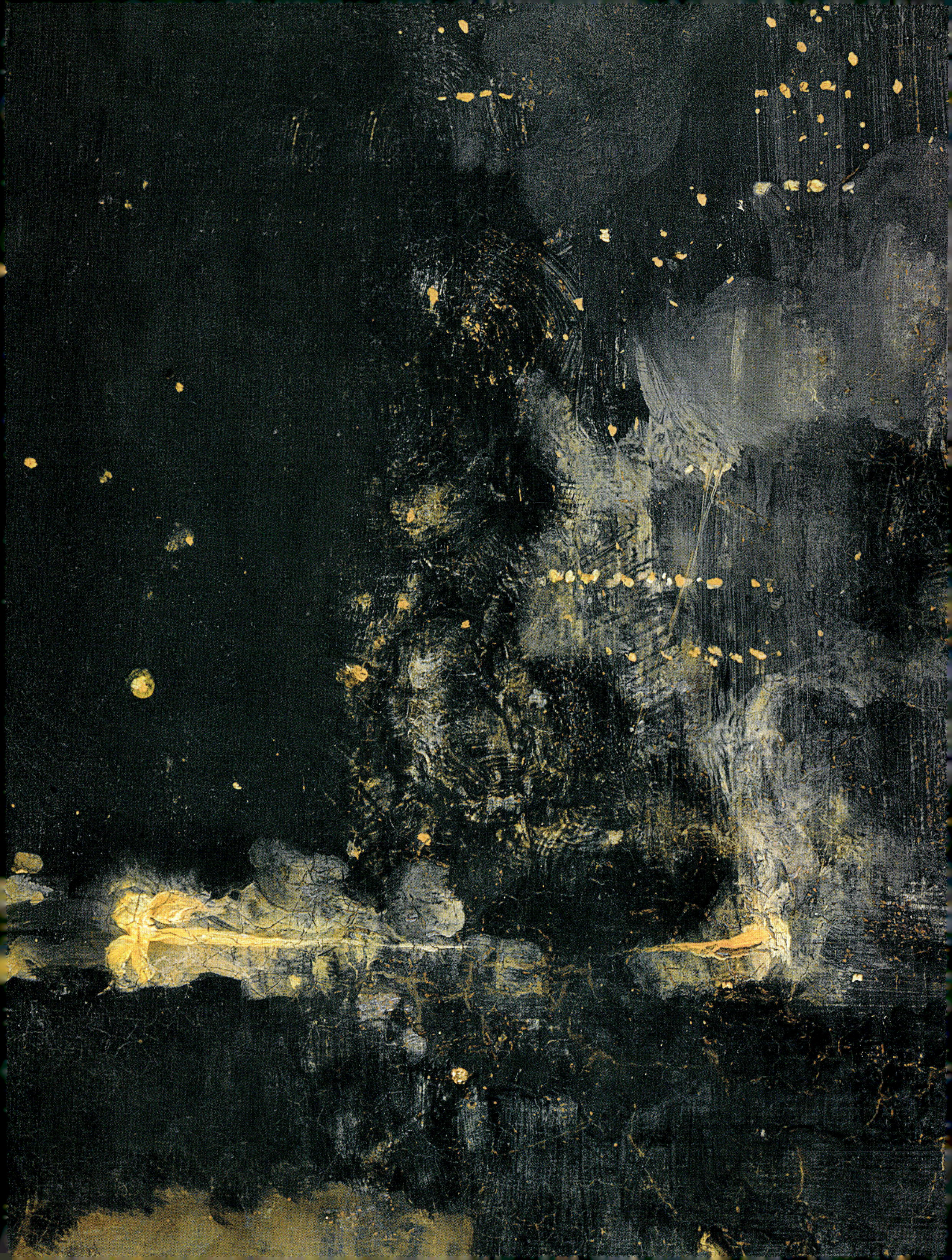

Introduction

In 1890 a short comic piece appeared in *Puck's Library* under the title "A Chapter in Art," in which the paintings stored away in a house's attic begin to talk. The main speaker in this exchange, a view of Mount Popocatépetl erupting, traces its career from fame to oblivion:

> When I first appeared in public, twenty-five years ago, I was the Artistic Success of the day. I am the work of an artist famous at that time. You may never have heard of him, for I believe he is now in the pork business in Cincinnati—but he was famous then. I was too good to be exhibited in the National Academy. I had a printed shrine in the innermost gallery of a great Art-Dealer. The critics came and bowed before me. They admired my glowing lava, the sunrise on my distant hills, my sparkling blue and white snow, my deep green forests and my bright blue sky. "Here," they said, "is American Art at one bound equaling and surpassing the Art of Europe. Here is the color of Titian, the touch of Rembrandt—" the grandeur of somebody else and the power of I don't know whom. A gentleman bought me. He had made a million in oil, and he paid seven thousand for me. He took me home to his magnificent mansion. He was just starting a picture-gallery, and he hung me there, under a magnificent catafalque of red cloth. People came and viewed me by special invitation. I was happy.
>
> But, alas, he went to Europe, and came back with a Schreyer, a Horace Vernet, a Kaulbach and an Achenbach. The moment I saw that Achenbach, I knew I was gone. He was two inches larger than me, all 'round. I came out of the catafalque—he went in. The next year a washy-gray Corot drove me out of the front parlor. I went into the dining-room, and was dislodged by a measly little black Rousseau. I went upstairs, and the march of art drove me from one bedroom to another—from the second story to third, from third to fourth.
>
> As the children grew up, I was passed from one to another. At last the youngest sent me to the attic, to hang in my place a water-color Whistler, with a salmon gray silk panel behind him.[1]

The fate of the Eruption, formerly acclaimed as the best in American art, is symptomatic of a radical change in American tastes in the late nineteenth century.

Fig. 10 detail

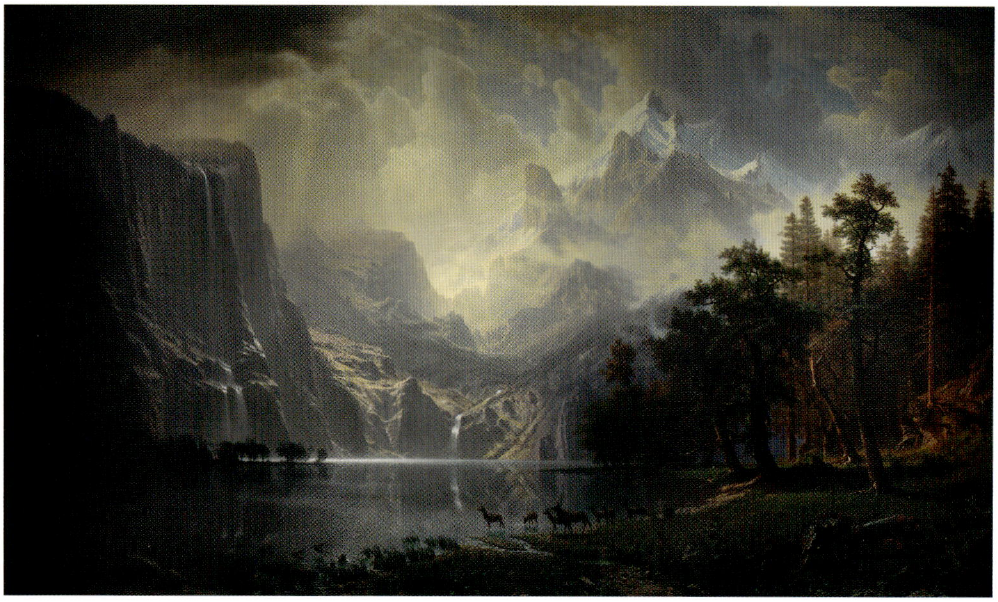

FIG. 1. Albert Bierstadt, *Among the Sierra Nevada, California*, 1868. Oil on canvas, 183 × 305 cm (72 × 120 1/8 in.). Smithsonian American Art Museum, Bequest of Helen Huntington Hull, granddaughter of William Brown Dinsmore, who acquired the painting in 1873 for The Locusts, the family estate in Dutchess County, New York (1977.107.1).

The decline of the painting, supplanted for the most part by European works, seems to point to the end of a certain notion of landscape painting associated with the definition of a national art for the United States. The multicolored, grandiose landscape of Popocatépetl brings to mind the favorite motifs of the leading American school of painting, the Hudson River School, which in the 1830s gave the United States an artistic legitimacy through a form of landscape painting that treasured spectacular views of majestic mountains, magnificent canyons, and verdant valleys illuminated by the setting sun. In celebrating the American continent's wilderness, artists of the Hudson River School contributed to the nationalist and imperialist discourse of their time: they supported the idea of Manifest Destiny, the belief that divine Providence would bestow America's extraordinary natural resources on the European settlers, so that they might found a new civilization on the continent.[2]

In highly detailed, colorful, large-format paintings, artists of the Hudson River School painted a natural world marked by the signs of divine presence, full of promise and ready to bow to the demands of its white conquerors (fig. 1). Those reading the piece in 1890 would have likely recognized the artist responsible for the Eruption—previously famous but now anonymous—as Frederic Edwin Church, a central figure in the Hudson River School, whose most celebrated paintings depict South American volcanoes.[3] Now, however, American landscape art, which according to mid-nineteenth-century commentators was a glorification of the new continent, had to step aside for a more cosmopolitan art and for landscapes where darkness and fog predominated: the German Oswald Achenbach is known for his night views of the Bay of Naples, while the Frenchmen Camille Corot and Théodore Rousseau produced intimist visions of hazy and shadowy landscapes (fig. 2). James McNeill Whistler personified the final phase of that change in perspective regarding landscape painting. An American living in Europe, he painted avant-garde canvases of the Thames and Venice shrouded in nocturnal darkness, a far cry from the glorious West of his predecessors (fig. 3).

The presence of Whistler's name on the list of works that dislodged the Eruption is significant. The generation

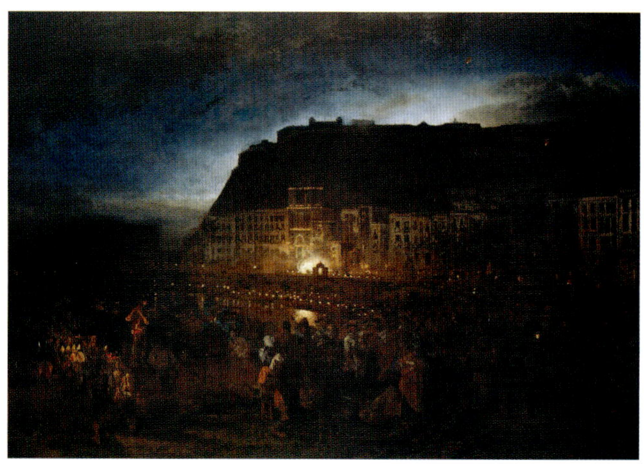

FIG. 2. Oswald von Achenbach, *Festival of Santa Lucia in Naples*, 1874. Oil on canvas, 141 × 197 cm (55 1/2 × 77 1/2 in.). Museumslandschaft Hessen Kassel, Neue Galerie, Städtischer Kunstbesitz.

FIG. 3. James McNeill Whistler, *Nocturne, Blue and Silver: Battersea Reach*, c. 1872/78. Oil on canvas, 29.4 × 62.9 cm (11 1/2 × 24 3/4 in.). Isabella Stewart Gardner Museum, Boston.

that succeeded the painters of the Hudson River School abandoned depictions of the American wilderness and its wide open spaces, devoting themselves almost systematically to an art that favored atmospheric effects, with a preeminent place given to nighttime. And the nocturnal landscape was primarily Whistler's domain. From 1866 to the mid-1880s, Whistler produced a series of night landscapes characterized by almost monochromatic abstraction: turning away from the political realism of his master Gustave Courbet, Whistler pushed his formal experimentation to an extreme form of art for art's sake. He thus gave new impetus to the centuries-old tradition of moonlight landscape painting. In the nocturnal landscapes of the great painters in that genre from the seventeenth and eighteenth centuries—Aert van der Neer and Claude Joseph Vernet, for example—the composition is laid out around a full moon. Lively scenes unfold below, featuring many human figures depicted in great detail. Their orderly arrangement is reminiscent of the classic seascapes of Claude Lorrain (figs. 4, 5). John Atkinson Grimshaw, an English painter and Whistler's contemporary, adapted these moonlights to the modern landscape of the London night illuminated by gaslight (fig. 6). Whistler, though he borrowed from these predecessors, also innovated by removing the sources of light, which are reduced to flickers or reflections, and immersed the human figures and the details of the landscape in a misty distance. He wanted to invent a genre in its own right, not just rework a certain style: indeed, on the advice of his client Frederick Leyland, Whistler borrowed the musical term "nocturne" from Frédéric Chopin to designate his moonlights.[4] From the 1870s on, the artist strove to have the nocturne recognized as his trademark. In a letter to his student Walter Greaves, Whistler, who was afraid that Greaves would copy him too faithfully, claimed his moonlights as his own invention and insisted that "never in the history of art had they been done."[5]

Despite the reservations expressed by Whistler, by the 1890s his nocturnes were being widely emulated: a search through the sales catalogues of paintings by American artists turns up more than three hundred works titled *Moonlight* or *Nocturne* between 1890 and 1917.[6] Some artists, such as Ralph Albert Blakelock and Charles Rollo Peters, specialized in night landscapes; Peters even

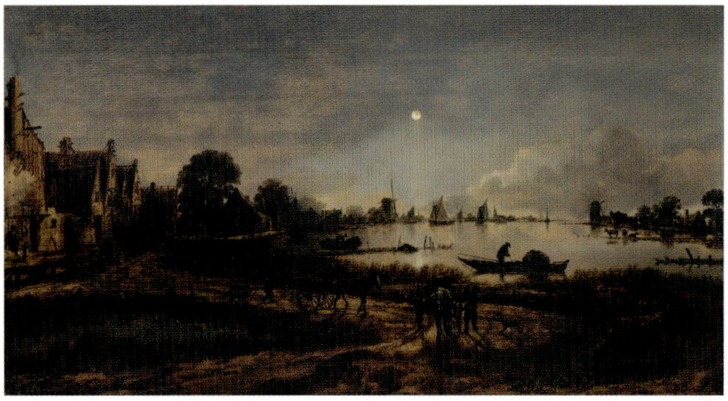

FIG. 4. Aert van der Neer, *River View by Moonlight*, c. 1640–50. Oil on panel, 55 × 103 cm (21 ½ × 40 ½ in.). Rijksmuseum, Amsterdam.

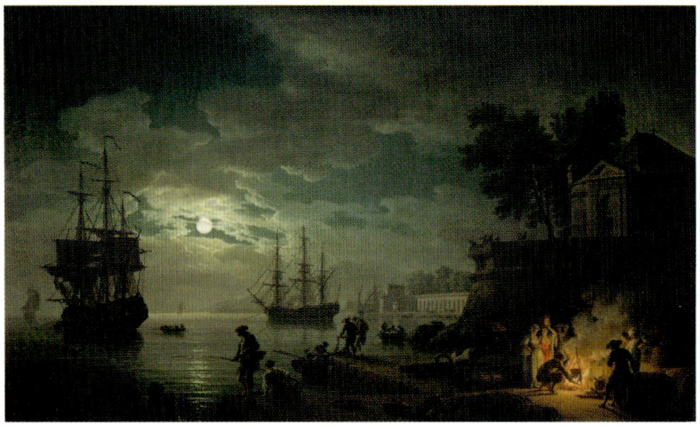

FIG. 5. Joseph Vernet, *Night, a Port in Moonlight*, 1772. Oil on canvas, 98 × 164 cm (38 ⅝ × 64 ⅝ in.). Musée de Louvre, Paris, France.

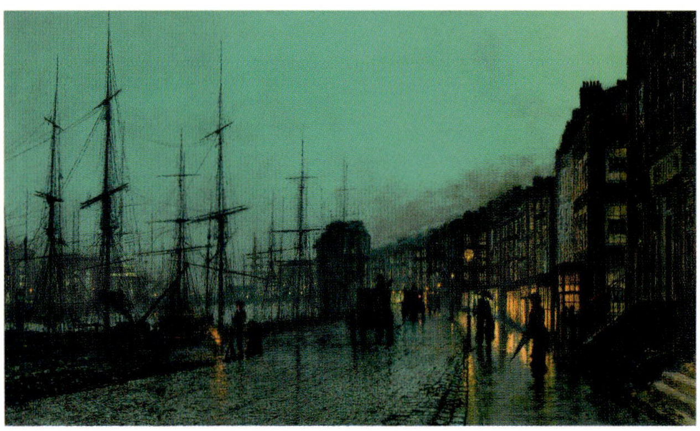

FIG. 6. John Atkinson Grimshaw, *Shipping on the Clyde*, 1881. Oil on cardboard, 30.5 × 51 cm (12 × 20 ⅛ in.). Carmen Thyssen-Bornemisza Collection, Museo Thyssen-Bornemisza, Madrid.

acquired the nickname "Prince of Darkness."[7] The genre was therefore distinctive enough to create an artistic personality and lucrative enough to support a professional career (figs. 7, 8). Its success was confirmed in 1913, when William A. Clark purchased one of Blakelock's moonlights for $13,900, at the time the highest price ever paid for the work of a living American artist.[8] Most American artists of the period understood the public appeal of night landscapes and adapted it to their own style. Artists already identified with particular themes, such as the illustrator Frederic Remington (who specialized in depictions of the Old West) and the realist painter Winslow Homer (who, beginning in the 1880s, devoted most of his oil paintings to fishing scenes set on the coast of Maine), applied the filter of nocturnal darkness to their pictures (fig. 9; see also fig. 53). As the ultimate proof of its popularity, the genre even became a joke among the young artists of the Society of American Fakirs of the Art Students' League. An article in the *New York Times* reports their salon parody of 1902: "'Oft in a Silly Night,' taken from R. A. Blakelock's picture, is the first winner. . . . A 'Nocturne' by Whistler is a favourite with the Fakirs. One of the take-offs is a mass of black ink, with a bunch of matches in place of the fireworks. Another shows a building burning dimly on a very dark night. A third consists of a couple of black cats on the back fence on a night so dark that they can't see their paws in front of them."[9]

What could explain such an infatuation with the night? The craze epitomized Whistler's success—as belated as it was sudden—in his native country. At the start of his career, in fact, his aesthetic commitment to art for art's sake and his provocative style had resulted in a mixed reception among American critics and the public. The extreme abstraction of his nocturnes aptly illustrated the artist's convictions. Whistler explored the entire range of aesthetic possibilities, combining visual and auditory perceptions in a sensorial experience that was as intense as it was harmonious, but he refused to attach any but formal values to his art. He had no interest in subordinating the ideal of beauty to moral precepts, or in using aesthetic refinement to "elevate" the intellect and the morals of the masses, or in allowing "devotion, pity, love, patriotism, and the like" (all "clap-trap" in his view) into his works.[10] Whistler therefore proposed a definition of the nocturne as an ascetic art, an almost scientific abstraction: "By using the word nocturne I wished to indicate an artistic interest alone, divesting the picture

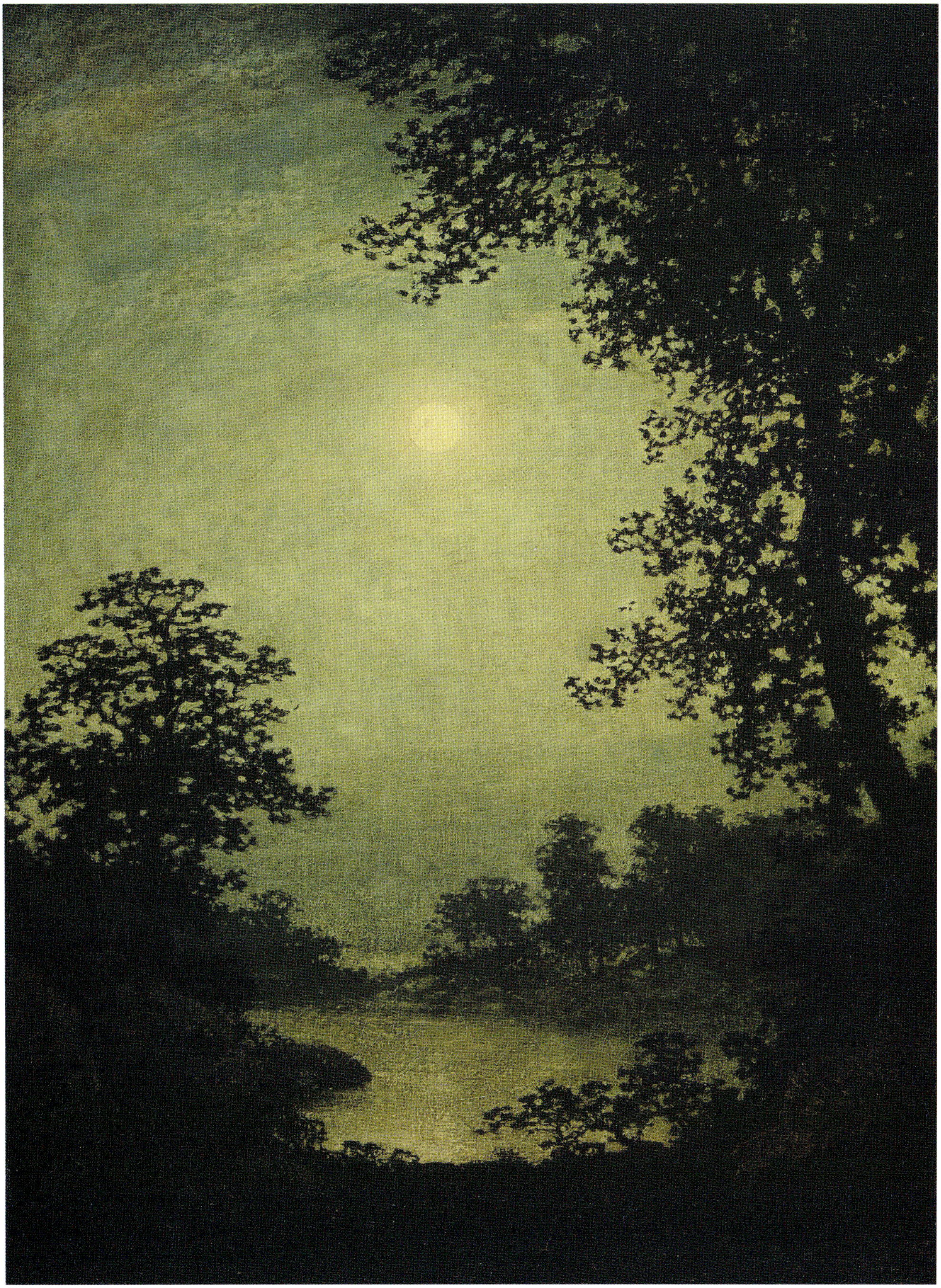

FIG. 7. Ralph Albert Blakelock, *Moonlight Sonata*, c. 1889–92. Oil on canvas, 77.2 × 55.9 cm (30 ⅜ × 22 in.). Museum of Fine Arts, Boston. The Hayden Collection—Charles Henry Hayden Fund (45.201).

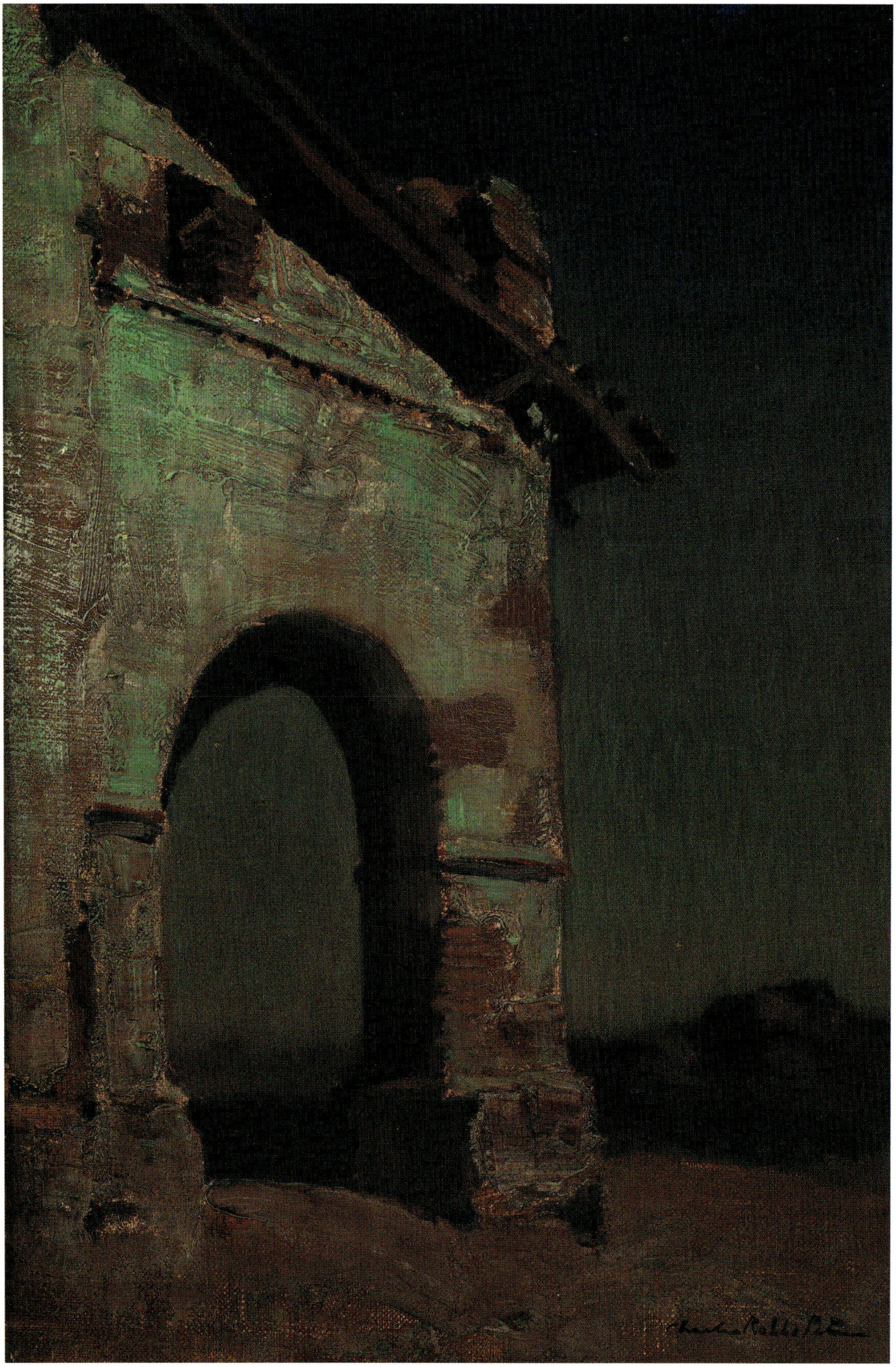

FIG. 8. Charles Rollo Peters, *San Fernando Mission*, n.d. Oil on canvas, 61 × 40.1 cm (24 × 15 3/4 in.). Crocker Art Museum, gift of William C. Wright, conserved with funds provided by the Historical Collections Council of California Art (1962.23).

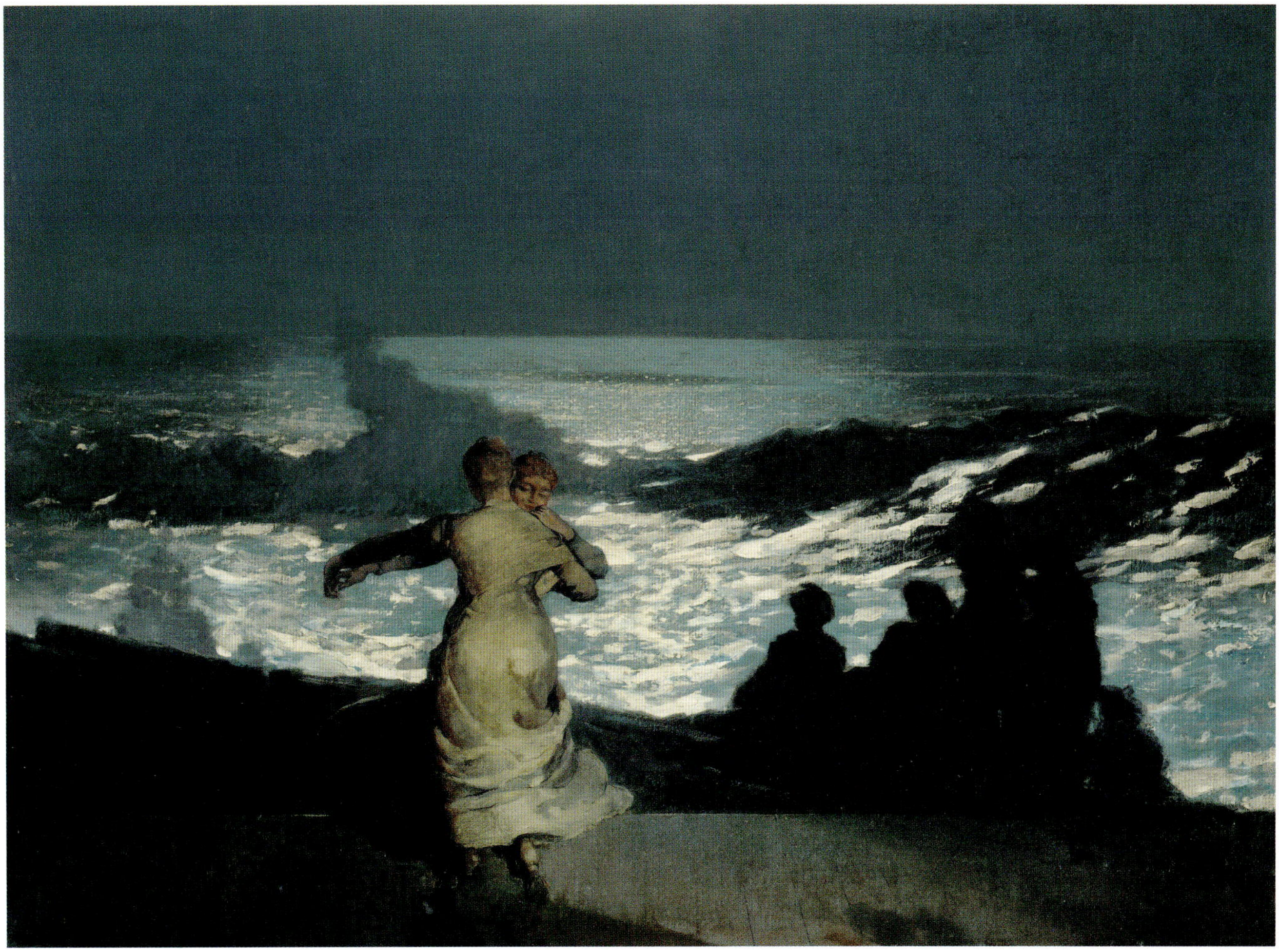

FIG. 9. Winslow Homer, *Summer Night,* 1890. Oil on canvas, 76.7 × 102 cm (30 1/4 × 40 1/8 in.). Musée d'Orsay, Paris.

of any outside anecdotal interest which might have been otherwise attached to it. A nocturne is an arrangement of line, form, and color first."[11] Joris-Karl Huysmans, in his portrait of Whistler, captured the intransigent formalism of his paintings. According to Huysmans, Whistler's nocturnes were "far from modern life, far from everything, at the far reaches of painting, which seem[s] to evaporate into invisible puffs of colors on these light canvases."[12]

Because of this radical aesthetic stance, Whistler was long regarded with suspicion in his home country.[13] In 1877, Henry James, who, unlike many of his compatriots at the time, could hardly be accused of provincialism, expressed a certain perplexity upon viewing Whistler's nocturnes: "Mr. Whistler's experiments have no relation whatever to life, they have only a relation to painting."[14] A year later, Whistler achieved notoriety when he sued the English critic John Ruskin for libel. Ruskin, outraged by the formal abstraction of *Nocturne in Black and Gold: The Falling Rocket,* had accused Whistler of mocking his audience: "I have seen, and heard, much of Cockney impudence before now; but never expected to hear a coxcomb ask two hundred guineas for flinging a pot of paint in the public's face" (fig. 10).[15] That lawsuit by a young American artist against one of the most respected figures of art criticism worked to Whistler's advantage, in that it made him better known in the United States. Nonetheless, because few of his paintings were exhibited outside Europe at the time of the scandal, the artist was generally greeted with incomprehension.[16] The major turning point in Whistler's career occurred in 1890, when the French government purchased *Arrangement in Black and Grey: Portrait of the Artist's Mother.*[17] That honor, rarely extended to an American painter, completely changed Whistler's reception in the United States. Previously considered a capricious artist of dubious taste, he now became one of the most prominent figures in American

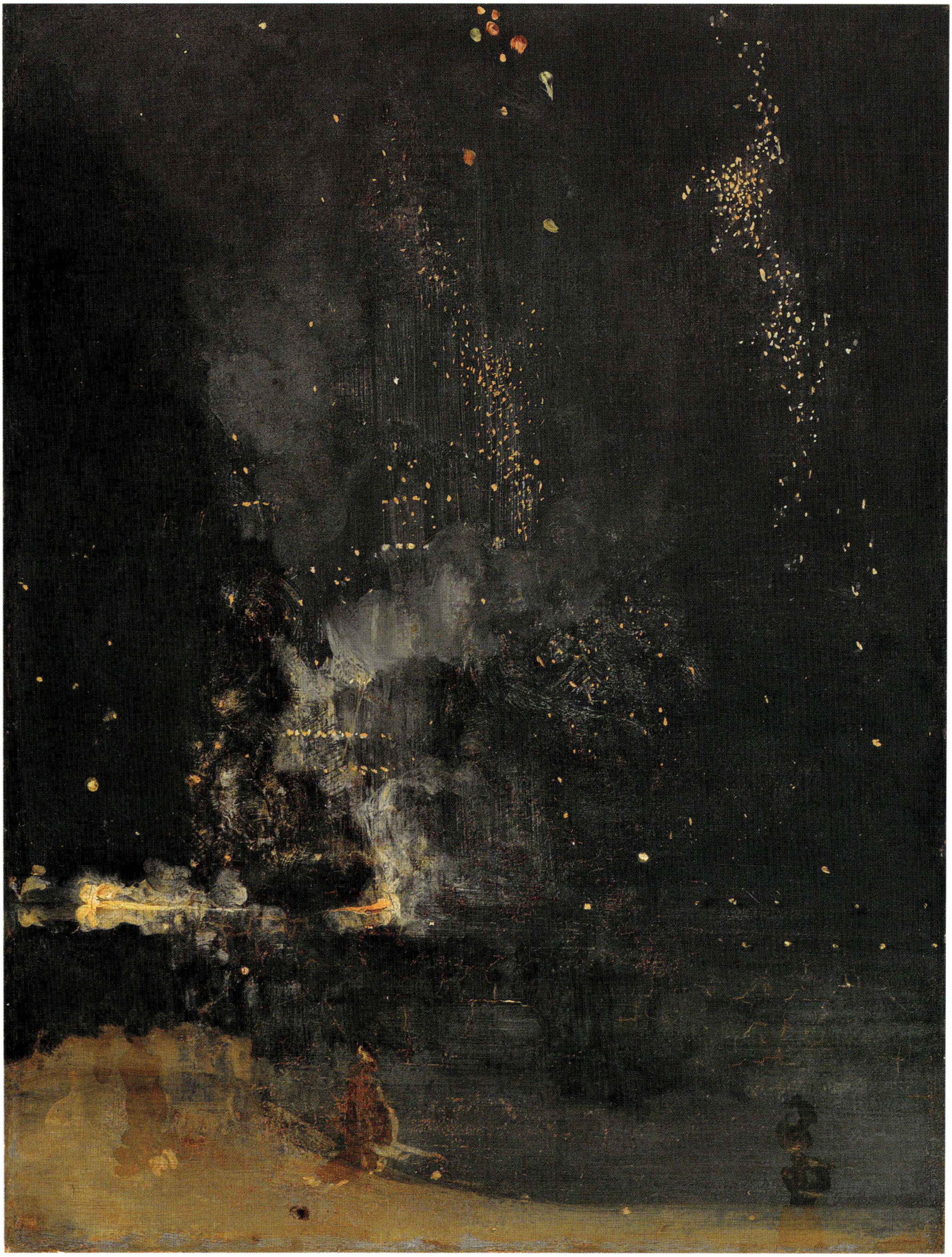

FIG. 10. James McNeill Whistler, *Nocturne in Black and Gold: The Falling Rocket*, 1875. Oil on panel, 60.2 × 46.7 cm (23 11/16 × 18 3/8 in.). Detroit Institute of Arts. Gift of Dexter M. Ferry Jr.

life, sparking admiration that would continue to grow over the years. Upon the painter's death in 1904, the "Whistler Memorial" exhibition in Boston, a veritable manifesto of the Whistleresque aesthetic, ushered the artist into the American canon and introduced his works to the general public. On the eve of World War I, Ezra Pound, in a poem titled "To Whistler, American," did not hesitate to erect Whistler into a national hero alongside Abraham Lincoln.[18]

Like impressionism, which was just beginning to be appreciated by the American public during this same period, Whistler's works took about twenty years to cross the Atlantic. It was only in the 1890s or later that the young painters who had followed the artist to Europe started to have a certain success among their compatriots. In 1894 the *Art Journal* declared of Whistler: "There is no man who has had a more far-reaching influence upon the younger generation of painters."[19] The critic John Van Dyke observed ten years later: "[Whistler's] pictures are widely scattered and are now being eagerly bought up by collectors. . . . His influence has spread far and wide with the schools of today, and every picture exhibition of the last dozen years has had its modicum of Whistleresque pictures."[20] In the case of landscape paintings, the artist's emulators did not form a school in the strict sense, but critics sometimes identified them by the term "tonalism," which echoed the association that Whistler, in adopting the term "nocturne," had established between painting and music.[21] His works served as a model for a variety of artists, from the painters who had known him in Europe and had followed his teachings there to those who, despite a style and aesthetic convictions very different from Whistler's, nevertheless showed signs of his influence. On the whole, the American artists were undeniably responsive, if not to Whistler's theories, then at least to the mark he left on the tastes and expectations of the public and of potential buyers.

◆ ◆ ◆

The vogue for nighttime, however, can be attributed not only to Whistler but also to a favorable cultural environment particularly consonant with the aesthetic strategies of the nocturne. In reality, the success of the nocturne can be explained by the many profound resonances—sometimes only implicit—between the night, with all the symbolism attached to it, and the changes affecting the era. In that sense, the nocturne must be understood primarily within its historical context: in the late nineteenth century, night, one of the rare phenomena of human experience that seemed truly universal and immutable, entered history. With the advent of electricity, night was suddenly vulnerable to technological conquest and assumed the dimension of a new frontier, similar to the one that was vanishing with the advance of capitalist civilization.[22] The cultural values of nighttime were thereby profoundly transformed.

In his *Electrifying America: Social Meanings of a New Technology, 1880–1940,* the historian David Nye addresses Paul Valéry's idea that "the general innervation of the world [by electricity] has more far-reaching consequences and a greater capacity to modify life in the future than all the 'political' events that have occurred between Ampère's time and our own."[23] Nye considers electrification in the United States, from 1880 to World War II, to have been a "social process" intimately connected to a whole series of historical phenomena, from urbanization to the restructuring of the market, from developments in literature and the fine arts to the advent of advertising and the leisure industry. Between 1880 and 1890, experiments in electric lighting multiplied: electricity began to appear in theaters and department stores; it was installed in the homes of millionaires; it illuminated a few fashionable neighborhoods in great cities, as well as national landmarks such as the Statue of Liberty (in 1886) and Niagara Falls (in 1907). Above all, electric lighting was deployed on a grand scale at the World's Fairs, allowing visitors to glimpse the brilliant future of American cities, the apotheosis of which would be the lights of Broadway, "the Great White Way" (fig. 11).[24] Nye, analyzing the baffled reactions of commentators on the international exposition's spectacle, advances the idea of an "electrical sublime" that profoundly altered the perception of the landscape: "Dramatic lighting made possible the revisualization of landscapes, filling them with new meanings and possibilities."[25] In the matter of electric lighting, the United States took a decisive lead over other Western countries at the dawn of the twentieth century. Even as nighttime underwent a more radical change in America than it did elsewhere, representations of the night in American art acquired a density of their own.

This night about to surrender to the assaults of technology took on a nostalgic cast when portrayed by the nocturne artists. In this context, the repetition of the nocturnal motif looks like a hostile reaction to change.

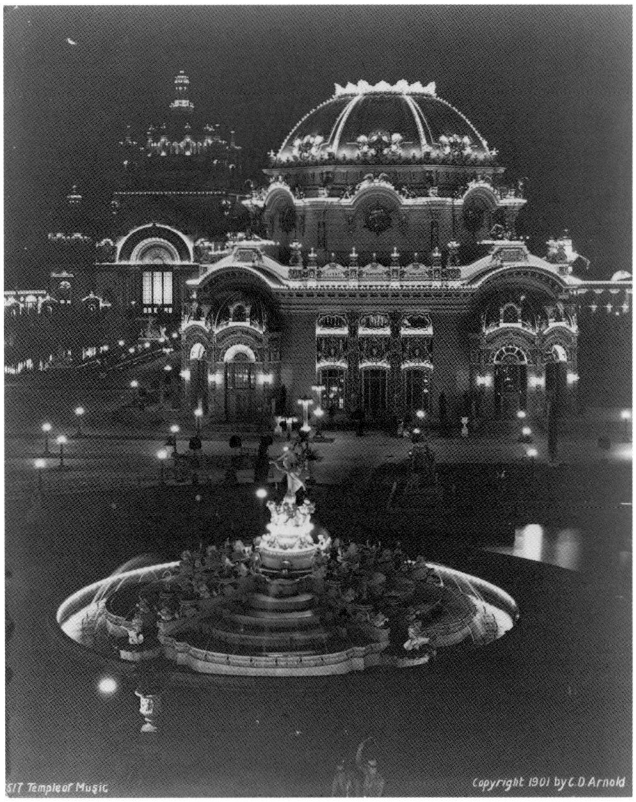

FIG. 11. Charles D. Arnold, *Temple of Music at Night, at the Pan-American Exposition, Buffalo, New York*, c. 1901. Photograph, 25 × 34 cm (9 ¾ × 13 ⅜ in.). Library of Congress, Prints and Photographs Division, Washington, D.C.

The darkness that artists sought to capture on their canvases sometimes acquired the opacity of a screen that kept modern reality at a distance. An oft-cited excerpt from the famous lecture "Mr. Whistler's 'Ten O'Clock,'" in which the painter describes nightfall in the industrial districts along the Thames, explicitly formulates the role of night: "And when the evening mist clothes the riverside with poetry, as with a veil, and the poorer buildings lose themselves in the dim sky, and the tall chimneys become campanili, and the warehouses are palaces in the night, and the whole city hangs in the heavens, and fairyland is before us—then the wayfarer hastens home; the working man and the cultured one, the wise man and the one of pleasure, cease to understand, as they have ceased to see, and Nature, who for once has sung in tune, sings her exquisite song to the artist alone, her son and her master—her son in that he loves her, her master in that he knows her."[26] Here Whistler is playing on paradoxes: the veil of night is revealing to anyone who knows how to see; conversely, the artist's gesture no longer shows but conceals. For Whistler, night covered with an enchanting darkness the modern landscape of factories and smokestacks that lined the banks of the Thames, transforming them into a vision ready to be reproduced by the artist. Night in and of itself was sufficient to turn the landscape into an image.

◆ ◆ ◆

But the nocturne was more than a melancholic reminder of a lost night or a screen concealing the advance of the modern transformations of the landscape. Although the radical changes in the visual representation of the night produced by the introduction of electric lighting were undeniably important, this immediate and almost self-evident context coexisted with more deep-seated motivations. Night fascinated American artists and their public because, through its representations, there circulated a set of cultural meanings that resonated profoundly with the everyday lives of Americans and with a modernity to which they sometimes struggled to adapt. Darkness proved to be a particularly fitting source of cultural representations through which to address a number of these new phenomena, whether scientific, technological, political, or social. The murkiness of the nocturne, for example, cast its spell over the American public at a time when the discovery of X-rays was calling into question the definition of the visible and the invisible. The conquest of the West was declared at an end in 1890, and American Indians suffered violent defeats in their last battles against whites. As it happened, the aesthetics of darkness was remarkably congruent with the idea of an Indian people destined to vanish. The play of shadows and silhouettes in the nocturne also gave a visible form to the new social relations, midway between anonymity and proximity, that Americans were discovering in urban life. These few examples show that the nocturne ought to be understood as an art in dialogue with its environment, one that reflected the deep-seated tendencies affecting that environment, and which in turn changed their direction.

This contextual definition of the nocturne, however, runs counter to its most common characterization: it was often considered, both by those who practiced it and by commentators, as a transcendent art that stood apart from its material context. Artists and critics repeated over and over again that nocturnes were works outside time, that they had no relation to their environment. In a treatise on landscape painting, the tonalist

Birge Harrison noted that two-thirds of American painters practiced the genre, a tendency he saw as the rejection of an environment bearing the stamp of modernity:

> Another cause of this universal return to nature is doubtless the fact that our lives are not, humanly speaking, so beautiful as they once were. . . . The advent of farm machinery has destroyed much of the pastoral and bucolic beauty of country life. . . . Even our buildings have deteriorated—at least from the artist's point of view; for the comfortable villa farmhouse of the present day does not cling lovingly to the soil and become part of the environing landscape, as did the spreading, low-hung buildings of our fathers. And so, to quench the eternal thirst for beauty, we must needs return once more to kindly nature, whose beauty is exhaustless and everlasting.

Harrison immediately qualified that invitation to paint nature. Artists ought not to celebrate wilderness landscapes, as the artists of the Hudson River School did. Rather, they should favor blurriness and darkness: "But, precious beyond all other things, [nature's] exquisite and ever-varying effects—that happen because of the change from night to day and from day to night again—are spread out always before us, an endless feast of beauty for those who have eyes to see and minds to appreciate."[27] Like Harrison, many nocturne artists professed a supercilious detachment from the social, economic, and technological realities of the age. One journalist distinguished between the country's artistic and its material development, contrasting a wholly atmospheric art to a reality whose contours were too sharp and whose colors too bright: "Art does not readily adapt itself to new conditions. It is tenacious of formulae and of established precedent and tradition; it harks back to the past, and lingers with the glamour and the dream. The kaleidoscopic changes in the action and color of the glaring present confuse the vision and the understanding, and impelled by his very nature the painter or sculptor retires to a world of the unreal in an enriched atmosphere of other times, rather than cope with the jarring motives of the day."[28]

Harrison's traditionalist tendencies were not unusual among nocturne artists, the vast majority of whom belonged to the white male elite living in the large urban centers of the United States, and whose political opinions were generally conservative. In pleading for a "universal return" to an "immutable" nature, where night would cover with an aestheticizing veil the least appealing aspects of the modern landscape, nocturne artists promoted an art that seems to have been chiefly reactionary.

◆ ◆ ◆

But darkness is never perfectly opaque, and night is always pregnant with ambiguous visions. The veil of night, because it allowed one to envision at a respectful distance what would be more difficult to consider directly, also opened a field of complex negotiations and contributed to the acceptance of a new cultural, social, and political environment. This dialectical relationship, which took shape through the artists' use of the nocturnal atmosphere, can be better understood in terms of the concept of "antimodernism" advanced by the historian T. J. Jackson Lears, who analyzes the fascination of American elites of the late nineteenth and early twentieth centuries with cultures diametrically opposed to their own, whether that meant the Catholic religion, medieval culture, or Asian art and philosophy. Subjected to the previously unknown pressures of a rapidly changing environment, members of the upper classes of American society tended to turn to cultures that offered them an aesthetic and spiritual escape. But Lears shows that, paradoxically, this fascination also allowed them to adapt better to the very thing they were attempting to flee: "Antimodernism was not simply escapism; it was ambivalent, often coexisting with enthusiasm for material progress . . . a complex blend of accommodation and protest."[29] That concept will provide a framework for analyzing the relationship between nocturnes and their historical context: representations of the night are characterized by a dual movement of rejection and acceptance, dissociation and adaptation, very similar to the attitude Lears describes.

The ostensible detachment nocturne artists displayed toward their environment has only rarely been called into question by critics and art historians, who in many cases merely repeat in their turn the rhetoric of the artists on whom they are commenting. Most of the texts devoted to the nocturnes point out their mysterious, poetic, and oneiric character, thus supporting the view that such paintings were impervious to their material context.[30] Some recent studies, however, have begun to revise that stereotype. To quote a few important examples: the catalogue accompanying the exhibition *Like Breath on Glass* analyzes, in the light of science and religion, the "art of painting softly" to which the nocturne belongs.[31] In *Painting the Dark Side,* Sarah Burns considers the moonlight painter Albert Pinkham Ryder from a new angle, contesting what she considers a sanitized interpretation of his nocturnes, and examines Ryder's "dirty pictures" within the context of a Victorian society obsessed with control and hygiene.[32] The three essays that accompany the catalogue for the National Gallery's 2003 exhibition of Frederic Remington's nocturnes view them from the perspective of the artist's professional career, the trauma of the Spanish-American War, the end of the conquest of the West, and the development of electric lighting technologies.[33] Finally, a recent exhibition entitled *Night Visions: Nocturnes in American Art, 1860–1960* at the Bowdoin College Museum of Art has provided a sense of the scope and depth of the nocturnes movement.[34] In the present book, I will continue and deepen these reflections and extend them to a large corpus of nocturnal images. My approach seeks to demonstrate that this corpus constitutes a coherent artistic movement and, beyond it, a particularly significant cultural phenomenon profoundly anchored in a pivotal moment of American history.

The connections I draw between the darkness deployed in the nocturnes and aspects of their historical context call for a reflection on the methods to be used here. My examination of artworks often lies halfway between art history and cultural history. I emphasize how the works are related to their environment, endeavoring to move beyond traditional hierarchies between the fine arts and the rest of "visual culture," that is, cultural images and products that do not belong directly to the fine arts but which constitute a veritable ecosystem within which artists move on a daily basis. Since my concern is primarily to explore the cultural values of nighttime, I will regularly consider, alongside nocturnal landscapes in the strict sense, works that may more readily be called "night scenes." These illustrate the artists' and the public's relation to darkness and will allow for a better understanding of the issues underlying the nocturne genre. I will also ground my argument in comparative analyses of advertising images, popular illustrations, and even scientific photographs. Consistent with the most recent contributions in the field of the history of American art, I will therefore pay attention both to the uniqueness and materiality of the works concerned and to their political content, as well as to the role these images played or aspired to play in American society. The position occupied by the image—whether an elitist work of art or a commonplace illustration for an advertisement—is in fact an integral part of its meaning. For example, in cases where formal blurriness was perceived as a mark of social distinction, the materiality of the image was inseparable from its conditions of production and diffusion and from its sociocultural status. I will therefore be obliged to consider the social tensions and power issues on display in the nocturnes, while also taking into account what the images, their creators, the institutions that promoted them, and the public that consumed them say about the role they played in the sociocultural sphere.

The chronological and geographical boundaries of this book should be understood as the porous borders of a diffuse movement. The vogue for the nocturne was part of a very cosmopolitan artistic trend. The works of American painters attest in the first place to their interest in Asian art and particularly in artists such as Utagawa Hiroshige, whose famous representation of Kyōbashi Bridge inspired Whistler's *Nocturne: Blue and Gold—Old Battersea Bridge* (figs. 12, 13). Incidentally, the views of the Thames painted by Whistler later influenced, in turn, the artist Kobayashi Kiyochika, who specialized in prints of nocturnal landscapes (fig. 14).[35] The appeal of the Orient is one of the most significant forms of antimodernism that Lears describes. In reality, the fascination of American elites with Japanese art, motivated by a rejection of Western modernity, sheds light on the American context as much as it evinces a real appreciation for Japanese art and culture. Another source of influence for the American nocturne at the turn of the twentieth century—or at least, a basis for comparison—was the European symbolist movement, which made nocturnal darkness one of its favorite themes. Given the growing circulation of works and reproductions by American painters in the late nineteenth and early twentieth centuries and their increasingly international careers, it is impossible to ignore the connections between American nocturnes and the symbolist movement. Notably, Whistler exhibited with Les XX in 1884 and 1888 and regularly associated with Stéphane Mallarmé in Paris.[36] But American artists seem above all to have fixed on the most conservative aspects of the movement. They had more of an affinity with the solitary and ethereal landscapes

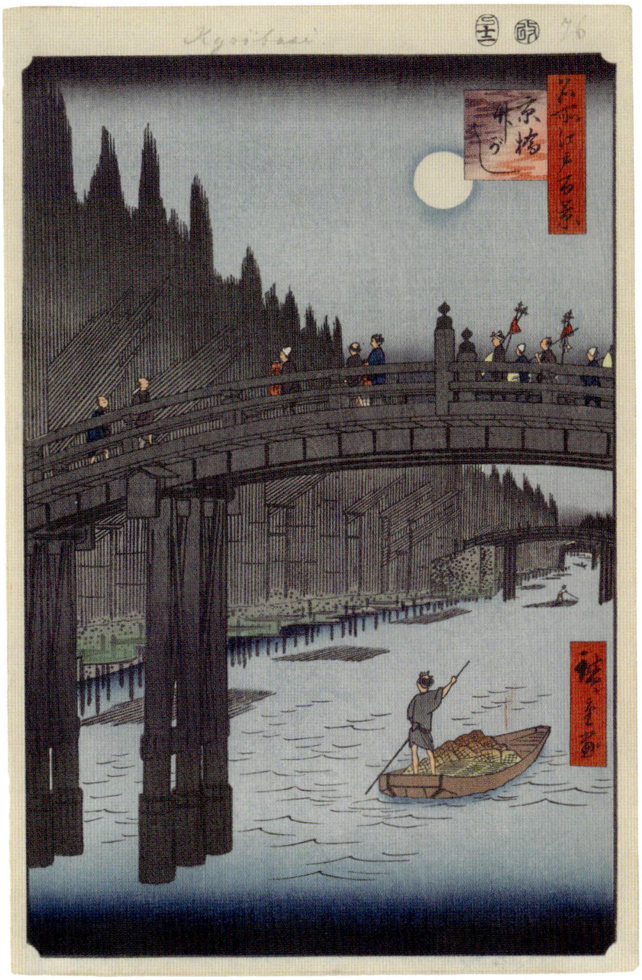

FIG. 12. Utagawa (Ando) Hiroshige, *Bamboo yards, Kyōbashi Bridge, No. 76*, from *One Hundred Famous Views of Edo*, 1857. Woodblock print, sheet, 36 × 23.5 cm (14 3/16 × 9 1/4 in.). Brooklyn Museum of Art, New York, Gift of Anna Ferris (30.1478.76).

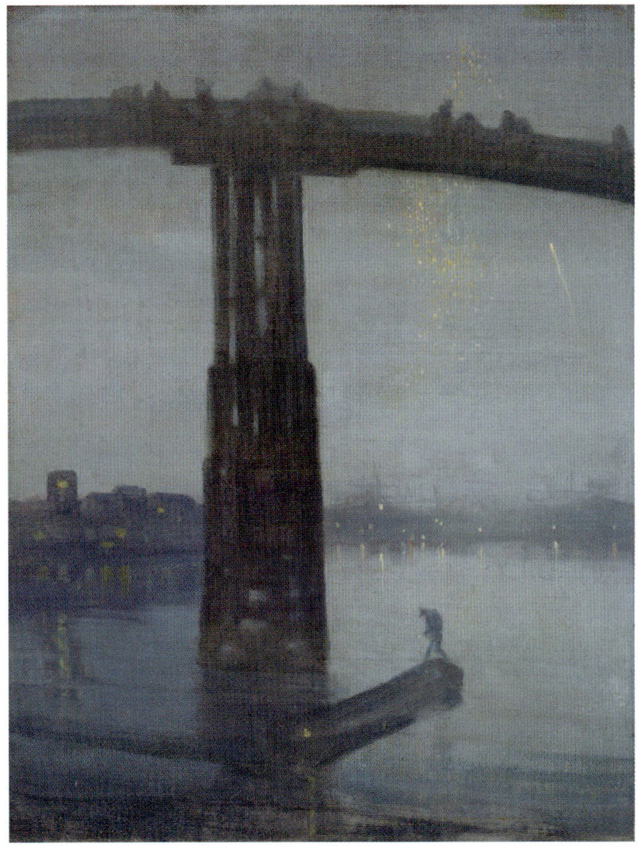

FIG. 13. James McNeill Whistler, *Nocturne: Blue and Gold—Old Battersea Bridge*, c. 1872–75. Oil on canvas, 68.3 × 51.2 cm (26 7/8 × 20 1/8 in.). Tate Collection, London.

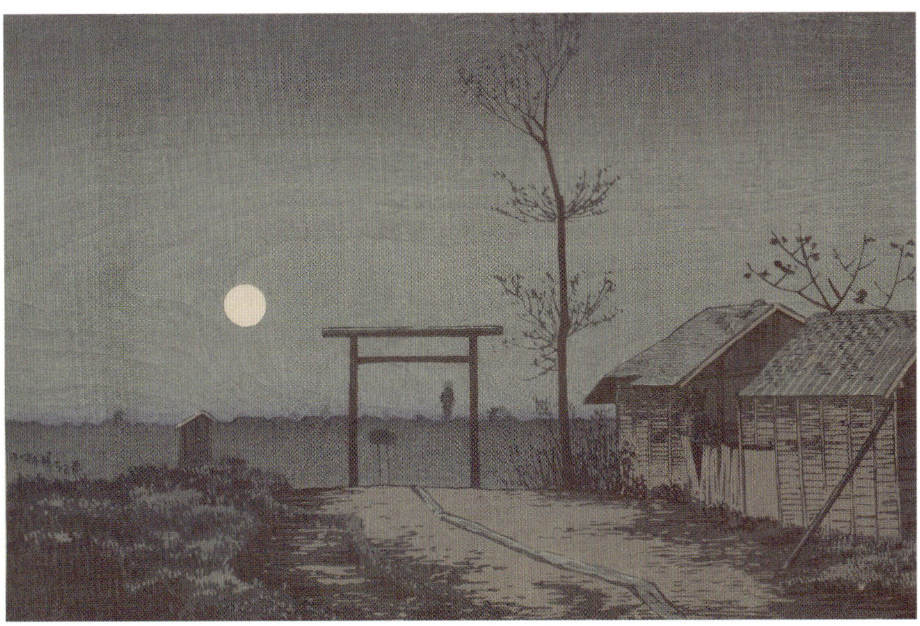

FIG. 14. Kobayashi Kiyochika, *Before Tarō Inari Shrine at Asakusa Ricefields*, 1881. Woodblock print, 21.2 × 32.1 cm (8 3/8 × 12 5/8 in.). Arthur M. Sackler Gallery, Smithsonian Institution, Washington, D.C. Robert O. Muller Collection (S2003.8.1174).

of William Degouve de Nuncques than with provocative visions such as Ferdinand Hodler's *Night* (figs. 15, 16).

Without neglecting the dialogue American artists maintained with nocturnal paintings from European and Asian cultures, I shall center this study on the role of the American nocturne in its own specific context. Like their predecessors, the artists active in the United States around 1900, as well as their critics, were very concerned with the "Americanness" of their art. Although the question was not new, it took a new turn in the late nineteenth century, when global exchanges were increasing. Many artists did not hesitate to spend a few years or even their entire careers abroad, and large-scale events such as the World's Fairs gave rise to an art market in which the various national schools competed.[37] The ambivalence that Whistler met with in the United States, ranging from rejection because he was too European to symbolic repatriation, was emblematic of that American identity, which fluctuated between an increased permeability to cosmopolitan influences and the need to continue to assert cultural preeminence through a few leading figures. I am less concerned here with determining how much American artists borrowed from their European or Asian fellows than with understanding what accounts for the extraordinary success of the nocturne in the United States during this period. Rather than attempt to establish subtle distinctions among national artistic movements, I have opted for a study restricted to the United States, but one that takes into account a broad historical

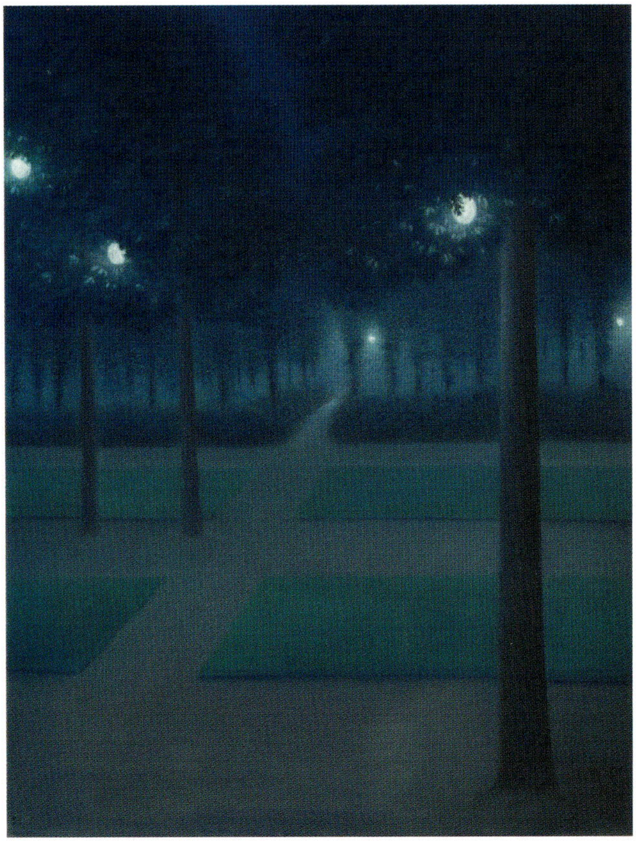

FIG. 15. William Degouve de Nuncques, *Nocturne in the Parc Royal, Brussels,* 1897. Pastel, 58 × 44.5 cm (22 7⁄8 × 17 1⁄2 in.). Inv. RF38999, Musée d'Orsay, Paris.

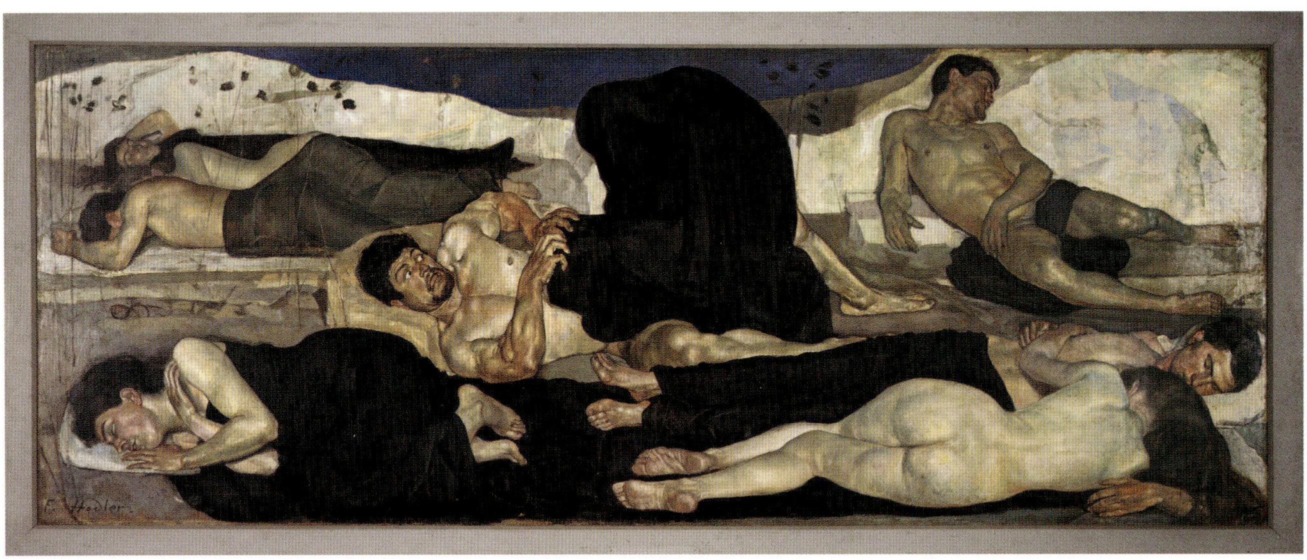

FIG. 16. Ferdinand Hodler, *Night,* 1890. Oil on canvas, 116 × 299 cm (45 5⁄8 × 117 3⁄4 in.). Kunstmuseum, Berne, Staat Bern.

field, extending beyond the realm of art history. This approach is founded on the principle that the vogue for the nocturne is to be explained in terms of its historical context. Certain aspects of that context will be shown to be specific to the United States, while others apply to Western cultures generally. In both cases, I will attempt to bring to light the deep-seated tendencies that inform artistic representations and to show how artistic representations, in turn, inflected these tendencies.

The dates chosen to define the period highlight the specificity of the American nocturne, by pointing out the intimate relationship between the movement and its historical conditions. The nocturne gained particular visibility in the early 1890s, when Americans discovered or rediscovered Whistler's oeuvre; it declined very sharply beginning in the mid-1910s, with the introduction to the United States, especially at the Armory Show of 1913, of a resolutely modernist art.[38] But these dates are significant for another reason: the year 1890 marked the official closing of the frontier that separated "civilized" America from the "wild" West, while 1917 marked the advent of a new phase in the United States' international politics. The enormous changes of that period form the three thematic axes around which I have organized this book. In Part I, I will consider nocturnes as a response to the incursions science and technology were making in the realm of the invisible and to the exponential growth of images. I will show how the nocturne artists sought to define a canon that distinguished them from other producers of images, by promoting an inward-looking vision that appropriated the recent discoveries of psychology. In Part II, I will explore how the medium of darkness became a metaphor for race, at a time when the United States was moving from the conquest of the North American continent to imperialism overseas, and when social tensions within the country were polarized around racial segregation and lynching. In Part III, I will examine the urban night, a space where identities and social relations were being refashioned in an environment subject to spectacular transformations. Although my approach is primarily thematic, I shall note a certain progression over the years. The nocturne allowed its beholders to adapt to modern realities, and that evolution in content is also apparent in the formal aspects of the genre. Rural moonlight landscapes, clearly traditionalist at the beginning of the period, gradually gave way to increasingly urban scenes, with aesthetic choices moving closer and closer to modernism. From the twilight of one century to the dawn of another, the night unfolding on the canvas acted as a transitional space.

PART I

Antivisions

The Redefinition of Vision by Science and Technology

The nocturne's antimodernism resides, first, in the ambivalent response it gave to the development of visual culture in the late nineteenth century. At a time when the visible and the invisible were being profoundly transformed by the various advances of science and technology, and when the image was gaining ascendancy in American culture, nocturne artists, in marking their preference for a realm that verged on the indiscernible, expressed mixed feelings toward the changes in the sphere of the visible.

That reconfiguration of the visible in both senses—what it is technically possible to see and what is accessible to the gaze on a daily basis—forced the nocturne artists to define a type of vision specific to their art. Even as they sought to detach themselves from a visibility aggressively asserted by science and technology, they were inspired by a different form of vision, one that was vague and inward-looking, for which they proposed a formal correspondence in their works. They dwelt on a darkness revealed, sometimes incidentally, by the spectacular discoveries and inventions of the time. In that sense, the nocturne introduced an atypical mode of vision, which expressly defined its role within the context of a visual environment in crisis: nocturnes, contradictory images that vexed the eye, were above all reactionary in the broad sense, encompassing both the political and the aesthetic. The nocturne, in conspicuously placing itself outside the field of the visible, raised a series of related questions: What is sight? What is representation? By what criteria may the various forms of vision and representation be distinguished? What is the artist's role in this new visual culture? Two intertwining threads emerge. The questions raised by the upheaval in the technological and scientific realm of vision often intersect those relating to the social status of the visual, of taste, and of the value of representation for individuals and society as a whole. The nocturne, in moving inward toward an art where less is seen, and even, strictly speaking, where there is almost nothing to see, imposed a new form of perceiving, consuming, and interpreting the image. Nocturnal landscapes, antivisions in the sense that they ran counter to their visual environment, nevertheless elicited an attitude that was much more complex than mere rejection. They fascinated the public because they put into play their affinities with the new zones of darkness paradoxically brought to light by progress. The nocturne, in becoming the image of a darkness resistant to ordinary modes of seeing augmented by technological advances, offered a vision it portrayed as truer and more profound.

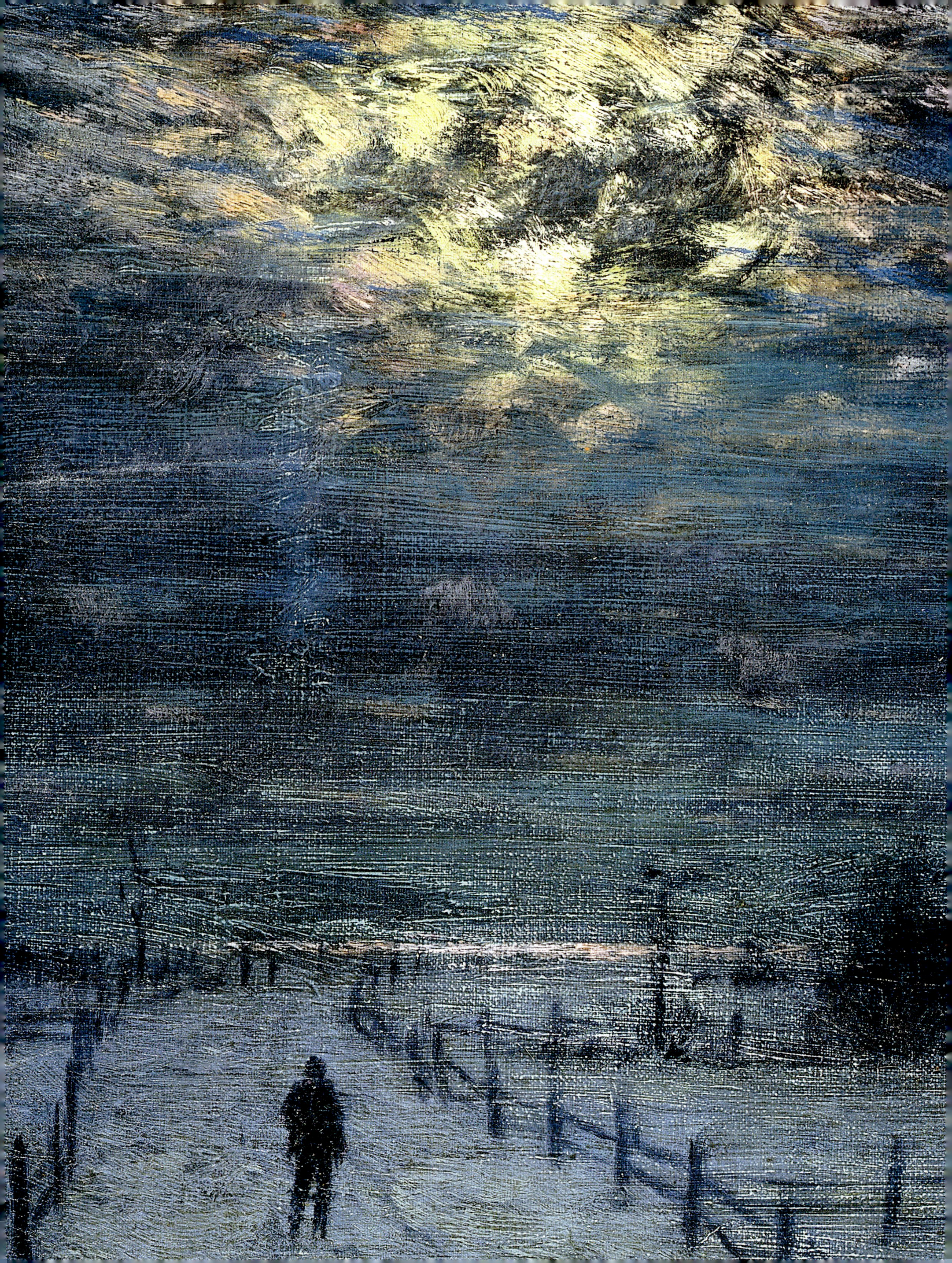

1 A Paradoxical Aesthetics

Whistler's radical formal practices and his highly polemical writings first prescribed the aesthetics of the nocturne genre. These prescriptions, adopted by his disciples and by critics, were erected into a systematic grid for interpreting the works of art. They promoted a paradoxical genre of painting, an antivision in the sense that the aesthetic codes that defined them rested on an almost systematic reversal of the traditional principles of landscape painting, a form of antipainting—beginning with the choice of darkness, which, with respect to almost the entire Western pictorial tradition, seemed to make no sense at all. Nocturnes, visual objects located at the limit of the perceptible, served to impede vision, thereby radically calling into question the beholder's relation to the work. In reconfiguring the space of the picture and its mode of perception, nocturne artists suggested a type of contemplation that might appear relatively esoteric. The nocturne, distinguished by its very indistinctness, was both directed against a certain practice of art and conceived as an exclusionary tool. The exclusion in question went beyond mere aesthetics, assuming social and political dimensions.

A PARADOX OF PAINTING

Painting the night is a self-contradictory exercise. The nocturne, in giving priority to darkness and indetermination, turned the principles of pictorial representation on their head. In 1435 Leon Battista Alberti had written in *De pictura:* "No one would deny that the painter has nothing to do with things that are not visible. The painter is concerned solely with representing what can be seen."[1] Before the nocturne painters relinquished their canvases altogether to darkness, the Western pictorial tradition had long rested on the equivalence between light and painting. The baroque chiaroscuro partly called into question that assumption—Nicolas Poussin supposedly said of Caravaggio that he had "come into the world to kill painting"[2]—but it maintained a certain balance between shadow and light, always kept together. In the late nineteenth century, the European avant-garde painters upset that equilibrium. When, in the mid-1880s, impressionism was introduced to the United States, the movement was immediately acknowledged to be an art of light. Critics welcomed one of the first American exhibitions of the impressionist school in words such as these:

Fig. 24 detail

FIG. 17. Herman Dudley Murphy, *Murano*, 1907. Oil on canvas, 50.2 × 77.5 cm (19 ¾ × 30 ½ in.). Private collection.

"A flood of white light streams from the walls of the South Gallery at the Fine Arts Building as one enters the sixteenth exhibition of the Society of American Artists. From the line well up the walls this blinding, dazzling whiteness springs to the eyes like the reverberation of the sun on long whitewashed walls in France or Italy." The critic, contemplating a canvas that depicted a sunlit garden, concluded: "The effect is one of electric lights. These young painters seem determined, like modern science, to teach the sun his place as a luminary that is well enough in his way, but no great shakes after all."[3]

Where impressionism exploited light to the point of artificiality, the nocturne opted for obscurity, a choice that marked a radical revision of artistic conventions. It ejected sources of light from the picture field or reduced them to faint glimmers. Darkness, formerly the negative pole of chiaroscuro, became the very subject of the painting, diffusing attention over a limited field of chromatic nuances and often refusing to offer a focal point for the eyes. The nocturnal landscape, in deliberately dissociating paint and light, thus not only challenged a long pictorial tradition but also and above all assaulted the modalities of vision underlying it. The nocturne artist affirmed that he could paint what is unseen and even what prevents sight, and that the product of his labor had to be considered from a point of view other than that of direct vision. That may account for the violent reaction of one of Whistler's critics, who denounced his nocturnes as "a contradiction in terms."[4] Herman Dudley Murphy's *Murano*, which exaggerated the already extreme principles of the Whistleresque nocturne, thus stands as a limit case of painting: the contours dissolve into a nearly monochrome landscape; the few points of light subtly suggesting a horizon line accentuate the blurriness and darkness more than they disrupt it (fig. 17). The work frustrates the gaze at least as much as it satisfies it and conceals more than it shows.

That new approach to landscape painting emerged within a particular historical context and revealed its underpinnings. Even as the nocturne constituted an unusual phenomenon within the pictorial tradition, the enthusiasm it generated was something of a paradox for

FIG. 18. James McNeil Whistler, *Nocturne in Blue and Gold: Valparaiso*, 1866/c. 1874. Oil on canvas, 76.4 × 50.7 cm (30 1/16 × 19 15/16 in.). Freer Gallery of Art, Smithsonian Institution, Washington, D.C. Gift of Charles Lang Freer (F1906.127a–b).

the culture in which it developed. The historian Neil Harris describes the turn of the twentieth century as a "visual age, the first time that the picture, the print, the cartoon, and the photograph had been produced on so large a scale. Newspapers and popular magazines, exploiting halftone pictures and photogravure, transformed their traditional appearance. And electricity's many marvels dazzled the eye."[5] The nocturne, by contrast, turned away from light and color, proposing a visual product distinct from the rest of images. As Americans were becoming aware of the massive presence of the visual in their culture, the nocturne artists partly rejected the usual notions attached to the production of images and declined, precisely, to represent them. At a time when American culture was beginning to discover itself through the mass image, the unusual practices adopted by nocturne artists appeared deliberately outmoded.

A THWARTED VISION

More than the choice of night as subject of an image, it is the aesthetic principles defining the nocturne canon that violated the traditional pictorial codes of landscape painting. Academic landscape painting, established by Claude Lorrain in particular, carefully arranged the space into clearly identifiable successive planes organized around

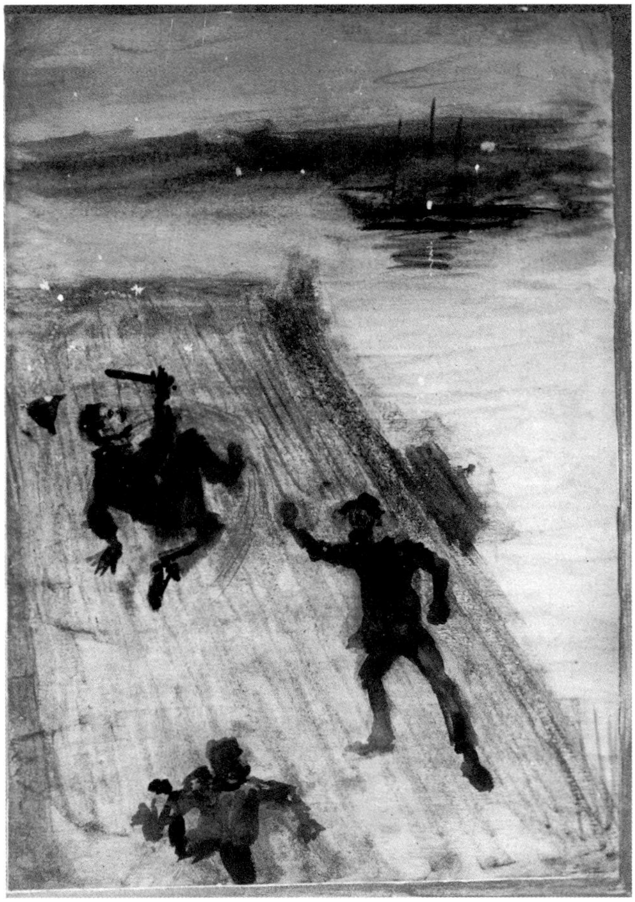

FIG. 19. Unidentified artist, *Knock-Turn, Paralyzo,* 1893–94. Ink on paper, 10.1 × 16.5 cm (3 × 6½ in.). Courtesy of the Pennsylvania Academy of the Fine Arts, Philadelphia. Dorothy and Kenneth Woodcock Archives.

a rigorous perspective: trees and colonnades framed the scene depicted, while the gaze was guided by various visual relays (figures, ruins, bodies of water) toward a horizon located in the center of the canvas. In the nocturne, by contrast, the uncommon, very spare composition and the extremely restricted palette emptied the landscape of its substance.

Landscape painting's conventions were called into question, first, through a revision of the composition's proportions, which became a shared formula for Whistler and his disciples. The horizontal, rectangular space of the canvas was divided up unequally to form a disproportionate relationship: either the horizon was placed very high, between a misty landscape or body of water and a sky reduced to a mere ribbon of color; or, conversely, the horizon was drawn very low, and the picture field was occupied by a vast expanse of sky. Courbet reportedly said of Whistler, when he was still a student, "Little Whistler has talent, but he always makes the sky too low or the horizon too high."[6] In either case, the horizon line is barely visible, and the two fields it is supposed to separate blend into each other in subtle tonal transitions. The nocturne, in neutralizing the foreground of the painting and eliminating the traditional contrasts—the visual reference points that create the illusion of depth—subjects the beholder to a disorienting spatial experience, a landscape that alternates between painted surface and dizzying precipice. A caricature of Whistler's *Nocturne in Blue and Gold: Valparaiso,* done by a young artist at the Pennsylvania Academy of the Fine Arts, targeted that very property of the nocturne, its way of turning spatial relationships on their head. In this illustration, called *Knock-Turn, Paralyzo,* the caricaturist lifted the veil of Whistler's serene night: concealed behind it are two men involved in a brawl, while a third, a police officer no doubt, moves in on them (figs. 18, 19). Beyond the comicality of this prosaic interpretation of nightlife on the docks, the title and the characters in the painting also satirically capture the sensation of disequilibrium produced by Whistler's deliberately out-of-proportion and unstable composition.

The "subject" of the landscape is itself often fluid, evanescent, formless. The tonalist artist Léon Dabo invented the term "airscape" to designate the conspicuous dematerialization of a landscape in which the land had become superfluous (fig. 20).[7] A good number of nocturne artists, imitating Whistler's views of the Thames, chose waterscapes with flat, unhindered perspectives (fig. 21). The optical properties of the water also thwart the gaze: whereas in Murphy's *Murano,* the sources of light reflecting on the water's surface allow one to determine the position of the horizon and to grasp the painting as a *landscape,* in Henry Ossawa Tanner's *Disciples See Christ Walking on the Water,* the play of reflections initially disorients the beholder, who must gradually reconstruct the scene's spatial organization (fig. 22). One of Whistler's critics had already reproached his nocturnes for confusing the beholder by failing to use solid elements of the landscape as reference points: "As pictures they are a dreamland of cloud, vapor, smoke; and so little subject have they that they are just as comprehensible when turned upside down."[8] The expanse of water reflecting the darkened sky thus functions as the opposite of a landscape, even as its obliteration. In that regard, it is not surprising, either, to find so many snowy landscapes

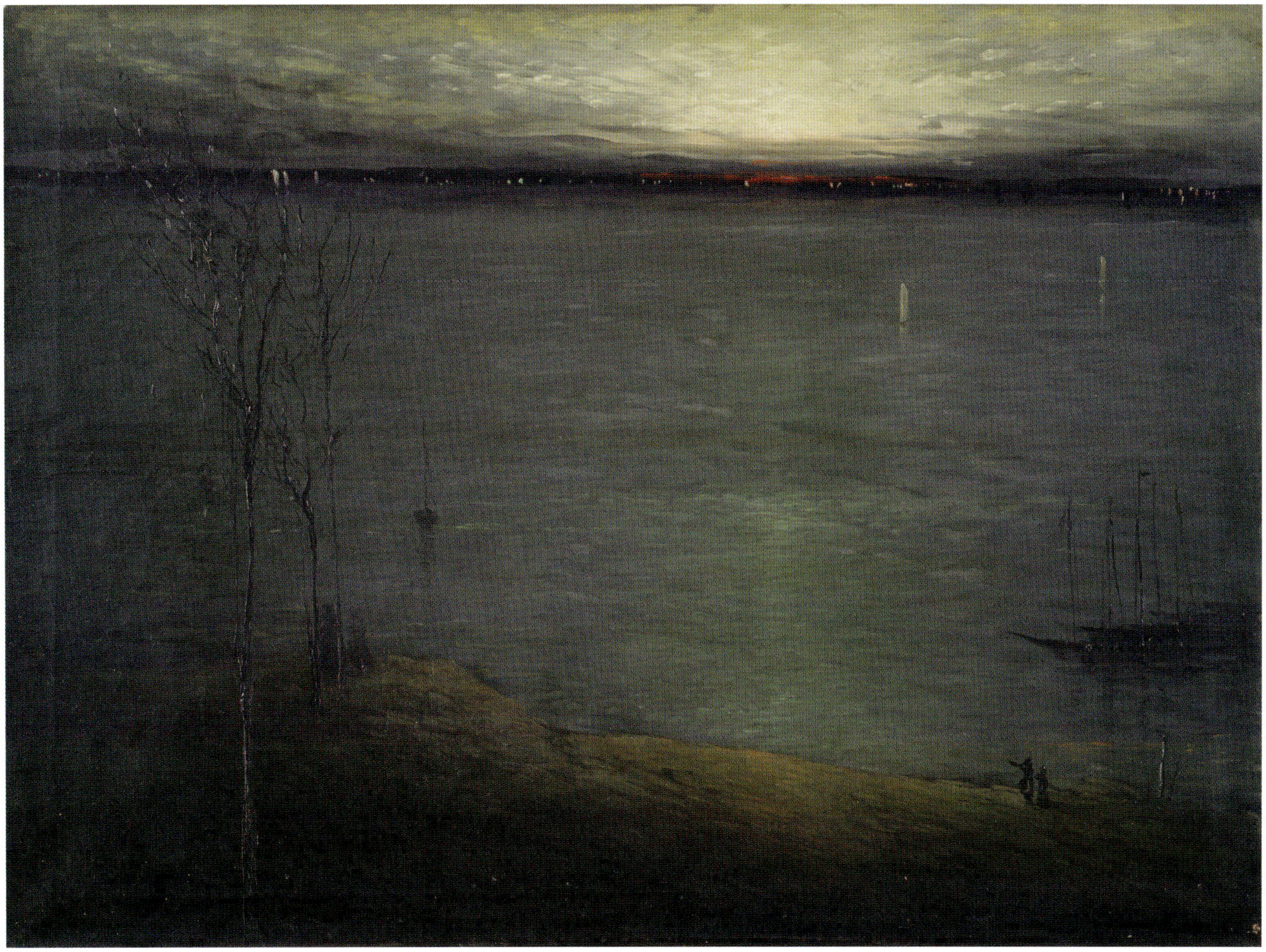

FIG. 20. Léon Dabo, *Roundout, New York*, c. 1907. Oil on canvas, 68.5 × 91.4 cm (27 × 36 in.). Indianapolis Museum of Art, Gift of S. O. Buckner, 07.18, imamuseum.org.

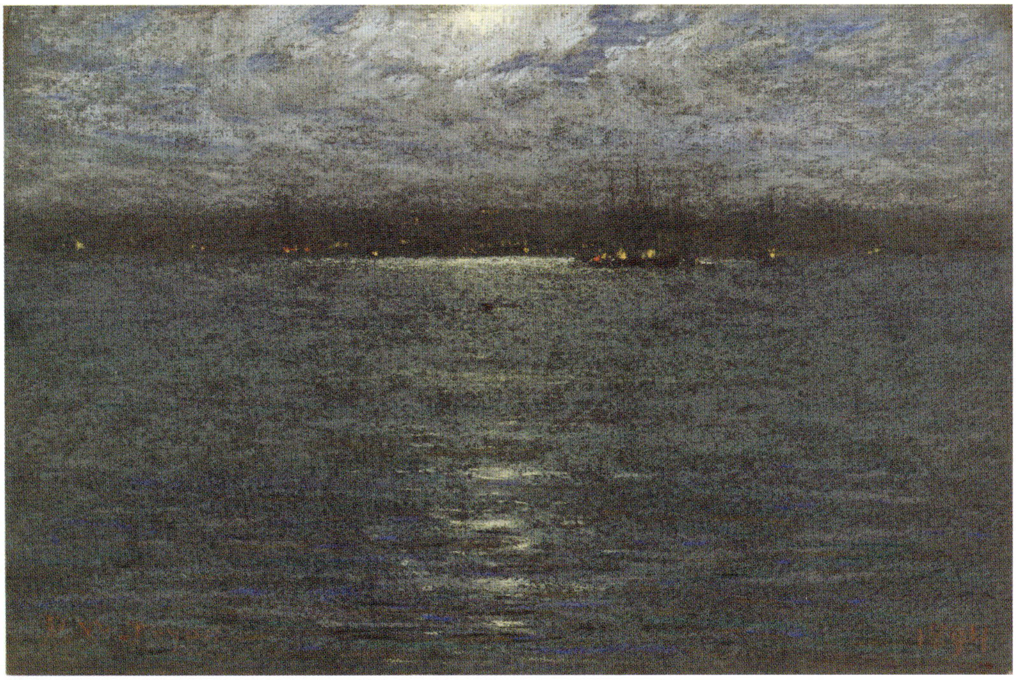

FIG. 21. Dwight William Tryon, *Night: A Harbor*, 1894. Pastel on brown paper, 19.2 × 19.2 cm (7 9/16 × 11 1/2 in.). Freer Gallery of Art, Smithsonian Institution, Washington, D.C. Gift of Charles Lang Freer (F1906.92a–b).

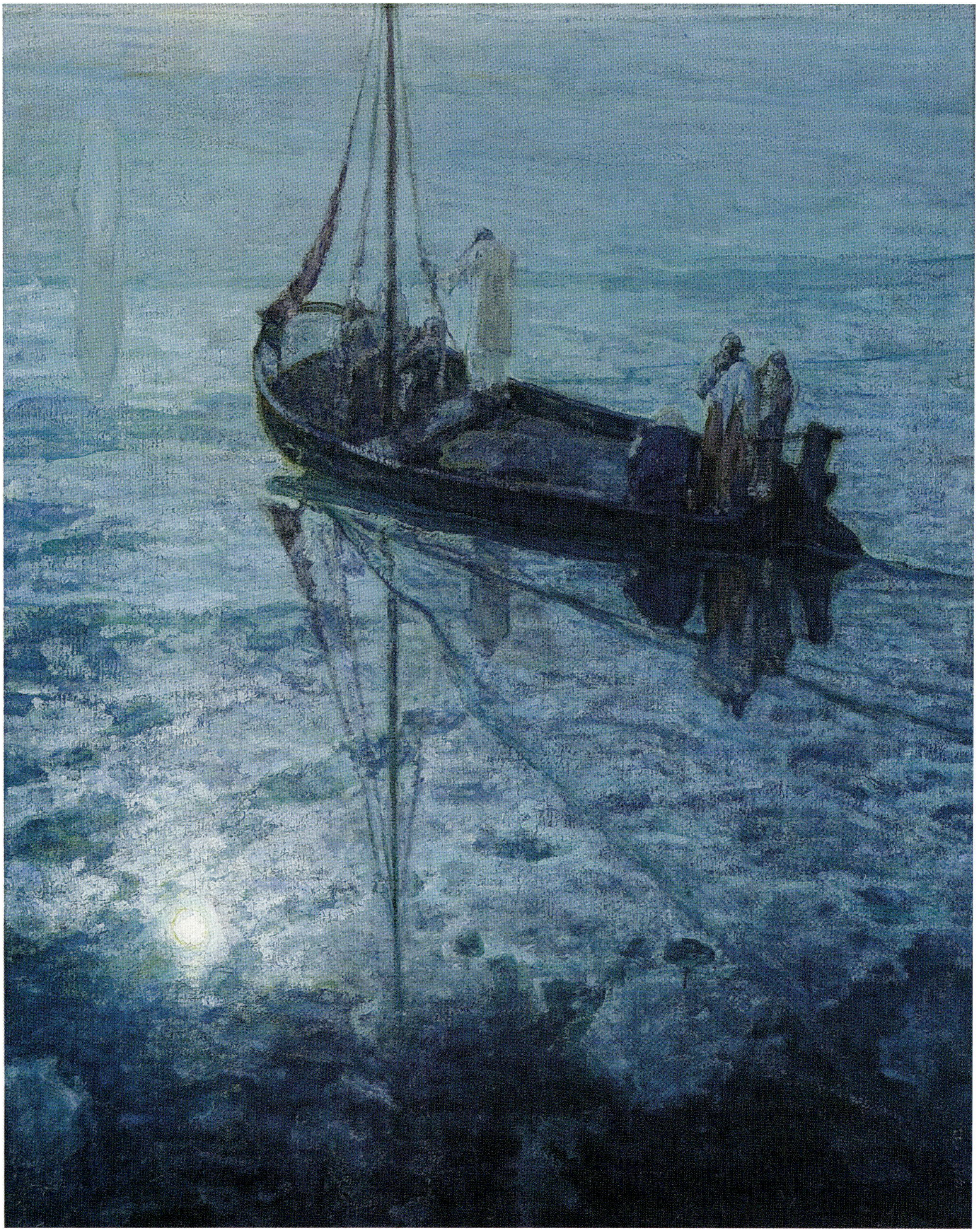

FIG. 22. Henry Ossawa Tanner, *The Disciples See Christ Walking on the Water,* c. 1907. Oil on canvas, 130.8 × 106.7 cm (51½ × 42 in.). Des Moines Art Center Permanent Collections; Gift of the Des Moines Association of Fine Arts, 1921.1.

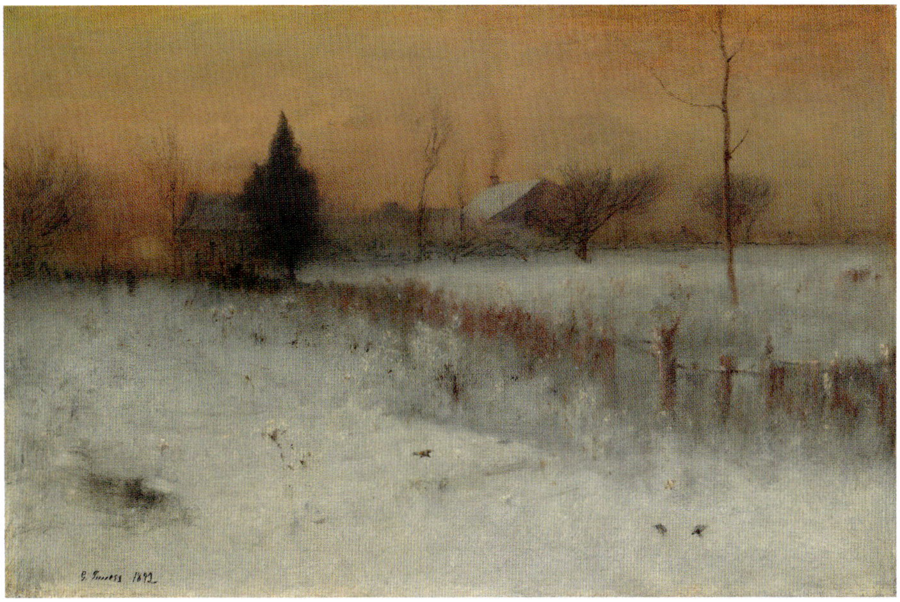

FIG. 23. George Inness, *Home at Montclair,* 1892. Oil on canvas, 76.5 × 114.3 cm (30 1/8 × 45 in.). Sterling and Francine Clark Art Institute, Williamstown, Massachusetts (1955.10).

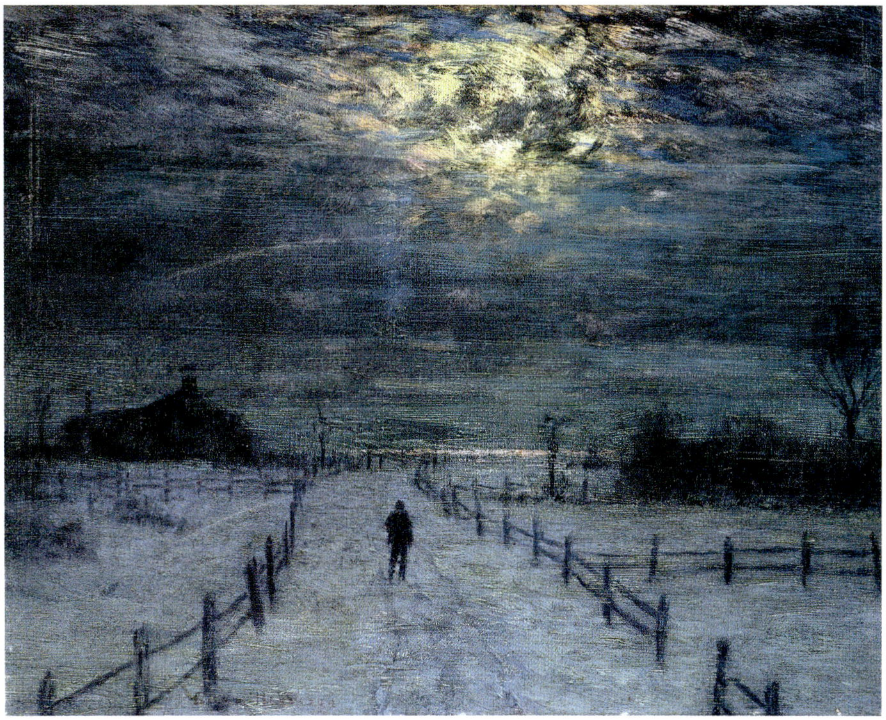

FIG. 24. Lowell Birge Harrison, *A Wintry Walk,* n.d. (before 1900). Oil on canvas, 42 × 51 cm (16 1/2 × 20 in.). Private collection.

among the nocturnes (figs. 23, 24). Snow covers over the details and, like water, increases the blurriness created by darkness. The dark of night is also often combined with the opacity of fog, which erases the shapes of things and diffuses the light. Hence the material qualities of the landscape, rather than filling the composition with distinct elements that guide the beholder's eye through the painting in a predictable narrative order, form as many screens which, on the contrary, tend to destabilize the gaze.

The details of the landscape, reproduced meticulously, even obsessively, by painters of the Hudson River School,[9] vanished from the works of the nocturne artists. In contrast to the factual and scientific vision of the landscape proposed by their predecessors, they preferred merely to suggest. In his treatise on painting, Birge Harrison enjoined his students to abandon the laborious precision of the previous generation: "See big! Grab the essential, and leave the little things for any foolish person who chooses to gather them up. To tell the truth, detail is so blatant, so insistent, that it takes years of hard training to see beyond it. . . . Always leave something to the imagination of the beholder." In pursuit of that aim, Harrison recommended exploiting the effect of night: "There is probably no better way of training the eye to simplicity of vision, than studying moonlight, for in moonlight effects, the broad masses alone are visible, and the shadows lie all over the picture in one big soft value. The lights are distributed in two or three values at most, and nowhere is there any detail."[10] The landscapes painted by Harrison himself (fig. 24; see fig. 135) favored views in which the atmospheric conditions obliterate the details, leaving only neutral surfaces on which he puts into play the tonal variations of restricted palettes.

Whereas, according to Harrison, some artists were sidetracked into gleaning the details of the landscape, the painter of nocturnes played a much more subtle game, appealing to the beholder's imagination. In opposition to the shrill insistence of an overly precise vision stood the soft value of the nocturne, congruent with a conventional contrast between scientific accuracy and poetic feeling. The painting's completeness, an issue that fueled many debates in Whistler's lawsuit against Ruskin, depended not on details but on the outside observer's participation. That meant seeing "beyond" the usual vision in two different ways, since to bypass detail was also to change the nature of the gaze. Night was put to work "training the eye to simplicity"; it functioned both as a subject and as a learning tool for the beginning painter. According to Harrison, one really learns to see by radically reducing the range of visual possibilities.

AN ALTERNATIVE MODE OF PERCEPTION

The nocturne, by refusing to render a factual and objective representation, by training the painter's eye over a long period of time, and by incorporating the beholder's active participation, rejects a vision in which everything is given directly, and thus shifts away from the effort of meticulous gestures and toward a concentrated gaze. It makes vision problematic by artificially reproducing liminal conditions of optical perception.[11] Pushing forms to the limit of perceptibility, it encourages the eye to move toward a different form of visual sensitivity: scotopic (night) vision, as opposed to photopic (day) vision. In scotopic vision, the eye is more sensitive to colors located at the high end of the light spectrum (blues and greens) and perceives more subtle variations of light in general. Given that it takes twenty to forty minutes for the eye to adapt to darkness and to make the transition from photopic to scotopic vision, the nocturne relies on a mode of perception that develops within a different temporality from day vision, requiring prolonged attention from the beholder. George Inness, who began his career as an artist of the Hudson River School before moving toward a more suggestive style liberated from detail, forced the beholder of his *Moonrise* (1887) to adjust her vision, so as to distinguish gradually the elements of the landscape (fig. 25). A beholder first has to fix her eyes on the glowing red moon, half concealed by foliage, then turn them toward the moon's reflection in the marshy waters in the foreground. It is only afterward that the colors animating the central strip of ground emerge, more solid but obscured by the twilight shadows. The final details of the painting—a human figure standing in a small boat in the middle of the canvas, and the roof of a house in the background—can be distinguished only after some time. Even as Americans were experiencing the pressures that modern life exerted on the use of their time, and as more and more voices were decrying the pace of that way of life, nocturne artists asked their beholders to step back from their daily lives and devote themselves to a kind of contemplation slowed down by the genre's formal limitations. More than a new genre, the nocturne introduced a new way of consuming art.

The nocturne compelled the beholder to occupy a particular temporal framework but also a space different from the one to which the late nineteenth-century American public was accustomed. The paintings of the Hudson River School promoted spectacular landscapes staged under theatrical conditions, with very large-format paintings designed to be exhibited to wide audiences, complete with special lighting on a grand scale and the rising of curtains. With impressionism, the American public discovered an art that disrupted that tradition, by revealing the artificiality of paintings. From one moment to the next, depending on the distance from which they are viewed, impressionist paintings are sometimes intelligible to the eye, while at others they dissolve into a formless chaos. The nocturne subverts conventional spatial relationships in a less provocative manner, by favoring the subject's immersion in a space reserved for individual contemplation. The nocturne artists thus re-created in part what Maurice Merleau-Ponty describes

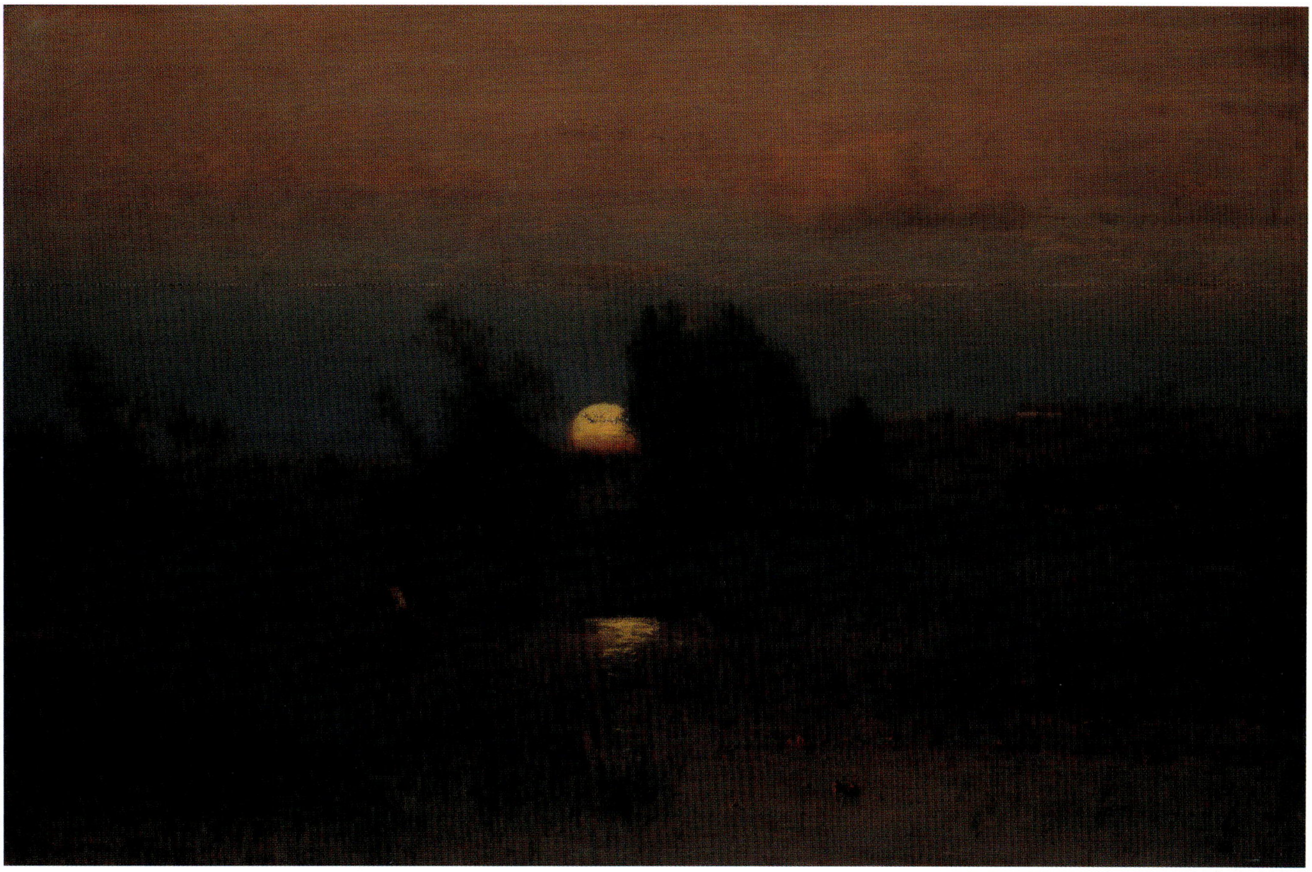

FIG. 25. George Inness, *Moonrise,* 1887. Oil on canvas, 51.4 × 77.5 cm (20 ¼ × 30 ½ in.). Yale University Art Gallery, New Haven, Connecticut. Gift of Teresa Heinz in memory of her husband, H. John Heinz III, B.A. 1960 (1992.5.13).

as a phenomenology specific to the night, which entirely absorbs the perceiving subject:

> When, for example, the world of clear and articulated objects is abolished, our perceptual being, now cut off from its world, sketches out a spatiality without things. This is what happens at night. The night is not an object in front of me; rather, it envelops me, it penetrates me through all of my senses, it suffocates my memories, and it all but effaces my personal identity. I am no longer withdrawn into my observation post in order to see the profiles of objects flowing by in the distance. The night . . . is a pure depth without planes, without surfaces, and without any distance from it to me.[12]

That dissolution of spatial reference points was most apparent when the nocturne was made to encompass an entire aesthetic environment. Whistler was a pioneer by virtue of the attention he paid to the exhibition of his paintings, extending the work beyond the limits of the canvas, crossing the barrier between the realm of the fine arts and that of the decorative arts. In particular, he was one of the first artists to design his own frames.[13] And that harmony between the work and its environment entailed much more than the canvases and their frames: Whistler conceived the display of his paintings as a creative work in its own right, designed to produce a total artistic experience.[14] He carefully chose the colors of the walls in his exhibition rooms and organized them by the same harmonious principles that governed his paintings. For example, he named his exhibitions *Arrangement in White and Yellow* (1883) or *Arrangement in Flesh Colour and Grey* (1884), on the model of the titles he gave his works.[15] The most fully realized example of that expansion of painting to dimensions that physically enveloped the beholder was no doubt the famous *Harmony in Blue and Gold: The Peacock Room,* created by Whistler in 1876–77 and installed in Charles Lang Freer's home in Detroit in 1904.

This *Harmony in Blue and Gold* is somewhat reminiscent of nocturnes from the same period: Whistler

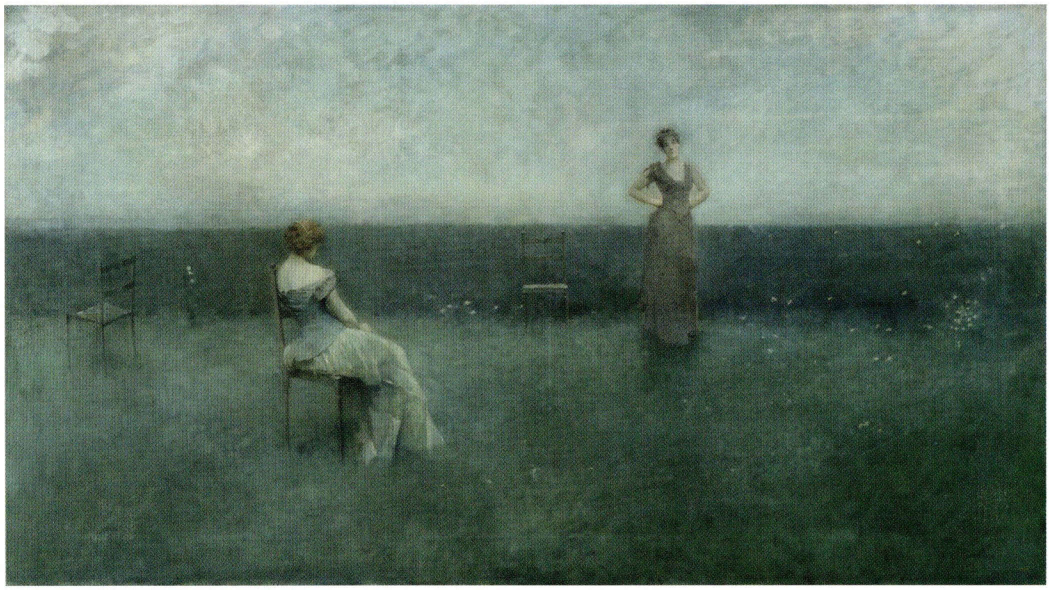

FIG. 26. Thomas Wilmer Dewing, *The Recitation*, 1891. Oil on canvas, 76.2 × 139.7 cm (30 × 55 in.). Detroit Institute of Arts.

chose the title *Nocturne in Blue and Gold* for six canvases, including three of his best known (*Nocturne in Blue and Gold—Old Battersea Bridge*, 1872–75; *Nocturne in Blue and Gold: Valparaiso*, 1866–74; and *Nocturne in Blue and Gold: Southampton Water*, 1872). From the bluish landscapes stippled with artificial lights to the decorations of *The Peacock Room*, the aesthetic principles were the same: they stipulated a different approach to the work, an almost literal absorption on the beholder's part. A critic of the exhibition *Arrangement in White and Yellow* noted the unexpected and somewhat disagreeable effect created by the mise en scène: "Sensitive guests felt threatened by the haze-suffused atmosphere, as though they might be overwhelmed by the ether rising in the room."[16] The beholder's relationship to the canvas was no longer a rational act of viewing that kept the object at a distance but rather a contemplation that engaged the subject beyond mere visual perception.

Nocturne artists demonstrated an increased interest in other forms of perception as well, particularly touch and hearing. In the first place, the nocturne's affinities with music reinforced the indetermination and expansion of perception. Charles Caffin points out the indirectness and allusiveness that the nocturne shares with music: "[Whistler] shunned the obvious, however brilliantly portrayed. Now the least obvious of the arts is music."[17] In a sense, the darkness of the canvas corresponds visually to the evasiveness and indirectness of music. There are many examples within the nocturne movement of an adherence to a paradigm establishing an equivalence between the musical and the visual, from the definition of "tonalism" to Blakelock's *Moonlight Sonata* (see fig. 7). A critic at the *Times* of London had already taken note of that analogy: the nocturnes, he said, "are illustrations of the theory, not confined to this painter [Whistler], but most conspicuously and ably worked out by him, that painting is so closely akin to music that the colors of the one may and should be used, like the ordered sounds of the other, as means and influences of vague emotion."[18] Thomas Wilmer Dewing's canvases, for example, regularly depict young women playing or listening to music. *The Recitation* is constructed like one of Whistler's nocturnes: the landscape, empty and indeterminate, is divided into three parallel bands in dark tones (fig. 26). A woman in evening dress—an incongruous but common refinement in Dewing's oeuvre—is shown in a state of absorption, her back turned to the beholder, listening to a singer who seems to hover in the middle distance. The distorted perspective of a chair, and a few flowers, indicated by a constellation of white spots on either side of the composition, further accentuate the impression of floating and indetermination, the "vague emotion" of the painting, to borrow the expression of the *Times* critic. *In the Garden (Spring Moonlight)* and *The Hermit Thrush* present the human figures, in *profil perdu* or with their backs turned, as engulfed in a landscape of imprecise forms (figs. 27, 28). The women are isolated from one another in contemplative attitudes, listening to the song of the solitary thrush. Hearing takes precedence over sight, and the beholder is invited to imitate the attitude

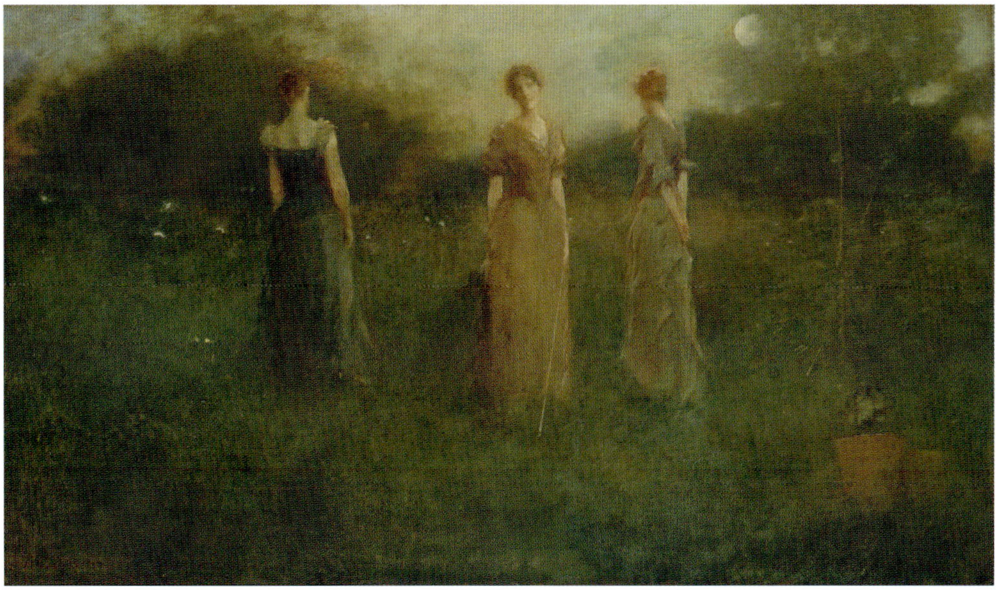

FIG. 27. Thomas Wilmer Dewing, *In the Garden*, 1892–94. Oil on canvas, 52.3 × 88.9 cm (20 5/8 × 35 in.). Smithsonian American Art Museum, Gift of John Gellatly (1929.6.37).

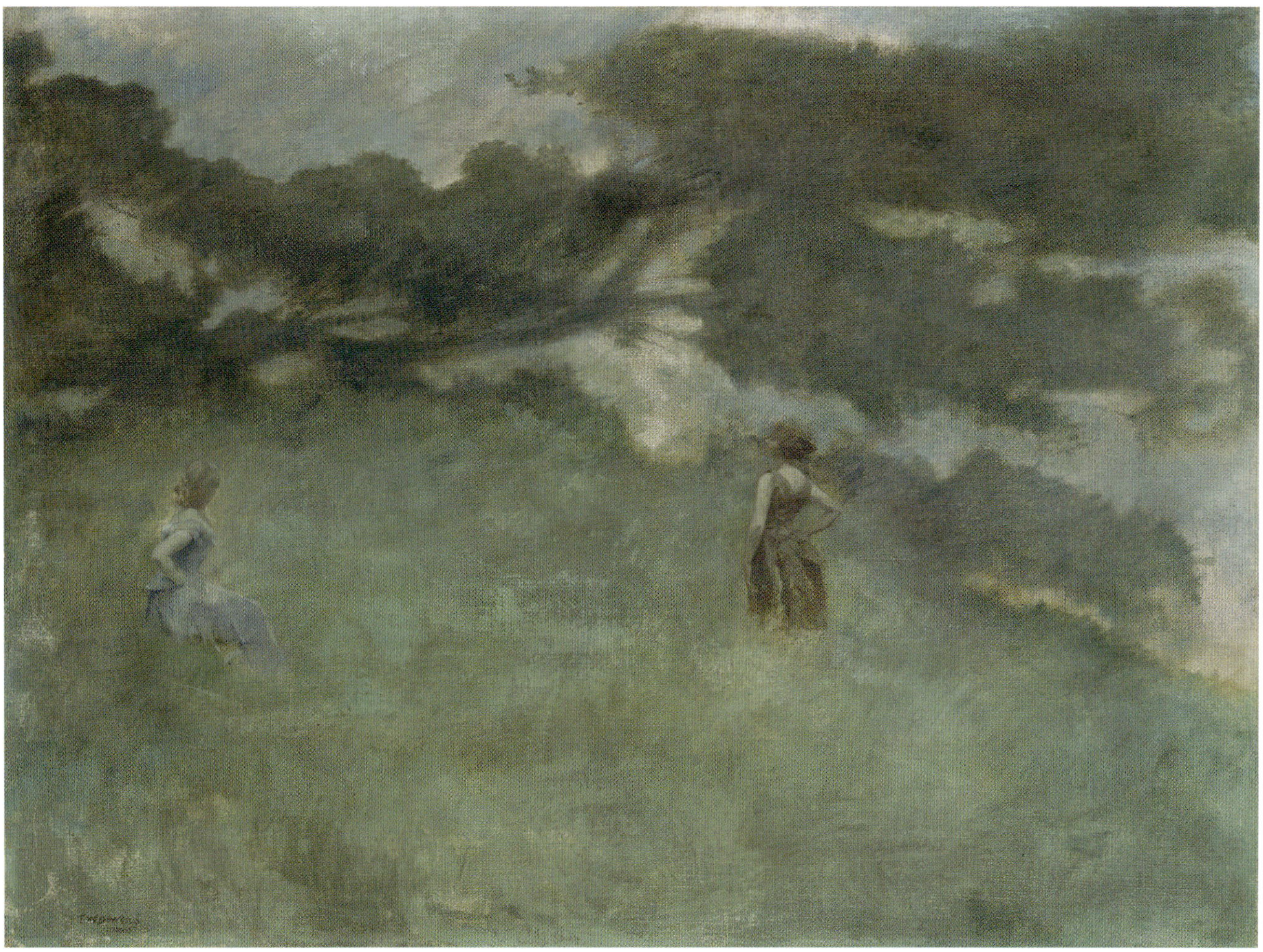

FIG. 28. Thomas Wilmer Dewing, *The Hermit Thrush*, 1890. Oil on canvas, 88.1 × 117 cm (34 5/8 × 46 1/8 in.). Smithsonian American Art Museum, Gift of John Gellatly (1929.6.39).

of the young women in the painting: though they listen and he looks, the beholder must adjust his eyes to the conditions of listening, because his aesthetic experience requires an intense attention and a continuous perception unfolding over time.

Finally, nocturne artists engaged the sense of touch, by working the coarse grain of the canvas to add a sensual dimension to the painting. Whistler and his imitators, in fact, chose canvases with a thicker weave, exploiting the texture to create a subtle diffusion of light, thus turning away from the "slick" surfaces of French-style salon painting. Whistler used a very fluid medium, a "sauce,"[19] into which the pigments were diluted, and which soaked into the canvas more than it covered it, leaving the details of the weft visible.[20] Dewing went so far as to stamp a motif imitating the weft onto the smooth surface of his decorative panels.[21] In 1894 a *New York Times* critic commented on the optical effects of the tonalist J. H. Johnson's textured canvases: "At first sight the impression given by his pictures is that of decided richness in colors, but a certain haziness and lack of definite outline. It is only upon longer examination that figures model out in their proper roundness and one perceives that drawing has not been neglected. In the method for oils now favored by many painters a dry, grainy quality is left that suggests pastel."[22] Here, the material properties of the canvas were exploited in a paradoxical manner: the light diffused by the irregularities of the painted surface transformed the rough, coarse canvas into a refined visual impression of overall softness. And in engaging the sense of touch in the beholder's imagination, the nocturne introduced a hybrid form of perception, a vision that, so to speak, felt its way along.

THE ART OF THE INEFFABLE

Just as nocturnes evade direct vision, they also shy away from discourse. In the course of his lawsuit against Ruskin, Whistler sparked the public's curiosity, and often hilarity, in expounding astonishing ideas. He admitted that he could not "describe" his painting *Nocturne in Black and Gold: The Falling Rocket*, and that to name it *View of Cremorne* "would certainly bring about nothing but disappointment on the part of the beholders."[23] A large share of the discussion during the trial turned on what the painting "represented." Whistler surprised the audience by publicly challenging any need for referentiality in art. He complained of the public's fondness for narrative and religious respect for titles: "Without baptism," he said ironically, "there is no . . . market."[24] The choice of the term "nocturne," proposed by his client Frederick Leyland, delighted Whistler, who reveled in the "irritation" it produced in critics and appreciated the fact that the title said "all I want to say and *no more* than I wish."[25] Whistler's biographer Bernhard Sickert declared of the artist's nocturnes: "They leave the critic nothing to say, nothing on which to expand."[26] Like Stéphane Mallarmé, with whom Whistler associated in Paris, the painter proposed an art "not set before the eyes but simply suggested," one that painted "not the thing but the effect it produces."[27]

Whistler, in refusing to let nocturnes refer to anything but themselves, liberated the work of art from its role as means to an external end and proclaimed its autonomy: "Nobility of action, in this life, is hopelessly linked with the merit of the work that portrays it; and thus the people have acquired the habit of looking, as who should say, not at a picture, but *through* it, at some human fact, that shall, or shall not, from a social point of view, better their mental or moral state."[28] Spiritual and moral elevation lies in the work itself and not in a "human fact" that the work might represent. Paradoxically, the desire to sanctify the work as an end also presupposes an arrested vision, confined within a restricted interpretive zone: nocturnes play the role not of transparent windows *through* which the beholder would see reality but of actual obstacles.[29] Kathleen Pyne connects Whistler's preference for a "semantic void" to a strategic positioning within the sociocultural sphere: "The indeterminacy of his forms conceived as slowly graduated tonal masses allowed for open-ended interpretations that catered to avant-garde taste, in distinction to the bourgeois demand for moralism and closure in art."[30] Paradoxically, the hermeneutic opacity suggested by the work's physical darkness has more to do with its very openness, its refusal to fix on a precise meaning. And in that play between openness and closure a third thing is at stake: the legitimacy of the beholder's gaze.

The aesthetic of the nocturne rested on a deliberately diffuse perception, which translated into an extremely vague critical vocabulary. Time and again, commentators looking at these paintings, which left them nothing to say, evoked "poetry," "the soul," "feeling," and the "mood" that pervaded the works, in a language that was itself imprecise. One of Whistler's biographers described a set of Whistler's nocturnal engravings as "sketches in black and white upon brown paper, of river subjects by night, studies drawn in the dark, by feeling not by sight."[31] Whistler advised his students to apply the paint as lightly as "breath on the surface of a pane of glass":[32] the artist's breath alone, his inspiration, sufficed to fabricate the work's substance. Moreover, Whistler, his disciples, and his critics refrained from defining too precisely the distinctive "feeling" of the nocturnes or the intention governing them—which likely explains why Ruskin and Frederic Remington suspected they were a hoax. Remington joked in his journal: "Whistlers [*sic*] talk was light as air and the bottom of a cook stove was like his painting."[33] Whereas the discourse surrounding the nocturnes seemed to have the transparency of self-evidence, requiring no commentary or explanation, the work remained opaque to the ignorant beholder, who was caught in the trap of the invisible.

At this point, aesthetics converged with sociocultural considerations. Indeed, the negation of vision that defined the nocturne rested in great part on a rigid elitism. Questions of visual perception were organized around a fundamental distinction, between those who could discern the work's artistic merits and those who literally saw nothing there. Remington, with a touch of insolence, proclaimed his ignorance after visiting an exhibition of Whistler's canvases in New York: "[I] saw some 'punk' Whistlers and how people can see everything in there I do not know," he noted in his journal.[34] Seeing the nocturne required a cultivated eye and put the beholder in a class apart: "There is a point where absence of definition in a picture becomes mere obscurity. Just where is this limit? To the commonplace person, the unimaginative, the matter-of-fact, it is reached as soon as any of the details are lost, any of the sharply defined edges blurred—details and edges—the obvious, in a word, being about all that a nature of this kind is capable of seeing and appreciating. A primitive person of this sort judges all things by their outside shell or husk. Remove that and he is hopelessly lost."[35] To distinguish the nocturne's qualities, in short, was to distinguish oneself. Because nocturnes demanded an unusual commitment on the beholder's part, and because they shirked a clear discourse linking them to familiar themes, their beholder was often reduced to trusting the artist or the critic, who took on the task of defining the norms by which the works were to be appreciated.

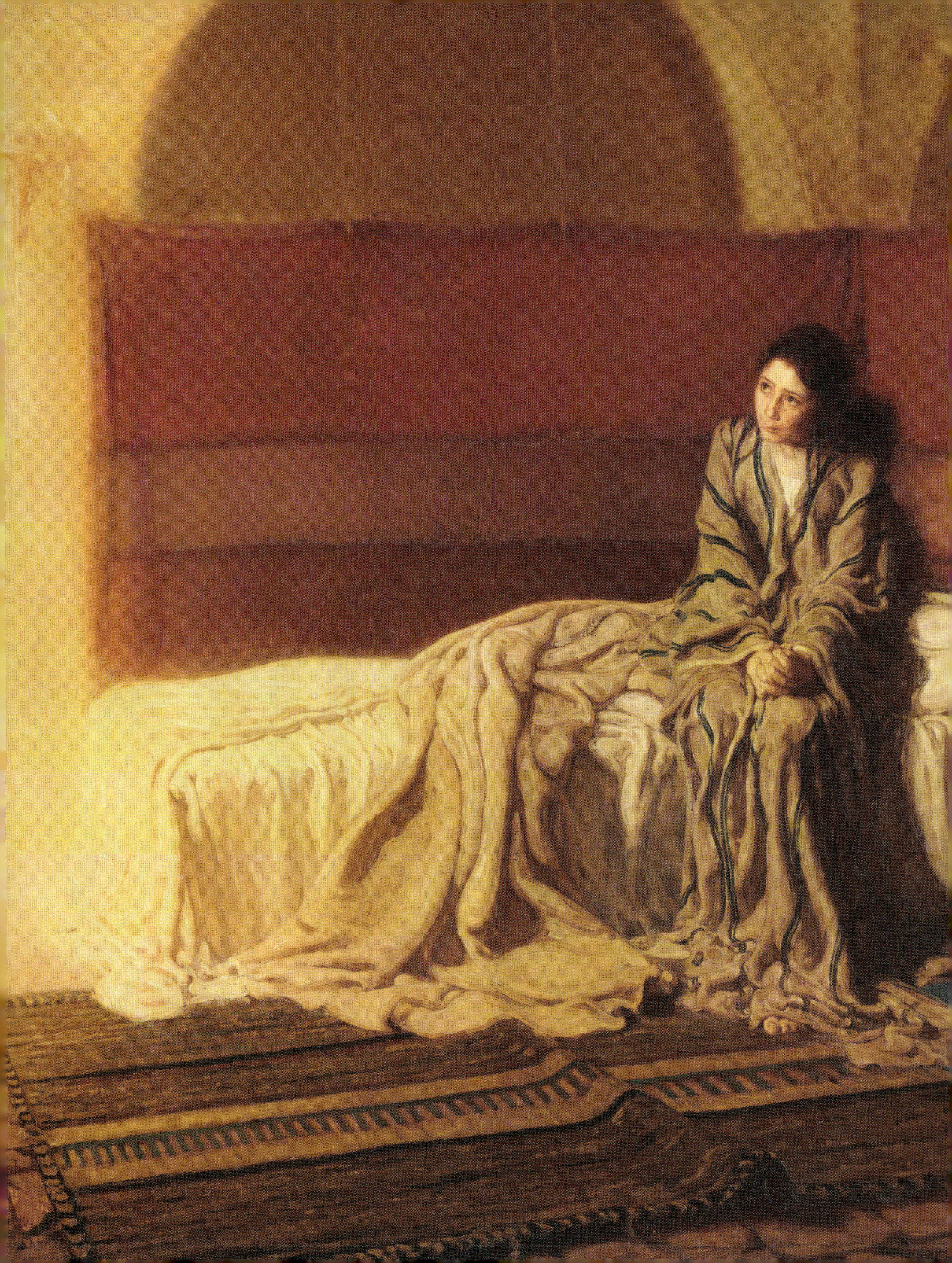

2 The Image in Crisis

Vision Questioned by Science and Technology

Aesthetic considerations formed only part of an entire cultural, social, scientific, and technological network in which the notions of darkness and vision assumed a new importance. Whistler's aesthetic—elitist, irrational, mystifying—produced or simply brought to light tensions that extended far beyond the sphere of sociocultural differences. The art of Whistler and his disciples prompted uneasiness in a large portion of the public, first, because it was a deliberately disorienting art, and second, because, at the dawn of the twentieth century, darkness and invisibility were becoming the particular domain of important philosophical, scientific, and ideological inquiries.[1] The nocturne primarily strove to redefine artistic contemplation, in reaction to a context in which the traditional parameters of vision were being radically altered. According to the historian Jonathan Crary, the status of vision evolved well before the invention of photography or the emergence of avant-garde painting in the late nineteenth century.[2] The eye, formerly perceived as an instrument of transparent transmission, came to be seen as a fallible organ, liable to be taken in by optical illusions. In that context, perception was increasingly understood as the workings of the mind, which had to complete, interpret, and put right the stimuli recorded by the eye. In the course of the nineteenth century, a shift occurred, therefore, from the notion of a clear, objective, rational vision to a complex and uncertain model, dominated by the observer's subjectivity. Crary demonstrates that the avant-garde painting of the 1870s and 1880s and the development of photography were not contributing factors to the mutations of vision, but rather symptoms of older changes. But though these "perceptual transformations" took effect in the early nineteenth century, it was not until the early twentieth century that they fully entered the collective consciousness and that their consequences began to be the subject of public debate. The nocturne reflected that new attention: it participated at least as much in a discourse on vision as in an evolution of the scopic regime per se.

REDEFINING THE VISIBLE AND THE INVISIBLE

The increased awareness of vision and its transformations is evident, for example, in the way the news of the discovery of X-rays spread: through images in the first place, especially the now-iconic photograph of the hand of Wilhelm Röntgen's wife. An article in the *Sacramento*

Fig. 32 detail

Daily Record-Union of October 25, 1896, summed up the impact of that scientific breakthrough on everyday perceptions of the visual. The article, taking up an entire page, describes the progress made in the use of X-rays since their spectacular discovery a few months earlier (fig. 29). Scattered over the page are numerous illustrations, from simple diagrams and engraved photographs to halftone prints of X-rays.[3] This is a significant example in many respects: the detailed article, published in a local daily newspaper, attests to the level of attention being given to discoveries affecting the field of vision; the large number of illustrations indicates that they were increasingly indispensable, taking precedence over the written word; their variety highlights the technological progress in image reproduction techniques and, at the same time, reveals the new habits of a large readership that could move easily from one type of image to another. Above all, the article demonstrates the infinite interconnections that existed in a visual environment revitalized, first, by the scientific discoveries touching on the sphere of vision, and second, by technological progress applied to the production and circulation of images.

The sudden expansion of the visible gave rise to a fair number of questions, however, and radical innovations were accompanied by a change of attitude affecting visual practices. The nocturne must be considered one of the avatars of that change. At a time when the infinitely large and the infinitely small, the previously unsuspected phases of motion, and the invisible depths of the body were shown to the masses in a spectacular manner, the return to darkness appears at first to have been an antimodern reaction, running counter to the technological and cultural history of its era, a refusal to bow to the new norms of the modern visual environment. It was by no means a frontal opposition, however. On the contrary, nocturne artists were also inspired by these technologies of vision and relied on them in their work. The nocturnes gave a visible form to that paradox peculiar to the history of science and technology at the time: the technologies of vision, far from eliminating the invisible, in reality shored up its existence; the developments of science and technology reinforced the idea of a realm that was unintelligible and inaccessible to the eyes.

Between 1890 and 1910, a series of scientific inventions and discoveries—in addition to X-rays—revolutionized the field of the visible. To cite only a few, the first inroads into radiography led to the discovery of the electron in 1897, closely followed by that of alpha, beta, and gamma rays between 1898 and 1900; photographic prints improved sufficiently to make the moon's geography visible, and photography also captured Halley's Comet for the first time in 1908; microscopy and microphotography revealed the minute details of forms invisible to the unaided eye, whose omnipresence Louis Pasteur and Robert Koch had just demonstrated; and the discovery of bacteria was followed by the even more disturbing exploration of viruses, such as the one responsible for yellow fever, identified between 1900 and 1902 (fig. 30). Eadweard Muybridge, in showing for the first time the position of a galloping horse's legs, caused a phenomenal upheaval (fig. 31). Not only was the understanding of motion called into question, so too was human eyesight. The microscope, the telescope, and chronophotography underscored the radical disconnection between human visual perception and technological vision.

Amid all these new instruments of vision, photography, which experienced what François Brunet has called its "second technological age" at the turn of the twentieth century,[4] played a crucial role in the technological and scientific reappraisal of vision. Often combined with other technologies (electric lighting and shutter releases, telescopic lenses), it was used primarily as a technique for recording the results of scientific investigations. The limits imposed by the first cameras—heavy devices with unwieldy photographic plates—confined scientific photography to immobile objects (such as those of archaeology), but the invention of lightweight, handheld cameras and, especially, of stable and easy-to-use negatives opened photographic investigation to the inconstant objects of the natural and human sciences.[5] Brunet points out, beyond the real technological progress, the institutional role played by photography in the late nineteenth century. No longer merely a research tool, cameras began to document scientific results, even for the general public, from ethnographic albums that attempted to catalogue the variety of human types to medical images to astronomical photographs. In that sense, the photograph became an "established image of science, its social sign."[6] The legitimacy of objective representation became the monopoly of the photographic image, at the expense of other forms of image production, whose status had yet to be redefined. A gap opened between a mode of seeing that was closely paired with knowing and all other ways of looking at images; by the late nineteenth century, that

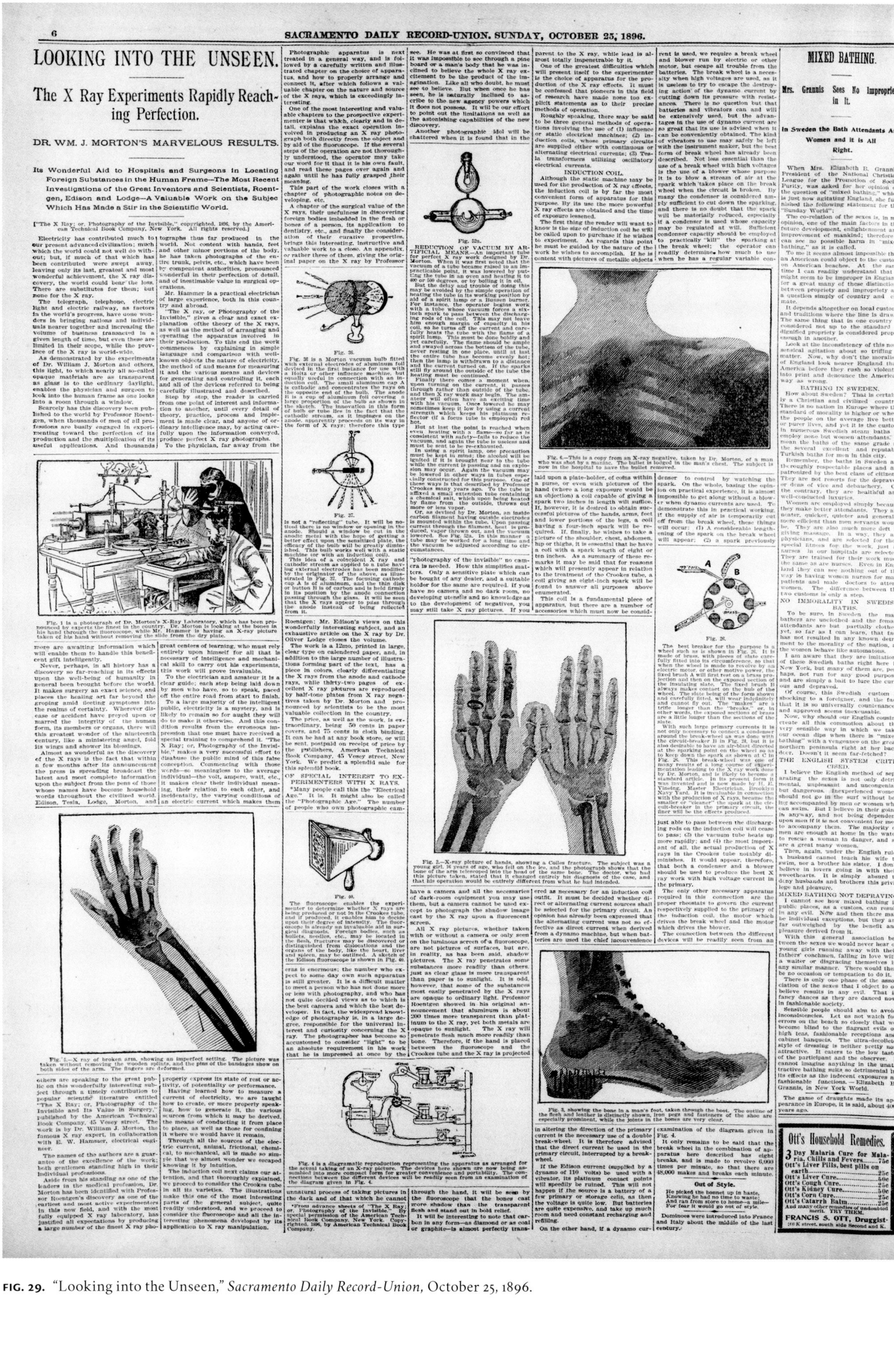

6 SACRAMENTO DAILY RECORD-UNION. SUNDAY, OCTOBER 25, 1896.

LOOKING INTO THE UNSEEN.

The X Ray Experiments Rapidly Reaching Perfection.

DR. WM. J. MORTON'S MARVELOUS RESULTS.

Its Wonderful Aid to Hospitals and Surgeons in Locating Foreign Substances in the Human Frame—The Most Recent Investigations of the Great Inventors and Scientists, Roentgen, Edison and Lodge—A Valuable Work on the Subjec Which Has Made a Stir in the Scientific World.

["The X Ray; or, Photography of the Invisible," copyrighted, 1896, by the American Technical Book Company, New York. All rights reserved.]

Electricity has contributed much to our present advanced civilization; much which the world could not well do without; but, if much of that which has been contributed were swept away, leaving only its last, greatest and most wonderful achievement, the X ray discovery, the world could bear the loss.

Photographic apparatus is next treated in a general way, and is followed by a carefully written and illustrated chapter on the choice of apparatus, and how to properly arrange and connect it, after which follows a valuable chapter on the nature and source of the X rays, which is exceedingly interesting.

One of the most interesting and valuable chapters to the prospective experimenter is that which, clearly and in detail, explains the exact operation involved in producing an X ray photograph both directly from the object and by aid of the fluoroscope. If the several steps of the operation are not thoroughly understood, the operator may take our word for it that it is his own fault, and read these pages over again and again until he has fully grasped their meaning.

This part of the work closes with a chapter of photographic notes on developing, etc.

A chapter of the surgical value of the X rays, their usefulness in discovering foreign bodies imbedded in the flesh or bones of a person, its application to dentistry, etc., and finally the consideration of their curative properties, brings this interesting, instructive and valuable work to a close. An appendix, or rather three of them, giving the original paper on the X ray by Professor

Fig. 52a.

REDUCTION OF VACUUM BY ARTIFICIAL MEANS.—An important tube for perfect X ray work designed by Dr. Morton.

INDUCTION COIL.

Fig. 1 is a photograph of Dr. Morton's X-Ray Laboratory.

Fig. 5.—X ray of broken arm, showing an imperfect setting.

Fig. 2.—X-ray picture of hands, showing a Colles fracture.

Fig. 6.—This is a copy from an X-ray negative, taken by Dr. Morton, of a man who was shot by a maniac.

Fig. 3, showing the bones in a man's foot, taken through the boot.

Fig. 4 is a diagramatic reproduction representing the apparatus as arranged for the actual taking of an X-ray picture.

OF SPECIAL INTEREST TO EXPERIMENTERS WITH X RAYS.

Out of Style.

MIXED BATHING.

Mrs. Grannis Sees No Impropriety in It.

In Sweden the Bath Attendants Are Women and it is All Right.

When Mrs. Elizabeth B. Grannis, President of the National Christian League for the Promotion of Social Purity, was asked for her opinion on the question of "mixed bathing," which is just now agitating England, she furnished the following statement for the "Sunday World":

The co-relation of the sexes is, in my opinion, one of the main factors in the future development, enlightenment and improvement of mankind; therefore I can see no possible harm in "mixed bathing," as it is called.

BATHING IN SWEDEN.

NO IMMORALITY IN SWEDISH BATHS.

THE ENGLISH SYSTEM CRITICISED.

MIXED BATHING NOT DEPRAVING

... its effects as the indecent exposures at fashionable functions.—Elizabeth B. Grannis, in New York World.

The game of draughts made its appearance in Europe, it is said, about 400 years ago.

FIG. 29. "Looking into the Unseen," *Sacramento Daily Record-Union*, October 25, 1896.

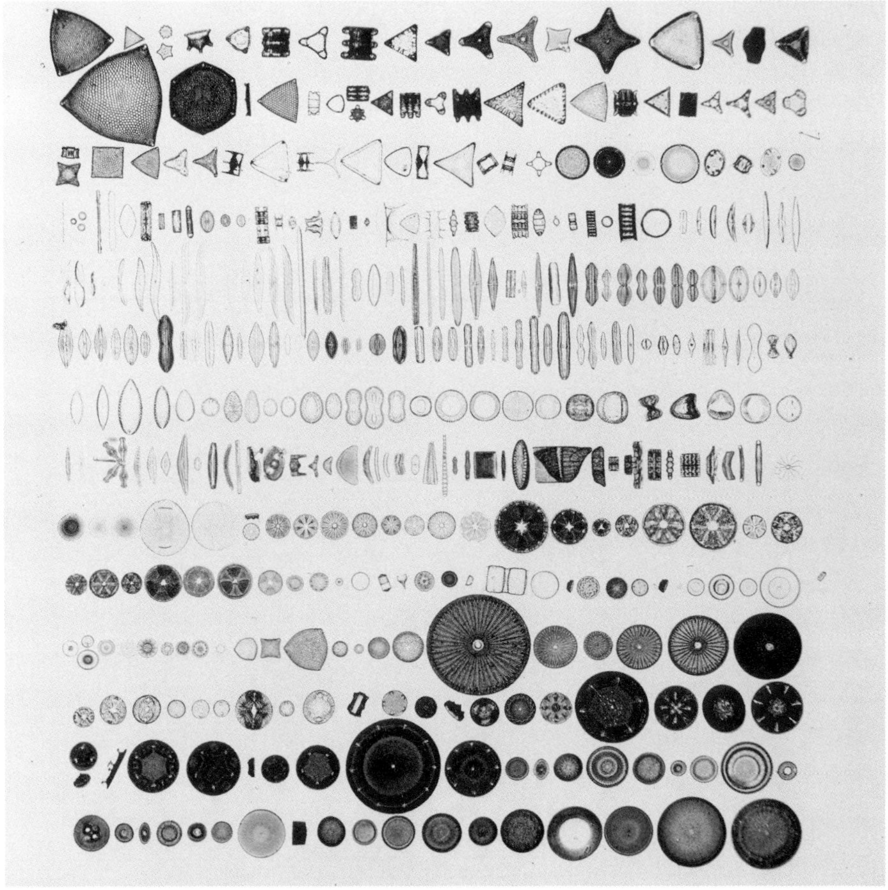

FIG. 30. Hans Hauswaldt, *Diatoms*, 1900. Photograph, 24 × 23.8 cm (9 7/16 × 9 3/8 in.). Albertina, Vienna—On permanent loan from Höhere Graphische Bundes-Lehr- und Versuchsanstalt, Vienna.

distinction had become a cliché. The nocturne's rejection of narration and mimesis can also be understood within that context.

The growing breach into the invisible introduced by technology and science had its share of ambivalence. The triumphant march of progress in the field of scientific vision was accompanied by an expansion in the realm of the invisible of at least the same magnitude. Indeed, the invisible seemed to grow in inverse proportion to the visible. Scientific and technological progress showed what remained to be discovered, as well as what had been discovered. Above all, it demonstrated that seeing is not altogether the same as knowing, just as knowing does not necessarily mean seeing. Photographs of the details of the moon's surface only underscored how far away its craters and valleys still were, and how little was as yet known about them. The illumination through photography of the moon's visible face only cast the hidden face deeper into darkness. Likewise, the radiation emitted by matter long remained an enigma, and the unexpected results of radiography revealed the ignorance as well as the knowledge of the scientists who made use of it.[7] For the general public, mystery was an integral part of the new advances of vision: the discovery of X-rays, for example, was announced in the press with headlines evoking an "invisible" or "dark" light. They thereby pointed to the fundamental ambiguity of that new instrument of vision, incomprehensible for the most part, which, though it revealed the invisible, itself eluded the eye. After a few years, radiography's damaging effects on health also became apparent, and its power was understood as not only imperceptible but also dangerous. X-rays, an unsettling discovery with multiple and unpredictable repercussions, resembled science itself, which had turned away from the positivist ideal at the end of the nineteenth century and which, above all, acknowledged its own lacunae. Behind the rhetorical division between a discerning scientific vision and the vision captured in all other images, science, in affirming both its triumphs and its limitations, articulated an equivocal discourse.[8]

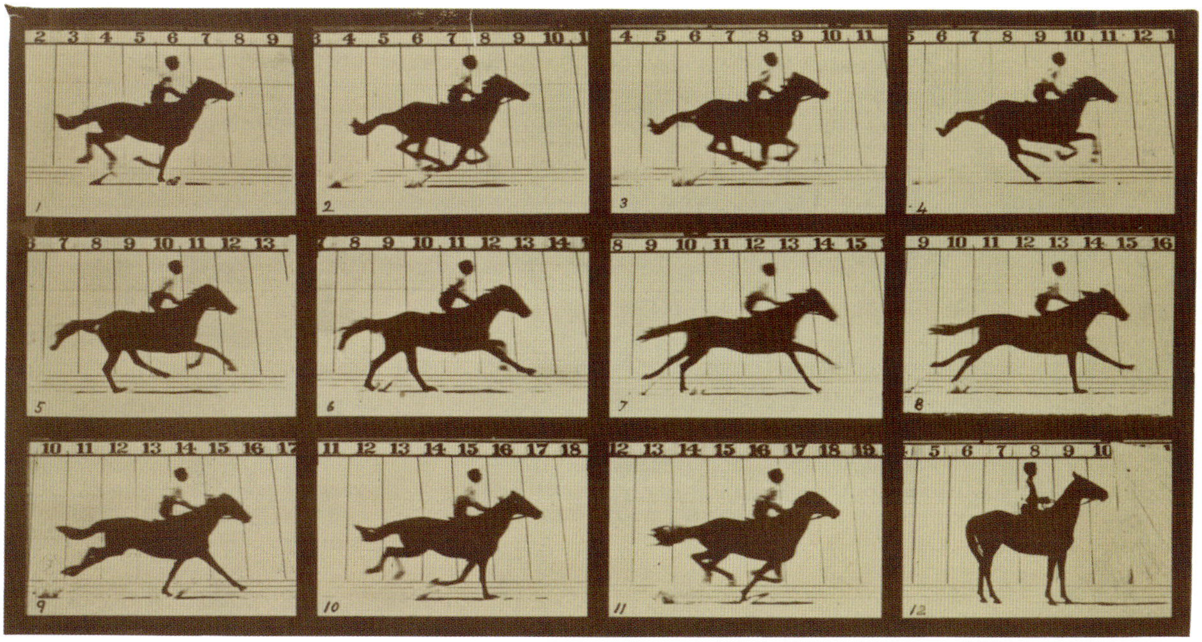

FIG. 31. Eadweard Muybridge, "The Horse in Motion," 1878. Albumen photograph. Library of Congress, Prints and Photographs Division, Washington, D.C.

THE DARK AND THE OCCULT, SCIENCE, AND TECHNOLOGY

Seeing, Believing, and Knowing

These multiple discoveries and inventions, in revealing the limits of knowledge, also toppled the hierarchy of beliefs. It seemed that everything was constantly being called into question; conversely, everything could also turn out to be possible. "No scientist can now say what is possible or what is impossible," declared a journalist in 1903, at the end of an article on radium.[9] The same confusion overcame the historian Henry Adams, when he was confronted with the latest technological and scientific innovations exhibited at the Exposition Universelle de Paris in 1900. Like Adams, his physicist friend Samuel Langley believed that this series of discoveries called positive science into question in a fundamental way. "He could see only an absolute *fiat* in electricity as in faith. Langley could not help him. Indeed, Langley seemed to be worried by the same trouble, for he constantly repeated that the new forces were anarchical, and especially that he was not responsible for the new rays, that were little short of parricidal in their wicked spirit towards science."[10] The disruptiveness and anarchy were such that Adams could henceforth conceive of modern science and technology only as a blind faith that renounced Cartesian clarity and rationality. The discoveries made in the decade preceding that moment of revelation, he noted, had the effect of removing the objects of science from the field of perception and even from objective measurement: "[Man] had entered a supersensual world, in which he could measure nothing except by chance collisions of movements imperceptible to his senses, perhaps even imperceptible to his instruments, but perceptible to each other, and so to some known ray at the end of the scale."[11] Physics, escaping the control of scientists, now lapsed into a bewildering metaphysics—"physics stark mad in metaphysics," concluded Adams, with the elliptical conciseness and verve of a magic formula. In the historian's eyes, modern science and the electric dynamo had supplanted the Virgin Mary as an "occult, supersensual, irrational" power.[12] Against all expectations, extreme modernity was now expressed in the terms of a medieval benightedness.

Conversely, science and technology tended to foster images of the irrational and the metaphysical. Even before Adams was confronted with the Paris dynamo, the

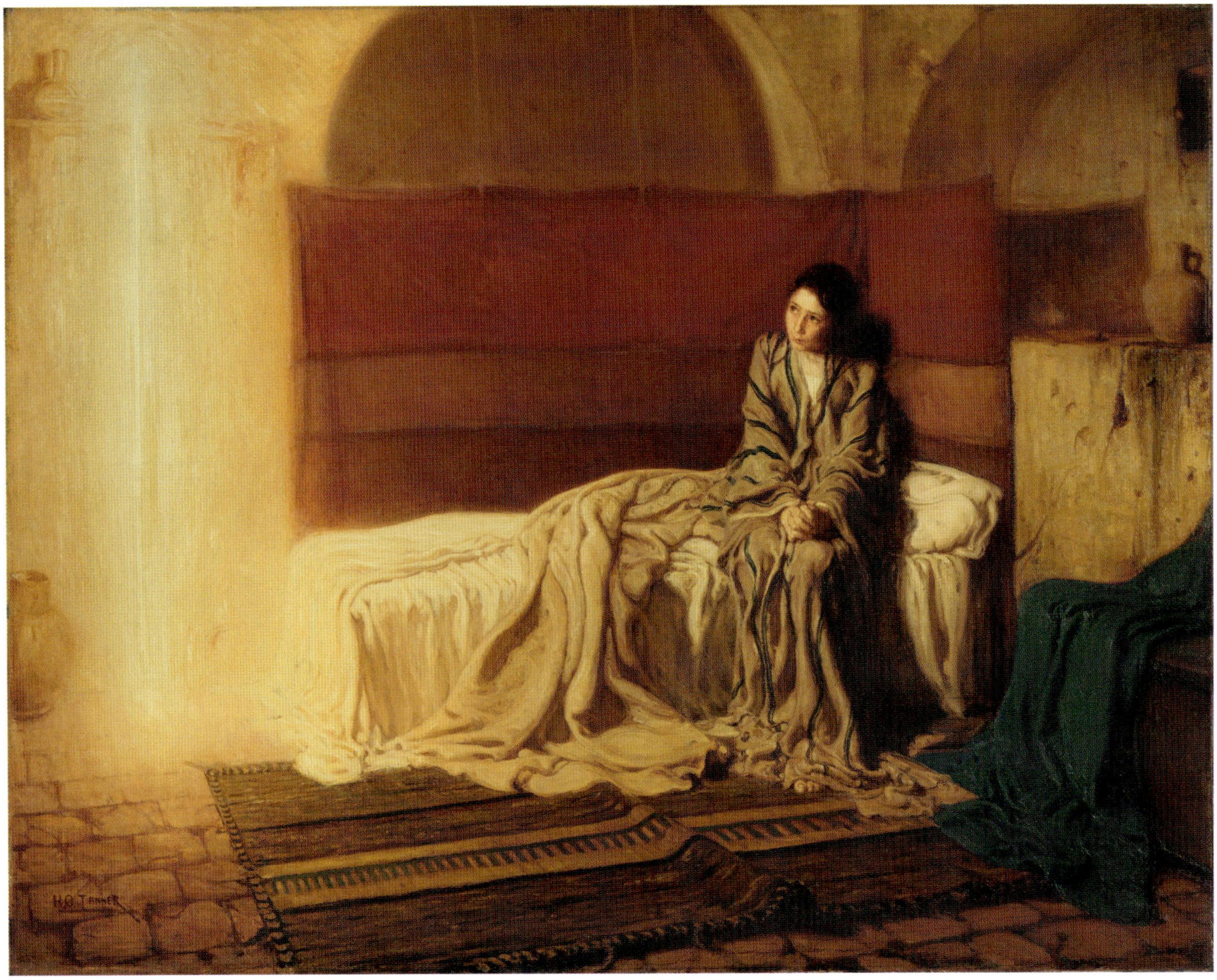

FIG. 32. Henry Ossawa Tanner, *The Annunciation*, 1898. Oil on canvas, 144.8 × 181 cm (57 × 71¼ in.). Philadelphia Museum of Art, gift purchased with the W. P. Wilstach Fund, 1899 (W1899-1-1).

painter Henry Ossawa Tanner erased the line between electric power and religious faith.[13] One of the rare African American artists to pursue a successful artistic career in the late nineteenth century, Tanner initially studied with the realist painter Thomas Eakins in Philadelphia, before choosing exile in France, where he painted religious scenes that clearly displayed Whistler's formal influence.[14] Tanner's *Annunciation*, painted in 1898, suggests that the artist's faith was in dialogue with the apparently supernatural manifestations of science at the time (fig. 32). The painting adopts the traditional iconography of the Annunciation, but with one major substitution. It was common practice—one still followed by James Tissot, who directly inspired Tanner (fig. 33)—to represent Gabriel as a winged human figure. Tanner confined himself to marking the angel's presence with a simple ray of light suspended in the void. That surprising shape, which emits an intense radiant energy, was a spectacle not unknown to Tanner's audience: its source is to be sought in the most recent advances of science and technology. In the years prior to the creation of Tanner's *Annunciation*, the engineer and physicist Nikola Tesla had organized spectacular demonstrations, during which he popularized his inventions, including, notably, a wireless lighting system that relied on high-frequency electricity. At the World's Columbian Exposition of 1893, for example, Tesla exhibited that innovation with all the gifts of a showman: visitors were invited to enter a dark room, hung throughout with black cloth, in which bulbs of various shapes and sizes were arranged on a table conspicuously free of electrical cable. Concealed on both sides of the room were plates through which Tesla ran high-frequency electricity, which created a magnetic field imperceptible to spectators. The electricity, in

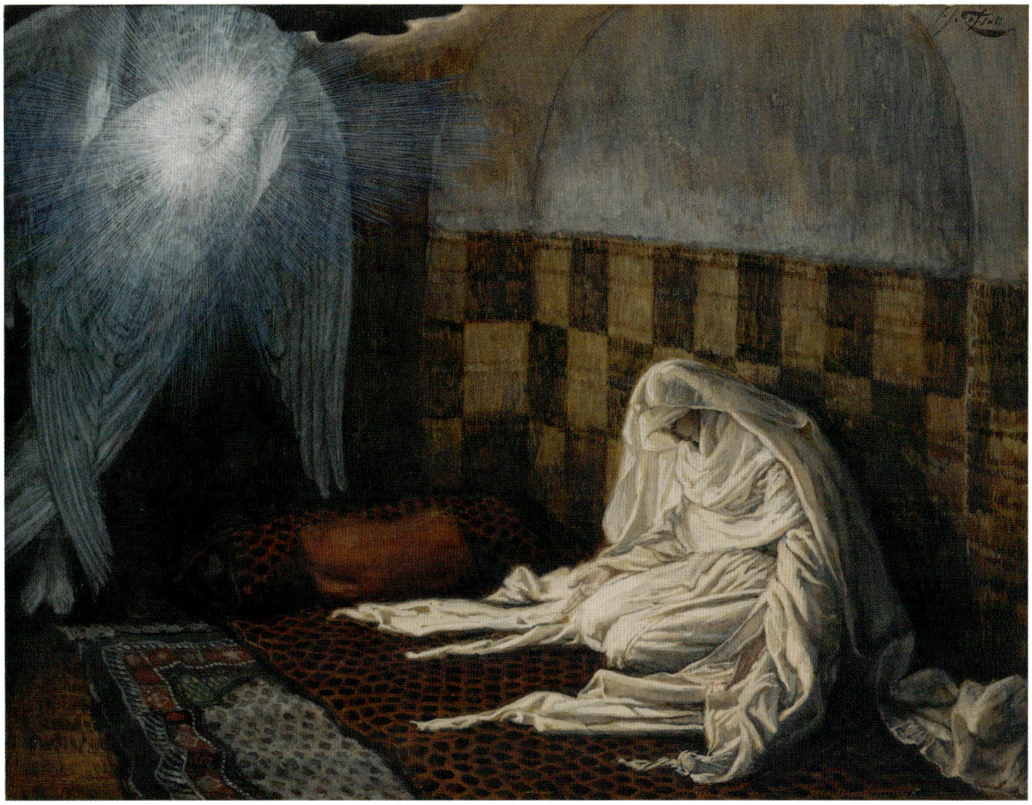

FIG. 33. James Tissot. *The Annunciation*, 1886–94. Opaque watercolor over graphite on gray wove paper, 17 × 21.7 cm (6 11/16 × 8 9/16 in.). Brooklyn Museum of Art, New York, Purchased by public subscription, 00.159.16.

stimulating particles contained in the bulbs, suddenly lit them up. It is possible that Tanner, who spoke at the exposition congress,[15] witnessed that demonstration or heard about it in the press. An article published in the popular magazine *Harper's Weekly* gives a measure of Tesla's popularity.[16] One of the many illustrations accompanying that long article, "Ideal Way of Lighting a Room," displays striking resemblances to Tanner's painting (fig. 34). The rhetoric used in the article indicates how easily images circulated between technology and religion: the subtitle, "Electric Lamp Fed from Space, and Flames That Do Not Consume," might bring to mind the biblical episode of Moses and the burning bush. Tanner thus brought together the two forces, modern and ancient, that Henry Adams would isolate a few years later in his *Education*. Here the Virgin, in an anachronism that speaks volumes, is brought face to face with the power of the electric dynamo.

The culture of Tanner's time provides many examples of that juxtaposition of the irrational and the scientific-technological.[17] Some of the big names in science on both sides of the Atlantic, such as the physicist William Crookes in England and the philosopher and psychologist William James in the United States, set out to explore paranormal phenomena. James was one of the founders

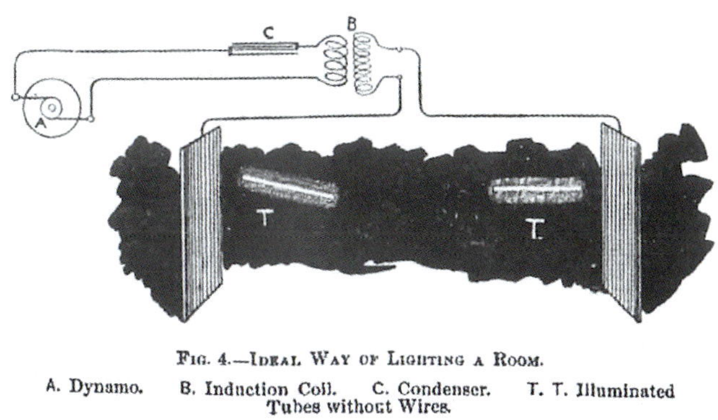

FIG. 34. "Ideal Way of Lighting a Room," *Harper's Weekly* 35, no. 1808, July 11, 1891.

of the American Society for Psychical Research, whose first president, named in 1885, was the mathematician and astronomer Simon Newcomb. Photography was commonly used to explore paranormal and supernatural phenomena, playing the role of "third eye," in Clément Chérioux's expression,[18] a "medium" in both senses of the word. A visual intermediary between technology and phenomena without a rational explanation, photography, in extending human vision, at the same time performed its function as an "image of science." It was both a recording tool and an instrument for disseminating the results of these investigations, to which it gave a

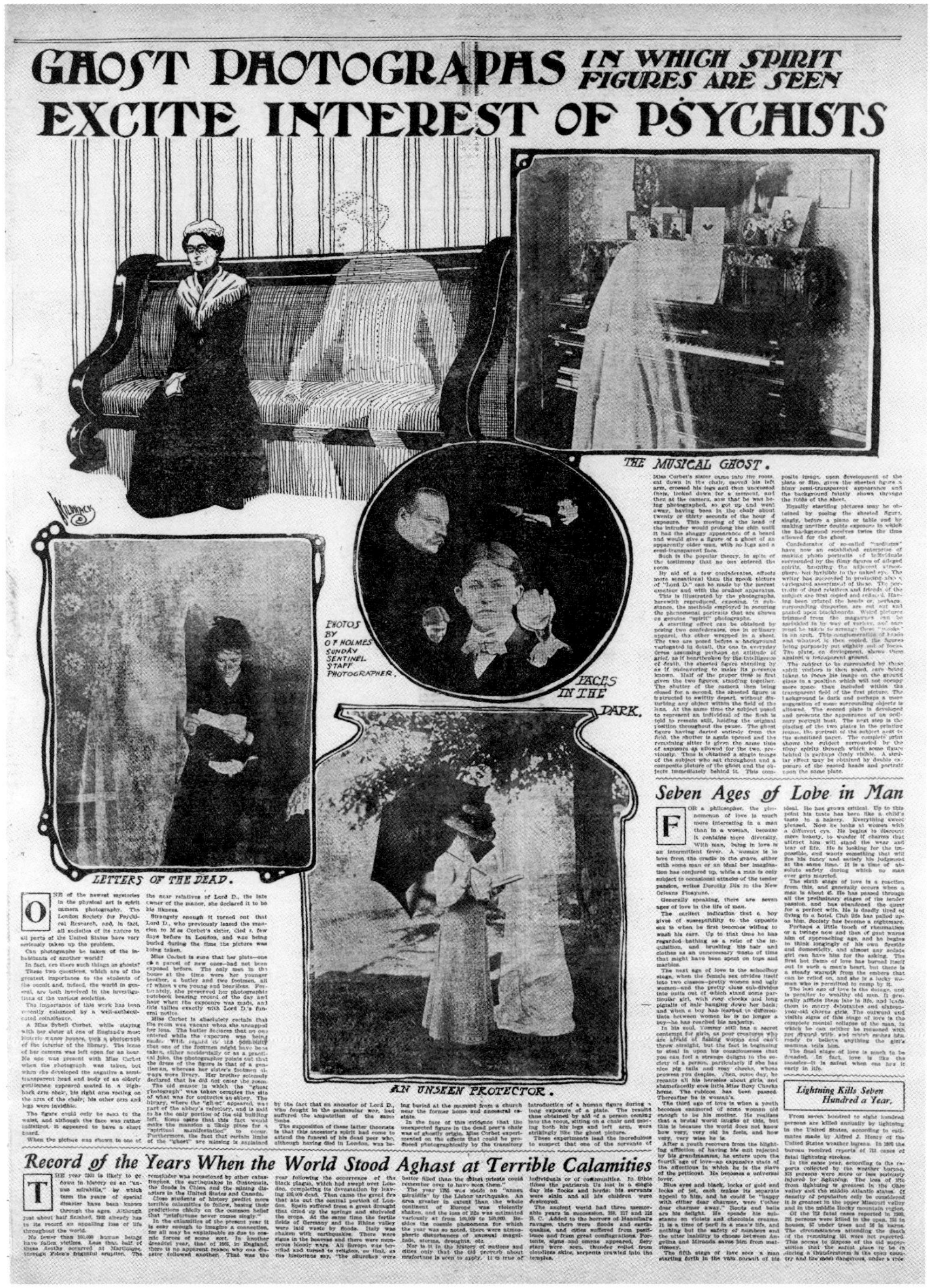

FIG. 35. "Ghost Photographs Excite Interest of Psychists," *Salt Lake Herald*, July 31, 1902.

scientific legitimacy, as indicated in an article on spiritualism: "However dim the light may be, which prevails in the average séance room, all appearing phantoms in their different stages of materialization are luminous enough to leave a distinct impression on the photographic plate, and with the help of the camera, the 'unerring eye of science,' such spirit photographs have often been taken and printed."[19] Photographs of supposedly supernatural phenomena circulated even in the local daily press (fig. 35). The historian Tom Gunning, comparing X-rays and spiritualist photography, shows how these two invisible "worlds" were connected. According to Gunning, photography revealed the strangeness of reality, even as it attributed a certain scientific authenticity to the supernatural.[20] The range of uses for photography in exploring occult phenomena was in fact very broad, encompassing fraud, playfulness, and serious investigation. For example, in the course of the 1860s–1870s the photographer William H. Mumler produced many prints showing ghostly silhouettes beside living persons.

Using a simple process of double exposure of the negative, Mumler launched a real and very lucrative craze for "spirit photography."[21] Another example of the extreme fluidity between science and occultism, which sometimes involved deception, was the hoax launched on April Fool's Day in 1896, a few months after the discovery of X-rays, by David Starr Jordan, a professor at Stanford University. He announced in *Popular Science Monthly* that he had captured a subject's thoughts on a photographic plate.[22] The article, which was intended to denounce sensationalism and bogus scientific experiments, at first sparked credulous enthusiasm. This was followed by indignation, directed more at the prank and its methods than at the mischief Jordan had originally wanted to condemn.[23] These examples expose a jumble of meanings: technological and scientific progress was perceived as an extension of vision with the naked eye, but also as a potential source of mystery, even mystification. They also indicate the broad spectrum that such imagery covered, from amateur spirit photography to the most advanced scientific articles on X-rays.

As a painter, Tanner navigated cautiously in these waters and adopted a perspective that called the act of seeing into doubt. The light introduced by Tesla and Tanner did not entirely dispel the darkness; on the contrary, in Tanner's painting, as in Tesla's demonstration, the beam of light emerges from a source whose mystery grows in proportion to its intensity. Tesla and Tanner both played on two opposite registers: hypervisibility (the spectacular, the miraculous manifestation) and opacity. In both cases, the scene established a contact (transmission of a message in Tanner's *Annunciation;* the message entirely contained in the medium of Tesla's bulb) that was obviously no contact at all. The transmission of intense and instantaneous energy occurred without any apparent connection; the angel remains an extremely strange figure, a fleeting presence whose message remains unspoken. The two scenes marked a leap toward the irrational that left Henry Adams so befuddled: Tesla's scientific demonstration undoubtedly confused visitors at the Columbian Exposition more than it instructed them; Tanner's canvas, in moving away from traditional iconography, deepened the religious mystery, even while making it eminently visible. The technological miracle dazzled beholders so much that it caused a kind of blindness. It patently announced the limits of their field of vision.

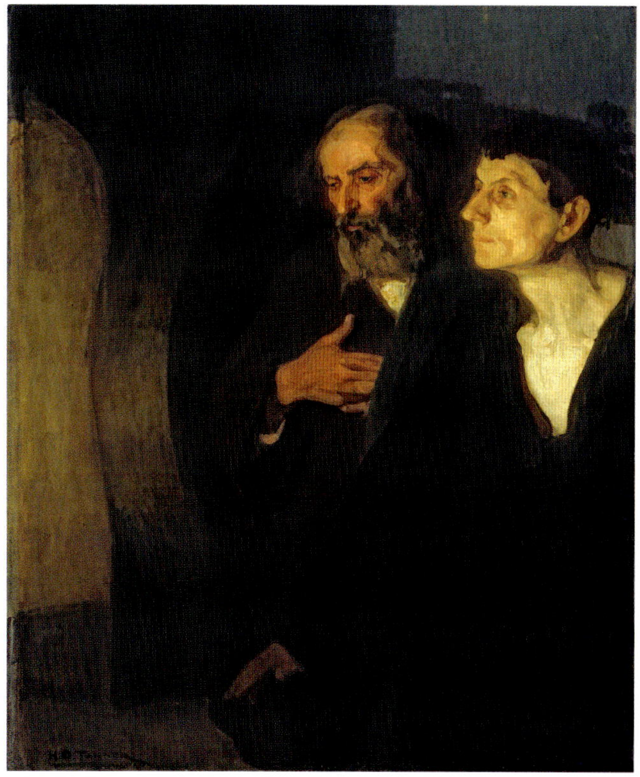

FIG. 36. Henry Ossawa Tanner, *The Two Disciples at the Tomb*, c. 1906. Oil on canvas, 129.5 × 105.7 cm (51 × 41 7/8 in.). Art Institute of Chicago. Robert A. Walker Fund (1906.300).

THE CONTINGENT GAZE

Beyond the single example of *The Annunciation,* Tanner's paintings reflect a complex relationship to the visible and the representable. Although his oeuvre contains more night scenes than nocturnal landscapes in the strict sense, Tanner, in returning repeatedly to darkness, regularly called into question the validity of sight. His paintings often depict characters witnessing a miracle in the middle of the night, one that remains outside the beholder's range of vision. In *The Two Disciples at the Tomb* (fig. 36), Christ's tomb lies outside the picture frame, but a light emanates from it, bathing the faces of the disciples approaching it, who are otherwise immersed in shadow. The beholder of the painting is reduced to looking at the others looking, while she herself remains in darkness, and the miracle (which, by definition, is an eminently *visible* phenomenon) is indicated simply by the streaming light. The distribution of darkness and light thus marks the division between the act of witnessing, immediate but inaccessible—and, above all, irreducible to pictorial representation—and the ambiguous position of a beholder kept on the periphery of the visible, in what is, in several different ways, an indirect relation to the event. I have already shown how *The Disciples See Christ Walking on the Water* (see fig. 22) entails several sorts of indirection: even its title places the beholder in a secondary position. The unusual point of view, the disorienting play of reflections—which are the only indications of the moon and a cloudy sky lying outside the frame—and the nocturnal atmosphere, underscored by a broad strip of dark water at the bottom of the painting, all constitute visual barriers between the beholder and the scene depicted. Within the composition, the characters' gaze is itself portrayed as imperfect and uncertain. The scene shows the disciples as they discern the presence on the horizon of a luminous silhouette, reminiscent of the vertical stroke of light representing the angel in *The Annunciation,* except that here the glimmer is much fainter. One of the disciples, turning his back on that apparition, hides his face in his hands, refusing to look. The miracle, observed directly by Mary in *The Annunciation,* is now the object of a problematic vision: the light fades and vanishes in the distance, as dazzling self-evidence gives way to ambiguity and uncertainty.

Tanner's visual strategies were a rethinking of religious painting and the role that the visual act of witnessing plays in faith. Tanner's painting, in which the miraculous is rendered at a remove, was situated within the context of a new scientific approach to the Old and New Testaments, which included philological research on the texts, archaeological excavations, and photographic documentation of the holy sites. Religion was increasingly approached by means of a positivist methodology—of which Ernest Renan was the best example in France, with his highly popular *Vie de Jésus* (*Life of Jesus*)[24]—and, in general, within a context where photography had radically redefined the truth of pictorial representation. Yet it was becoming more and more difficult to paint Gospel scenes without lapsing into an iconography that was both naïve and conventional, or into a realism that could be perceived as inappropriate or even shocking.[25] Tanner abandoned any direct representation of miracles, wagering instead on suggestion, relatively abstract forms, and the distance that the nocturnal atmosphere allowed. In other words, he avoided two pitfalls, realism and conformism, by adapting Whistler's precepts to religious painting.

But Tanner's reticence extended beyond the matter of religious witnessing. It was also a result of new reflections on human vision. If, for example, one compares *The Annunciation* and *The Disciples See Christ Walking on the Water* to a third painting, *And He Vanished Out of Their Sight,*[26] created the same year as *The Annunciation,* the question of visual perception takes a more specific turn. The disciples of Emmaus have just come to understand that the man with whom they were sharing their meal is Jesus. At precisely that moment, he vanishes, leaving nothing behind but a vertical light comparable to the one in *The Annunciation,* but more faintly drawn. It seems that, between the blinding flash of light in *The Annunciation* and the barely visible trace of a similar phenomenon in *And He Vanished Out of Their Sight,* only a few seconds have passed. In the first painting, the apparition is rendered in all its radiance; in the second, the painting records only its afterimage in the disciples' eyes. Upon closer inspection, in fact, we find that the stroke indicating the sudden absence of Christ is modeled on the type of impression that persists on the retina after it is dazzled by light. The general public took a great interest in the phenomenon of the afterimage throughout the nineteenth century.[27] In 1890, it was well enough known to become the implicit subject of a pseudoscientific fiction: the *New York Times* published an account of the experiments of one Dr. Gabriel, a scientist specializing in optics who bears the name of an archangel. The doctor has succeeded in capturing the ghostly image of his recently deceased wife. The story, taken from an apocryphal letter written by Dr. Gabriel, tells how, with the assistance of a system of colored lenses, the young doctor manages to perceive the "ultra rays" that constitute the apparition. Dr. Gabriel, his powers of perception enhanced by means of that technology, captures an image more faithful than a photograph. But that vision is so intense that it leaves an impression on his retina itself, obliterating any other form of visual perception. By means of science and technology, Dr. Gabriel's fiction reactivated the topos of the blind clairvoyant: "For a moment I was dazzled by a brilliant flash of light; then, clothed in indescribable colors, I beheld the face of my dead wife. . . . Impulsively I sprang towards her, throwing aside the lenses in my ecstasy. They fell upon the floor, shivered to atoms. Yet the brilliant image remained before me in all its loveliness. . . . Before long I awoke to the fact that I was blind to everything but my wife's image. This remained permanently before me, but not in its original hues—still more beautiful tints gradually

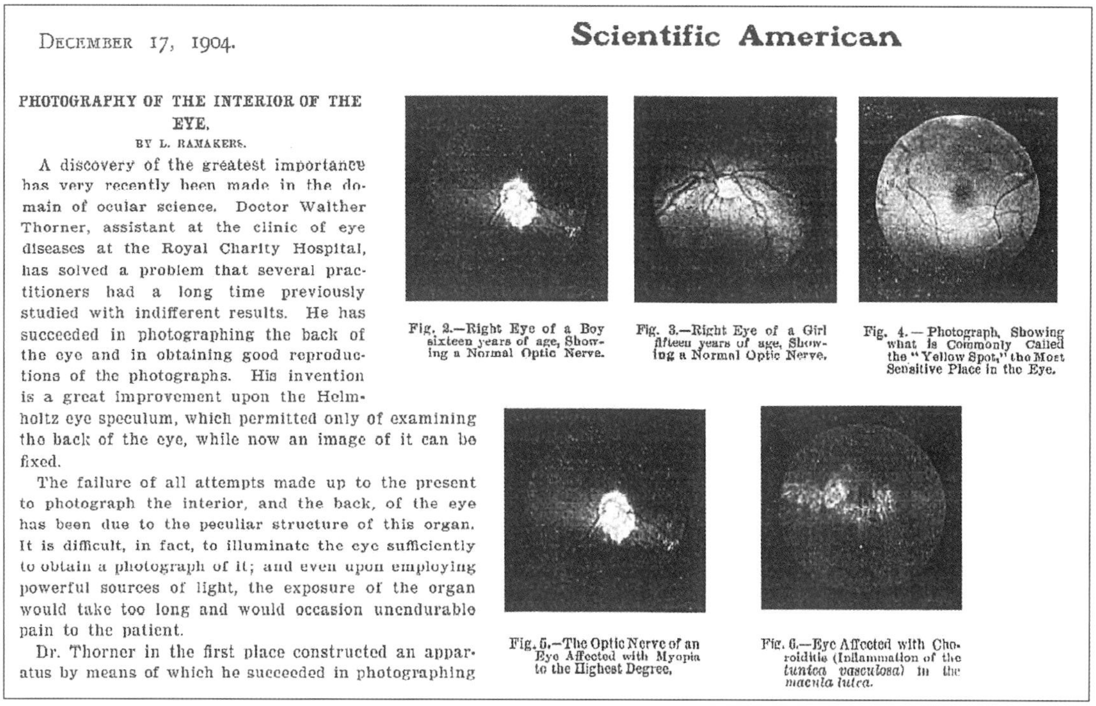

December 17, 1904.

Scientific American

PHOTOGRAPHY OF THE INTERIOR OF THE EYE.

BY L. RAMAKERS.

A discovery of the greatest importance has very recently been made in the domain of ocular science. Doctor Walther Thorner, assistant at the clinic of eye diseases at the Royal Charity Hospital, has solved a problem that several practitioners had a long time previously studied with indifferent results. He has succeeded in photographing the back of the eye and in obtaining good reproductions of the photographs. His invention is a great improvement upon the Helmholtz eye speculum, which permitted only of examining the back of the eye, while now an image of it can be fixed.

The failure of all attempts made up to the present to photograph the interior, and the back, of the eye has been due to the peculiar structure of this organ. It is difficult, in fact, to illuminate the eye sufficiently to obtain a photograph of it; and even upon employing powerful sources of light, the exposure of the organ would take too long and would occasion unendurable pain to the patient.

Dr. Thorner in the first place constructed an apparatus by means of which he succeeded in photographing

Fig. 2.—Right Eye of a Boy sixteen years of age, Showing a Normal Optic Nerve.

Fig. 3.—Right Eye of a Girl fifteen years of age, Showing a Normal Optic Nerve.

Fig. 4.—Photograph, Showing what is Commonly Called the "Yellow Spot," the Most Sensitive Place in the Eye.

Fig. 5.—The Optic Nerve of an Eye Affected with Myopia to the Highest Degree.

Fig. 6.—Eye Affected with Choroiditis (Inflammation of the *tunica vasculosa*) in the *macula lutea*.

FIG. 37. "Photography of the Interior of the Eye," *Scientific American* 91, no. 25, December 17, 1904.

eclipsed the others, probably their complementary colors."[28]

The epilogue to the *New York Times* story describes Dr. Gabriel's friends performing the doctor's autopsy and using a photographic process to develop an image imprinted on his retina. This example illustrates that the physiology of vision was not only a very active area of research in the late nineteenth century but also a subject highly appreciated by the general public, who found the aberrations and errors of vision—hallucinations, mirages, the miraculous recovery of sight, and so on—particularly appealing. The same theme was explored fairly often in various forms, from popular science to sensationalist pseudoscience: the rumor that the retina recorded, in a more or less lasting manner, the images seen by the eye fascinated the press and fueled much speculation. The tabloid press claimed that this discovery made it possible to identify a murderer based on the image imprinted on the victim's retina. During this same period, *Scientific American* published the first photographs of the interior of the eye (fig. 37).[29] The same year that the account of Dr. Gabriel's experiments appeared, William James described the phenomenon of the afterimage in his *Principles of Psychology:* "As a rule sensations outlast for some little time the objective stimulus which occasioned them. This phenomenon is the ground of those 'after-images' which are familiar in the physiology of the sense-organs. If we open our eyes instantaneously upon a scene, and then shroud them in complete darkness, it will be as if we saw the scene in ghostly light through the dark screen."[30] Tanner's paintings depict, precisely, spectral lights perceived through the filter of darkness. The gesture of shrouding the eyes in obscurity, rendered as the darkness of the canvas, initiates a withdrawal to a kind of inward vision firmly rooted in the physical subject. Consciousness of a vision detached from its external referent was a veritable commonplace in the late nineteenth century: its embodied and subjective nature was emphasized, its inadequacies continually pinpointed. The physiology of vision had thus become sufficiently well known by the turn of the century to be among the themes commonly discussed in lessons and manuals for art students and art lovers. Hermann von Helmholtz's writings on optics were widely circulated, for example, in the collection *Popular Lectures on Scientific Subjects,* which was reissued more than ten times between 1890 and 1917. Michel Eugène Chevreul's and Ogden Rood's books on color were standard references for American artists of the period.[31] The painter Birge Harrison was also able to discuss Daltonism and the limited spectrum of human vision in a book on painting intended for a broad readership: "We are all born color-blind. The most perfect eyes in the world cannot see one-quarter of the colors which are known to exist in nature. Those of us who are fortunate, it is true, are able to differentiate with reasonable exactness the three primary colors which go to make up our limited human color-scale—but what about the tones which certainly exist above the ultra-violet band and below the infra-red?"[32] In short, the nocturne artists, in choosing to restrict their palette to one extreme of visual perception, playing with their beholders' sight, embraced that notion and opted for a limited, contingent, subjective, and embodied vision. Their works, located at the far reaches of the perceptible, were in dialogue with increasingly familiar reflections on the question of human vision.

GEORGE INNESS AND THE SCIENCE OF COLOR

George Inness provided a unique response to these questions. Like Tanner, he combined a scientific approach to vision with a religious interpretation. As several studies devoted to the painter have shown, throughout his career Inness developed an aesthetic methodology sustained by a symbolism based on his readings of the philosopher and theologian Emanuel Swedenborg.[33] Although many critics during that era and some art historians, notably Rachael Z. DeLue, pointed out the artist's "idiosyncrasy," it is important to emphasize his very strong ties to the art circles of his time: he dispensed advice to many young artists who visited him in his New York studio, and later, in Montclair, New Jersey;[34] expressed his views frequently in the press; and regularly exhibited with his fellow artists, in particular, at the National Academy of Design, of which he had been a member since 1853, before founding the Society of American Artists in 1878.[35] By the end of Inness's life, his paintings, which tend toward twilight or nocturnal atmospheres, were considered some of the best examples of tonalism, and the artist was one of the "poet painters"[36] very prized by collectors such as Thomas B. Clarke, alongside nocturne painters such as Dwight William Tryon.[37] Around the turn of the century, Inness's misty landscapes, and especially the works he left behind upon his death in 1894, some of them unfinished, were particularly resonant for a public that had embraced the aesthetic of the nocturne.[38] The painter Childe Hassam, for example, in a letter to the gallery owner Roland Knoedler, lauded one of the many moonrises painted by Inness, saying that in his view "there are only one or two other moonlight pictures that I know of in art that can rank with it, one by Whistler, and the small picture of a waning moon by Millet."[39] Although Inness began to paint moonlight landscapes well before the vogue for the nocturne, and though he died at the start of the period under study in this book, he shared the sensibilities of his age and partly shaped the aesthetic of his younger fellows. The attention he gave to optical perception also illustrates his place within the intellectual debates of the time. As indicated in an interview he granted to *Harper's Weekly* in 1882, he was one of the first artists to call into question the principle of a scientific and rational vision, and to offer his public a vision that extended beyond the given: "When we know how imperfect the human eye is when compared with the eyes of some insects, although it is so wonderful, why should we undertake to say that states do not exist of which we have no physical perception, and can have none?"[40] For Inness, indeed, art was a sensory experience but also a sort of metaphysical exploration. In his view, painting was theology "gradually resolved into a scientific form,"[41] a science regulated by highly developed geometric and mathematical arguments.[42] His view was inspired by Swedenborg's theory of correspondences, according to which disparate realities can be linked together through a series of symbolic transfers. There would thus be a spiritual counterpart to the physical world, the two united in such a way that the state of one can affect that of the other.[43] In an article Inness published in the *New Jerusalem Messenger* (the publication of the Swedenborgian church), writing both as a man of faith and as a professional, he put forward his interpretation of color, consistent with the Swedenborgian theory of correspondences: "It is generally known that there are three of what are called primitive colors, but it is not generally known that one, namely, red, is positive, and apparently the parent of the two others, blue and yellow. Of these latter, blue presents an idea of what is spiritual and appears like something intangible."[44] Inness was referring here to a sermon by the Reverend Jonathan Bayley, published in the journal the previous year, which was devoted to a biblical verse from Numbers, in which God asks Moses to bring a blue ribbon to the children of Israel.[45] According to the painter, the definition of "warm blue" proposed by the minister was incorrect. Inness claimed that, rather than a blue mixed with red, as Bayley suggested, it was a blue complemented by the other two primary colors: blue tinged with red verges on a purple corresponding to royalty, while blue augmented by yellow tends toward green, the color of the natural world: "But tinge blue with both and the greatest warmth is obtained without altering its value as blue at all, and not only so, but it will in this condition bear a greater amount of white, which corresponds to light and wisdom, without loosing [*sic*] its value as pure blue, than even the purest blues. . . . The blue ribband of Israel is warmed with orange, the color of ripeness . . . the color of the pure, celestial flame that warms while it illumines. Seeking for God, the rational is developed, loving humanity, the scientific is built up. Faith in the Lord joins them in harmonious union and is a 'blessing for both.'"[46]

Moonrise, which Inness painted in 1887, can be interpreted in the light of that elaborate science of correspondences: the sky, traversed by a "blue ribband" in its center, is also tinged with the orange colors of the setting sun and of the moon. Parallel to the green band of vegetation, which in Inness's theory corresponded to the natural order, the blue of the sky would embody a spiritual order. The moon, revealed between two dark masses, illuminates the sky, thus appearing as a symbolic force that reorders the landscape and gives it a more profound meaning. In this landscape filled with uncertainty, where water and earth mingle in an unstable foreground, and shadows obscure the forms contemplated by the solitary figure, the blue of the sky illuminated by its complementary colors assumes the aspect of a literally "metaphysical" horizon, symbol of the faith that guides the believer. Correspondences merge fluidly in that "harmonious union," as Inness combined in a single gesture the natural and the spiritual, the visible and the invisible, art and science.

ELECTRICITY AND MOTION PHOTOGRAPHY: THE "POSITIVE DISCORDS" OF WINSLOW HOMER'S *SUMMER NIGHT*

The choice of nighttime may appear to distance the object or to appeal to a world beyond vision; yet at the same time, darkness exacerbates the problems of visual perception. That is particularly the case in Winslow Homer's *Summer Night,* painted in 1890 (see fig. 9). Ordinarily, Homer's work was acclaimed by critics as a virile and realistic vision of America. *Summer Night,* however, received rather mixed reviews—a sign that the painting did not fulfill its audience's expectations. This rather romantic canvas, which shows two women waltzing by the water's edge while a group in silhouette, seated on the rocks below, look at the moonlight reflected on the ocean, is different from Homer's usual genre scenes, in which weather-beaten fishermen or hunters struggle against the elements. Here the figures are not toilers of the sea but tourists, come to spend the summer at Prout's Neck, a small vacation town on the Maine coast where Homer set up his studio. Critics seem to have had difficulty viewing this painting as an instance of the painter's trademark "realism," with many characterizing it instead as a poetic and imaginative work.[47] One critic called the painting a "spiritual entity,"[48] while another saw the two dancers as "young witches of Endor," advancing a very nonrealist interpretation of the scene: "Their phantom-like appearance might mean the impersonation of death or folly or what not."[49] Many commentators, on the other hand, still insisted on the canvas's fidelity to reality, as did Homer's biographer William H. Downes: "The genesis of *A Summer Night* is easily divined. It is a virtually literal transcript of a scene which Homer saw in front of his own studio at Prout's Neck. The platform is the only part of the composition which did not exist in the real scene. The girls were dancing on the lawn. As usual, the artist painted exactly what he saw."[50] Somewhat contradictorily, however, Downes also read the painting as a very Whistleresque "harmony in a minor key,"[51] seemingly indicating that the main interest of the artwork was not, in his eyes, its down-to-earth realism. The very qualified success of the painting, which, despite Homer's persistence, found no buyers among his usual clients (it was ultimately acquired by the French government ten years after its creation), also indicates a certain uneasiness on the part of Homer's American public. The catalogue entry for the painting on the website of the Musée d'Orsay, where it is now held, translates the conflicted impressions that Homer's contemporaries perceived: "This nocturne, set along the oceanside, transcends the observation of reality by means of an acute sense of poetry and mystery"; it "perfectly expresses [the] synthesis" between "realism and symbolism."[52]

The trouble Homer's critics had in categorizing the painting stemmed from unresolved contradictions that deeply undermine the composition. Tellingly, reviewers were quick to identify the couple of dancers as one of the major incongruities of the painting.[53] "[Homer's] figures do not interest us, and we almost wish them out

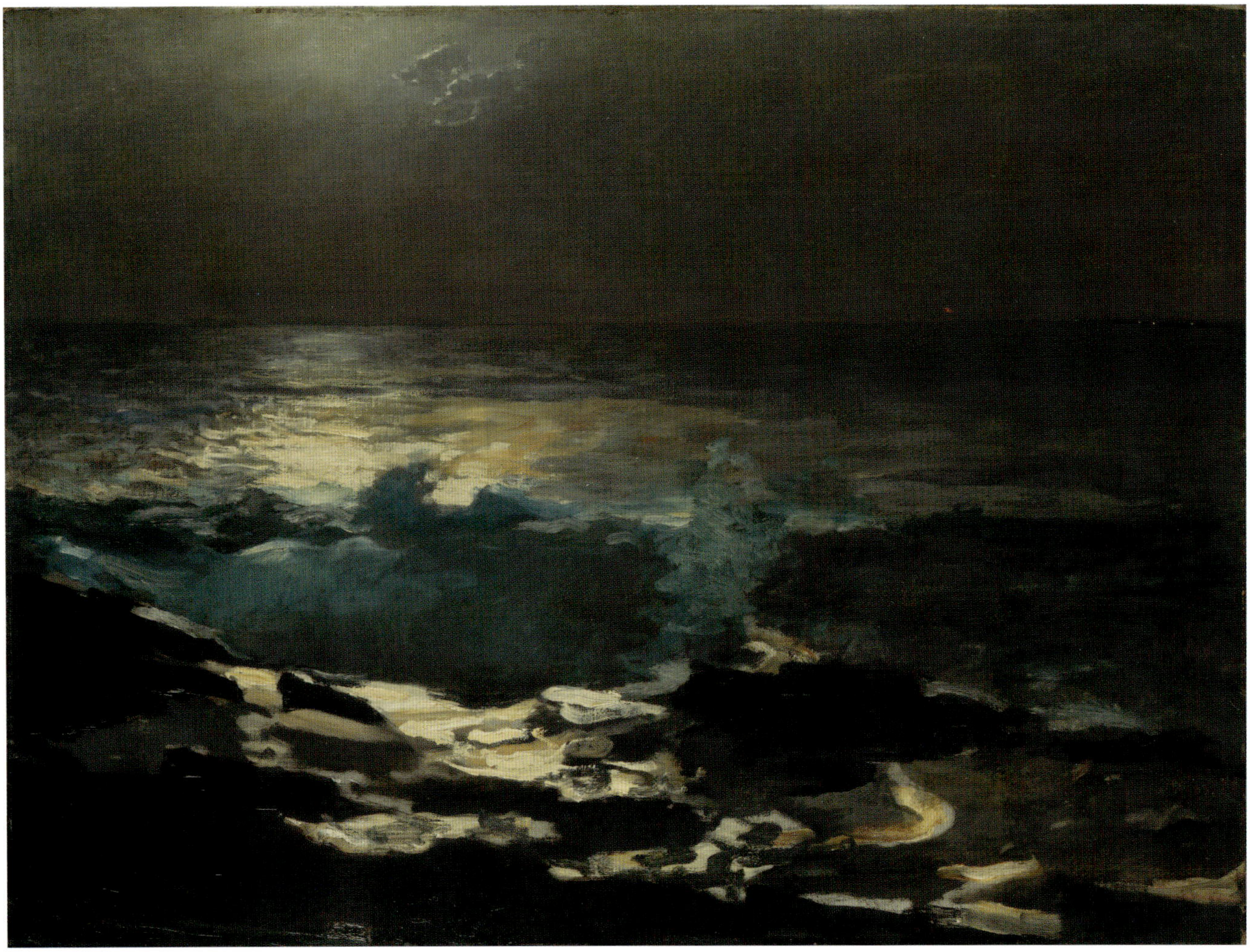

FIG. 38. Winslow Homer, *Moonlight, Wood Island Light*, 1894. Oil on canvas, 78.1 × 102.2 cm (30 ¾ × 40 ¼ in.). Metropolitan Museum of Art, New York. Gift of George A. Hearn, in memory of Arthur Hoppock Hearn, 1911 (11.116.2).

of the way that we might more wholly enjoy the sea,"[54] noted a journalist for the *New York Sun*. A reporter for *Art Amateur* echoed this view: "The painting would be much more impressive if the figures in the foreground were left out."[55] Homer undoubtedly heeded these remarks when he painted *Moonlight, Wood Island Light* four years after *Summer Night*. That landscape adopts the same point of view, but without human figures (fig. 38). The review in the *New York Times* clearly shows that the young women's presence in *Summer Night* was a departure from pure realism: "The dancing girls . . . are not carried to the point of realism that some artists teach. We do not find the artificial light flaming over them, but whether this is intentional or not is not easily seen. It may be that Mr. Homer is not up to that trick; it may be that he judged such realism inexpedient considering the bizarre effect of dancers who decline to be rendered motionless by the splendor of the scene."[56]

However odd they may seem in the composition, though, the pair of dancers merely attracts attention to two more fundamental problems in the painting: first, its handling of natural and artificial light; and second, its representation of movement. As the *New York Times* critic pointed out, the source of artificial light illuminating the dancers lies outside the frame, hidden. So too the moon: we see only its reflection on the water's surface. The light projected onto the young women, so intense that it plunges the silhouettes in the background into an artificial darkness, very probably comes from outdoor electric lighting, no doubt an arc lamp. Prout's Neck did not have an electric lighting system before the early twentieth century, but it is likely that the owner of the hotel next to Homer's studio, an innovative entrepreneur, equipped his property with an independent generator, a practice common at tourist establishments in the region.[57] And even if this was not the case, Homer certainly saw the effects of electric arc lighting in the streets of Portland, about a dozen miles from his studio. From 1885 on, the city was a testing ground for Thomas Edison's firm and one of the first cities in the United States to be equipped with an entirely electric public lighting system.[58]

The introduction of artificial lighting in Homer's painting raises several delicate questions and challenges the artist's reputation of fidelity to nature. Lighting conditions impacted, in the first place, Homer's artistic practice. They posed an obvious dilemma: either he painted immediately from life, but to do so he had to make use of artificial lighting; or he painted by daylight, but in that case he had to paint from memory and no longer from life. Homer, who commented only rarely on his process, mentioned precisely the subject of lighting ten years after painting *Summer Night*. He explained that the paintings of the great masters could be created only in the studio, because "you can't control the thing out-doors." Yet, in the same interview, he also claimed that "this making studies and taking them home to use them is only half right" and that "it is impossible to paint an out-door figure in studio light with any degree of certainty." In Homer's view, only natural light allowed the artist to obtain a scene that possesses verisimilitude, one in which the transitions remain invisible. Conversely, the studio made shapes and shadows jump out and gave the impression of a "made picture."[59] The various accounts of how the painting was created bear witness to that contradiction inherent in the realist artist's process. One of Homer's biographers, for example, told of the evening that had inspired the subject for *Moonlight, Wood Island Light*. Homer, contemplating the moonlight, is said to have had a burst of creativity. He grabbed his painter's tools and proceeded to work outdoors until dawn. "The picture called *Moonlight, Wood Island Light* was the result of that impulse and four or five hours' work. Like his other moonlight pictures, it was painted wholly in and by the light of the moon, *and never again retouched*."[60] This last statement occurs only a few pages after the description, quoted above, of how *Summer Night* was composed. There, in the same breath, Downes explained that the platform on which the young women were dancing was an addition by Homer and that the artist painted "exactly what he saw." The myth of a spontaneous, faithful and immediate relationship of the painter to his subject-matter does not resist confrontation with the reality of its creation here: the existing studies for *Summer Night*[61] indicate that the painting probably resulted from a series of takes in different lights, so to speak, forcing Homer to make compromises with realism and to create a picture that is "only half right."

This conflicted process might explain why Homer left the sources of light outside the frame of the painting—to attenuate, precisely, that impression of artificiality. Yet, the jarring effect of the two coexisting lights still irked some commentators, who struggled to reaffirm the work's coherence: "[*Summer Night*] is a renewal of the painter's favorite attempt to harmonize two lights in one picture, but this time the artist resolved not to spoil his unities [*sic*] by pushing to any excess one of his extremes, so that the two girls who dance in the foreground in the glow of the illumination that streams from the house are carried just far enough to give value to the immeasurable moonlit sea that stretches far beyond. It is probably not possible to paint moonlight on the ocean better than it is done here."[62] But the presence of the dancing girls, caught as they are in the electric glare, only reveals the artificiality of the composition, and introduces what the critic of the *Art Amateur* called a "positive discord" with the background landscape.[63] The introduction of harsh artificial light transforms the space of the image, alters the perspective, and turns the pictorial representation on its head. It shatters the unity of the image into several disarticulated planes, several "unities," to use the awkward phrasing of the *Art Interchange* reporter. It flattens the figures in the background and reduces them to mere silhouettes, while at the same time highlighting the pair of dancers in an almost phantasmagorical manner. Like luminous apparitions projected on a dark screen, the two young women take on a spectral appearance: they seem to belong to an ambiguous space, located between the moonlit landscape and the viewing space occupied by the beholder of the painting. It is not surprising, then, that critics singled them out. Standing on a platform whose edge is parallel to the bottom of the frame, they give the impression that they occupy a different plane from the rest of the landscape, or even that they inhabit a different picture. The disjunction between the foreground and the landscape in the background could lead us to think that the two dancers are in front of a painted decor, which,

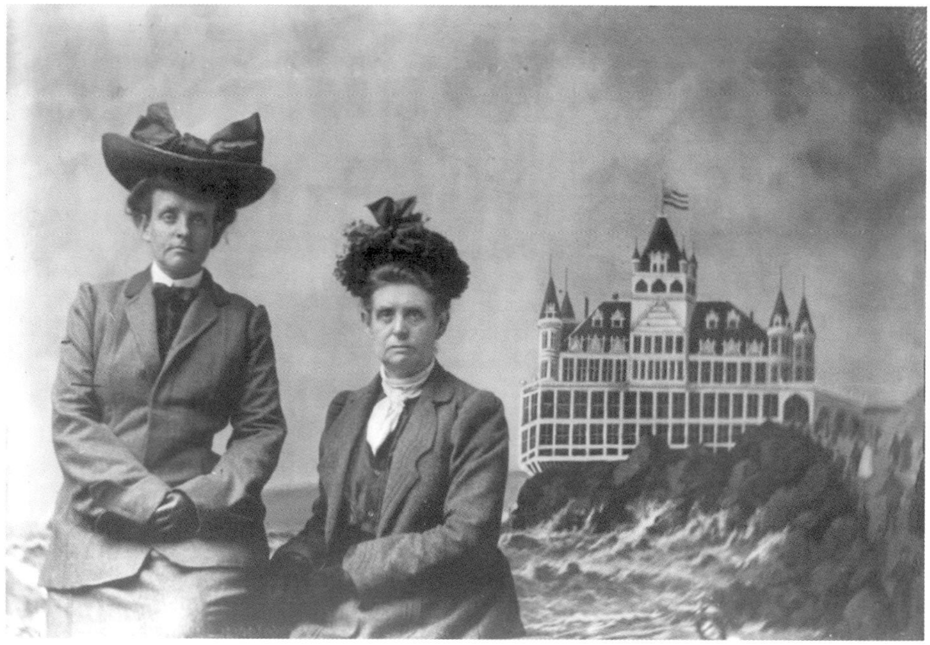

FIG. 39. *Frances Benjamin Johnston, with Maddie (her mother), 1903, with a painted backdrop of the Cliff House in San Francisco, California, 1903.* Tintype. Library of Congress, Prints and Photographs Division, Washington, D.C.

combined with the artificial light, would suggest theatrical sets or those used in photo studios. The use of such decors was a particularly widespread practice at the turn of the twentieth century.[64] At holiday resorts, for example, tourists could have a photo of themselves taken in front of a set evoking the region's landscape or local curiosities (fig. 39). *Summer Night* has the same mediated relationship to the natural landscape as such tourist photographs, and the discontinuities in its composition (its creation in several distinct stages, its visual incoherence) make for an equally artificial image.

Homer's dancers, arrested in their waltz, draw attention to a second dilemma in the painting, namely, the representation of movement. Here, photography might have interfered with Homer's realism. The painter was no doubt familiar with the experiments of Eadweard Muybridge, who in 1886 published hundreds of photographs in his *Animal Locomotion* and also projected them as slides at lectures, addressed to artists in particular, in all the large cities on the east coast.[65] It is difficult to imagine how Homer could have failed to see these astonishing images or to take into account Muybridge's revelations about movement before painting *Summer Night*. The two girls frozen mid-movement seem to replicate Muybridge's studies on dance (fig. 40), while the waves, captured as they break against the rocks, bring to mind his photographs of human figures splashing in water or pouring from pitchers.[66] The regularity of the shape of the waves even suggests a chronophotographic interpretation of the painting: rather than read the two bursts of sea spray as one simultaneous movement, we may understand them as the recording, in the same image, of two successive moments of a single wave. Similarly, the two young women seem interchangeable enough to be perceived as one dancer viewed at two different stages of the waltz. Just as the ambiguous lighting tends to make the various elements of the composition appear disjointed, the capturing of movement produces the impression of jerkiness and incompletion. In contrast to the fluidity suggested by the music and the ocean, Homer's canvas is able to capture reality only by freezing it, to render movement only by its opposite. Muybridge fascinated his audience not only by meticulously dissecting the various phases of bodies in motion but also by reconstituting, with the aid of the zoopraxiscope, the illusion of that motion. Homer, on the contrary, was limited by his medium. The "bizarre effect" of the young women's presence, as perceived by the *New York Times* critic, comes not only from the fact that they "decline to be rendered motionless" by the spectacle of the ocean but perhaps also, and even more so, from their remaining oddly suspended between motion and motionlessness.

In this case, the intrusion of technology destabilized pictorial realism. Under pressure from new visual phenomena such as electricity and photography, realism in painting seemed to be becoming an increasingly perilous exercise. With *Summer Night*, Homer's hesitant efforts in

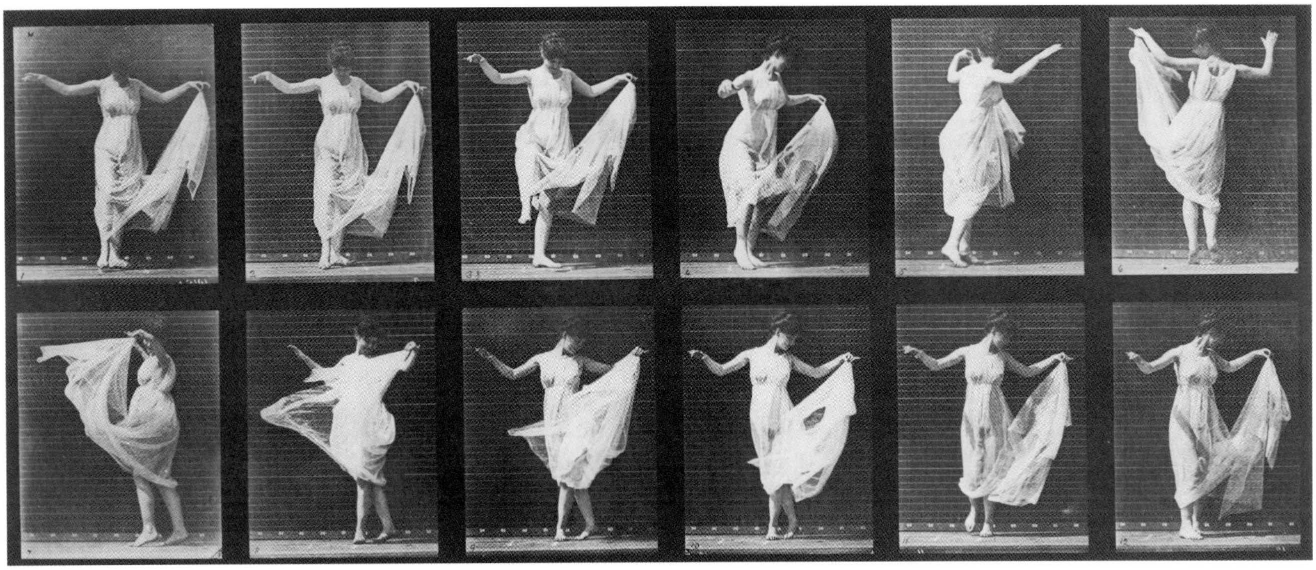

FIG. 40. Eadweard Muybridge "Dancing—Fancy," c. 1887. Phototype. Library of Congress, Prints and Photographs Division, Washington, D.C.

the direction of a direct and realist representation paradoxically culminated in an unreal image filled with disjunctions. Yet some of Homer's critics interpreted these difficulties and incoherencies as elements that contribute to the poetry and mystery of the painting: its fundamental ambiguity allows it to be reinvested with poetic values. The art historian Nicolai Cikovsky Jr. writes that the works Homer produced from the 1890s onward moved away from an overly simple and direct realism and shared with European symbolist works the propensity for suggestion. In Cikovsky's view, the "affinities" of *Summer Night* with the European movement explain why the painting was exhibited in the symbolist gallery of the Musée d'Orsay.[67] By virtue of their ambiguous location, the dancing girls invite the beholder to step away from a realist interpretation, and make the painting an open work, a potential image.[68] As if to add to the work's ambivalence, the dancers, while highly visible in the streaming electric light, simultaneously suggest a certain withdrawal into invisibility and darkness, a refusal to see, underscored by the closed eyes of the girl facing the beholder. Technological advances forced Homer to retreat into darkness, as both a refuge and a visual compromise: in that play between light and darkness, *Summer Night* oscillates permanently between the visible and the invisible, without ever really committing itself to one or the other. In that sense, the painting is a symptom of a certain discomfort on the part of artists in an environment where the conditions of vision and representation were being profoundly altered by the incursion of technology.

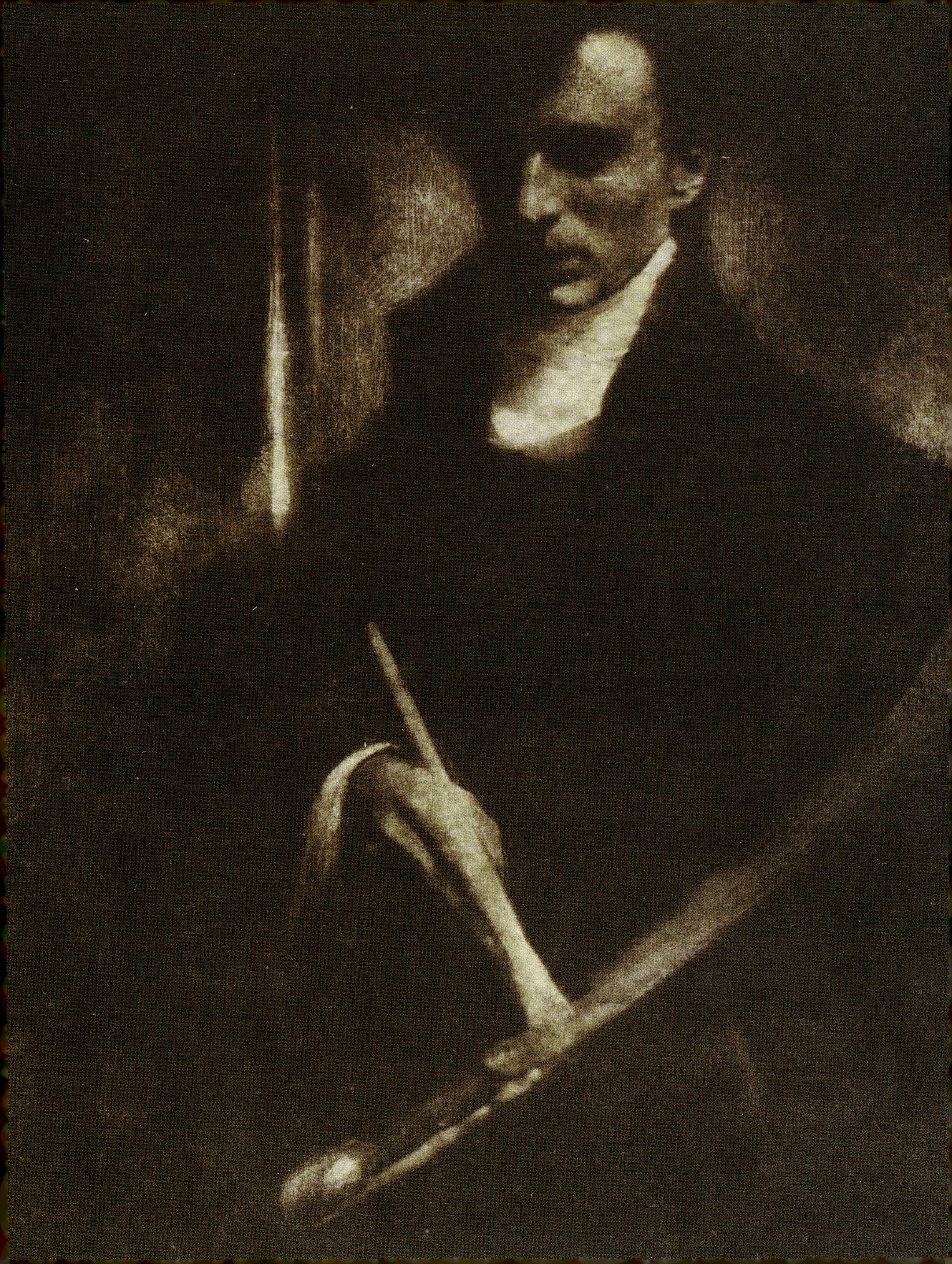

3 The Work of Art in the Age of Mechanical Reproduction

Not only did the field of the visible expand through the discoveries of science and technological innovations, it was also profoundly transformed by them on a daily basis. At the dawn of the twentieth century, people saw *better,* thanks to increasingly precise and effective technology; but they also saw *more,* given the greater reproducibility of images. Among elites, image reproduction technologies, viewed as a factor in the leveling of cultural values and the upheaval of the social order, produced a certain anxiety. Photography in particular played an essential role in that reconfiguration of the conditions of vision. Artists, confronted with that emblematic medium for mechanically reproducing images, strategically used the nocturne's codes to situate themselves (artistically, sociologically, and economically) within the ever-expanding economy of images. The nocturne aesthetic was seen as a guarantee of the uniqueness and authenticity of works of art. Ironically, that defense of elitist values against the profusion of commercial mass images proved to be a profitable economic strategy, which contributed toward imposing the nocturne on the market.

Fig. 45 detail

THE PERILS OF THE MASS IMAGE

The "Kodak Moment," the Beginnings of Cinema, the Halftone, and the Rise of Illustration

Advances in photography introduced changes that went far beyond scientific practices and their promotion among the general public: they transformed the public's relationship to the image, its production, and its consumption. George Eastman's genius in launching Kodak cameras was that he snatched photography away from its most skilled practitioners, by separating picture-taking from the development process, certainly the most technically complex aspect of the activity. Amateurs were invited to "press the button," and the Kodak firm would "do the rest" (fig. 41). From simplified and inexpensive cameras to intensive advertising campaigns to the establishment of a vast network of development laboratories readily available to the public, Eastman rolled out a whole commercial system intended to revolutionize the field of photography. Significantly, the Kodak camera became one of the first products of mass consumption whose manufacture was completely standardized.[1] In 1895 Eastman launched the Pocket Kodak with a five-dollar

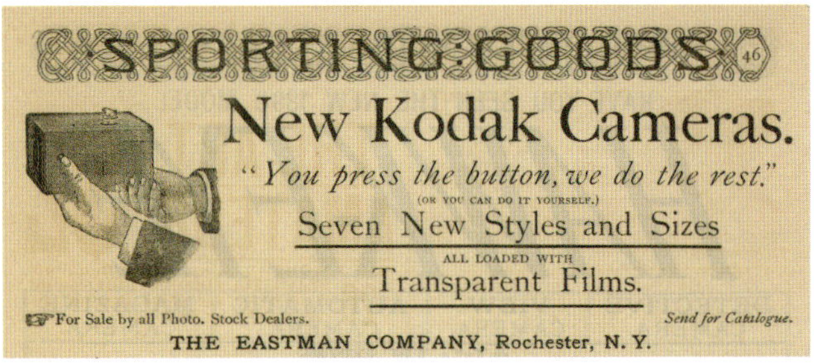

FIG. 41. Kodak, "You Press the Button, We Do the Rest." Advertisment, 1890. Emergence of Advertising in America, 1850–1920, David M. Rubenstein Rare Book & Manuscript Library, Duke University, Durham, North Carolina.

price tag; five years later he introduced the one-dollar Brownie, a camera designed especially for children. Cameras were sold preloaded with film and, when the film was used up, they were sent to development laboratories; the labs then printed the negatives and reloaded the cameras. Kodak commercials shattered the image of the photographer as seasoned professional. They featured children and women—including the famous "Kodak girl"—to demonstrate the universal accessibility of an "artless art" whose simplicity would guarantee its success. The wager paid off: the Kodak firm increased its sales fourfold between 1889 and 1899, then again between 1899 and 1909. It dominated the American market and monopolized the global market, as amateur clubs and specialized publications multiplied. The impact was so great that Eastman went down in history, creating what historians, borrowing from one of Eastman's own advertising campaigns, have called a "Kodak moment," an era that, with the triumph of digital photography, has only just ended.

At the dawn of the twentieth century, cinema was still in its infancy; the lighting techniques and special effects that would allow nocturnal scenes to appear onscreen were not developed until after World War I. It was only with film noir in the 1940s–1950s that night would become a theme of aesthetic importance. From its early days, however, cinema contributed indirectly to the transformation of spectators' vision. It added a new dimension to the image, allowing it to develop over time and to be repeated ad infinitum. The wonderment at a medium that constantly displayed its manifold effects was typical of the fascination during that period for the booming growth of images and the increase in their visual potential by means of technology. Tom Gunning understands the early years of cinema in terms of the development of an "exhibitionist" practice of the image, one with little interest in narrative, concerned primarily with the entertainment potential of the moving picture.[2] He compares that "cinema of attractions" to the amusement parks and mass entertainment that developed in the last decades of the nineteenth century. Cinema was in fact originally associated with fairground attractions and popular entertainments, like those provided by P. T. Barnum. Very short films were shown in individual coin-operated machines or in vaudeville theaters, where they served as interludes between various live shows. Gradually, some theaters came to devote most of their programming to films. These show palaces targeted a wide, working-class audience: the low price of admission, often only a nickel, made for their success. These nickelodeons became so popular that, by 1910, more than fourteen thousand projection rooms existed in the United States.[3] Film, in a much more visible manner than any other kind of visual production, introduced a collective form of image consumption. Its enormous impact on American culture was not yet perceptible in the early years of the twentieth century, but it is now possible to assess its role in the revolution of images that marked the period.

The halftone, also an extension of the photograph, was introduced by Georg Meisenbach in 1886. It revolutionized reproduction techniques. In the halftone process, a fine screen placed in front of the lens decomposes the image into a series of easily printable dots. That innovation made it possible to print text and illustrations together, avoiding recourse to hand engraving or the insertion of stand-alone plates. In the early 1900s, a process was developed that allowed images to be printed in simple but bright tones, based on combinations of the three primary colors.[4] Thanks to the halftone process, the use of illustrations grew exponentially, and images quickly disseminated via various media, from newspapers to advertisements. Illustrated magazines such as *Harper's Monthly, Collier's, Scribner's,* and *Ladies' Home Journal* greatly increased their circulation in the 1890s, and the rapid expansion of daily illustrated newspapers made the fortune of magnates such as William Randolph Hearst and Joseph Pulitzer.[5] Illustrated magazines published special issues on particular subjects: it became common, for example, to publish a "Christmas number," in which illustrations were more plentiful and of better quality than in the regular issues. The big names in journalism also engaged in the lucrative practice of publishing books of images, assembling the works of particular illustrators and then selling them as more or less limited editions.[6] The number of halftones in books also increased spectacularly, whether these were souvenir albums for the world's fairs, guidebooks for tourists, educational works, or illustrated novels. Advertising quickly seized on that new technology, saturating the daily lives of Americans with posters, packaging materials with pictures on them, and advertising cards. Images, offered as gifts in the form of illustrated cards published in series on popular themes (occupations, traditional costumes of the world, African animals) now took on a dual function: they were not only the medium for a commercial message but objects desirable in and of themselves.

Increased demand offered unprecedented professional opportunities to artists who specialized in illustration. The turn of the twentieth century, now considered a golden age for illustration, thus witnessed the ascent to the rank of celebrities of artists such as Howard Pyle, N. C. Wyeth, Charles Dana Gibson, and Maxfield Parrish. Their names sold the books they illustrated at least as much as those of the authors.[7] These famous figures also attracted and provided on-the-job training to an entire generation of young illustrators, whose professionalism was ensured by the creation of such institutions as the Society of Illustrators, founded in New York in 1901. Within the class of illustrators personalities emerged, but their "signature" lay more in a specialized theme than in a personal style. For example, Edward Kemble focused on genre scenes depicting African Americans; Howard Pyle had a near monopoly on pirate stories; Charles Dana Gibson became famous for his fashionable young women, the "Gibson Girls"; and Frederic Remington was the artist to turn to for depictions of the American West. This professional specialization was a mark of the illustrators' participation in a capitalist economy with an increasingly sharp division of labor, where each task was part of a broader system of production. Another measure of the success of commercial illustrators lay in the scorn sometimes heaped upon them by easel painters, who embraced the notion of an art elevated above daily life, stamped with the unique seal of individual and creative genius. In their view, the commercial illustrator, even when he did not work for an advertising firm, did not have the independence of the "true" artist. His subjects, and often the execution of them, were assigned at the editor's whim, and the editor's main concern was to please the largest

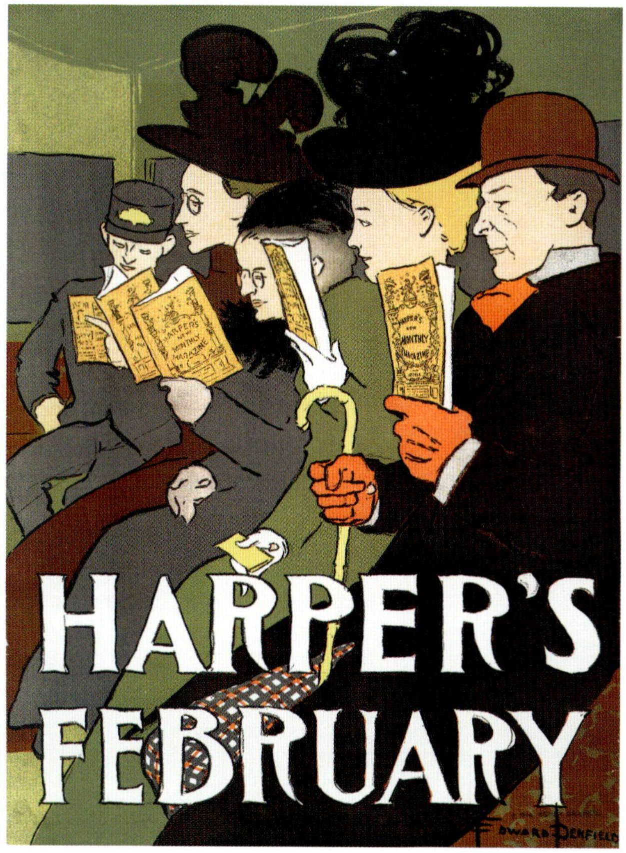

FIG. 42. Edward Penfield, *Harper's New Monthly Magazine* February 1895. Color lithograph, 49 × 35.5 cm (19 ¼ × 14 in.). Art & Architecture Collection, Miriam and Ira D. Wallach Division of Art, Prints and Photographs, The New York Public Library, Astor, Lenox and Tilden Foundations.

readership possible. That tendency toward "mediocrity" gave rise to contempt on the part of the cultural elite.[8]

An advertisement for *Harper's Monthly* in February 1895 shows how omnipresent images in the public space were in people's daily lives and how much more aware people were of that presence and its impact on society (fig. 42). The ad depicts five characters aboard a train or streetcar, each engrossed in an issue of *Harper's*. Ironically, the mise en abyme points out a discrepancy between the cover of the magazines in the illustration—a yellow sheet dominated by text and the arabesques of its frontispiece—and the advertisement, which celebrates the visual richness of the magazine's actual content: a bright-colored image, different for each issue. The identical magazines, marking out the illustration like yellow flags, guide the eyes through the image as through the physical and social space of the car, symbolically linking the elegant man in the foreground to the ticket inspector in the background, by way of three female figures of different classes and ages. Readers are confronted with an image offered for individual consumption but one that is, at the same time, standardized and multiplied ad infinitum. The image becomes both the obstacle that separates the individuals, completely absorbed as they are in reading their magazines, and the common denominator that unites the anonymous members of a socially heterogeneous group.

Against the "Tyranny of the Pictorial": The Triple Threat of the Proliferation of Images

The invasion of the social space by images clearly gave rise to a certain mistrust. The proliferation of images resulting from technological progress was seen by a large number of commentators as not only an aesthetic threat but also an intellectual and moral one. Many voices rose up against the "tyranny of the pictorial," which was supposedly debasing art, good taste, the country's intellectual vigor, and even its morals.[9] An article by Charles L. Congdon titled "Over-Illustration," for example, attacked that multiplication of images, asking a multitude of questions of an aesthetic nature.[10] The author organized cultural productions into a conventional hierarchy: the first half of his argument was devoted to the reaffirmation of the primacy of the letter over the image; then, pausing to consider the various types of illustrations, he distinguished between the fine arts and the mechanical arts. "Photography is a cheap and convenient resource, but the utmost care and skill cannot make it much better than a manufacture. Its want of originality is a necessity. Its merits are its economy, and the rapidity of execution of which it is capable, together with that superficial fac-simile resemblance which finds favor in uneducated eyes."[11] The photograph, an imperfect substitute, was only the most obvious example of the intellectual poverty of the image in general. Congdon was especially alarmed by the concessions the press of his time was making to "the limited intellectual capacity of readers." Journalists seemed to be convinced that "the eye could be made to do the work of the mind."[12] Congdon was worried about the growing predominance of image over text and, as a result, of the hold the image had over the beholder's mental activity. Images spoke to the inferior portion of the intellect, or worse, overrode other faculties, such as the imagination. The "originality of impression" seemed increasingly difficult to defend in the face of a visual empire encroaching a bit more every day on the reader's freedom.

That invasion of private space by images also assumed a different form: not only did images penetrate everywhere, but they also promoted the circulation in the public sphere of what had until then remained private. In a founding text of American law, which for the first time established the concept of privacy and the need for laws to protect it, Samuel Warren and Louis Brandeis focused primarily on the image and its new technologies: "Recent inventions and business methods call attention to the next step which must be taken for the protection of the person, and for securing to the individual what Judge Cooley calls the right 'to be let alone.' Instantaneous photographs and newspaper enterprise have invaded the sacred precincts of private and domestic life; and numerous mechanical devices threaten to make good the prediction that 'what is whispered in the closet shall be proclaimed from the house-tops.'"[13] At a time when the separation between the domestic and public spheres was becoming institutionalized,[14] images, with their accelerated circulation, were perceived as disruptive agents. The urban setting in particular intensified the role of vision in social relations. The advertisement for *Harper's Monthly* suggests that, in a common space shared by isolated and anonymous individuals, only visual clues allowed one to decipher social identities. The gaze, mediated by the image—the printed image or one's own self-image—became the principal connection between individuals. The remaking of the sphere of the visible around that mediation was the occasion for many commentaries, in which, notably, the visible and the invisible were paradoxically linked. Distracted consumers of images, blind to their surroundings, were also in dangerous proximity to their neighbors. The mass circulation of images raised the risk that private space and public space would collapse into each other, combining hypervisibility and invisibility, an intensification of the visual and an incapacity to control all its particulars. That alliance of the visible and the invisible took a disturbing form with, for example, the increasingly discreet cameras developed by Eastman and his competitors. These devices were depicted in an illustration by Ferdinand Keppler called *The Peeping Toms of the Camera,* which was published on the cover of *Puck* magazine in 1891 (fig. 43). Here it is clear how technology was radically altering the social nature of vision. The young bather in Keppler's illustration is the

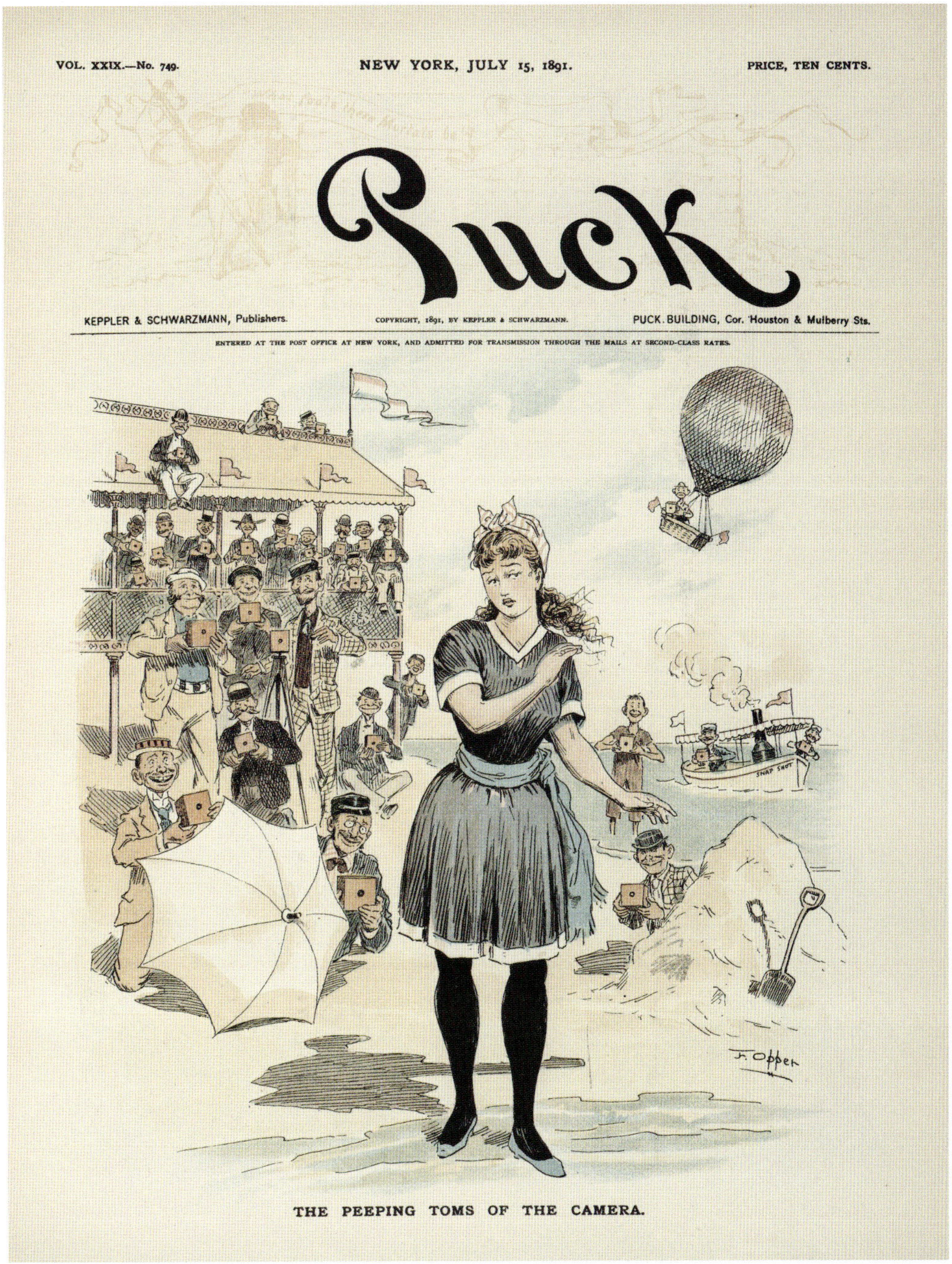

FIG. 43. Joseph Ferdinand Keppler, "The Peeping Toms of the Camera," *Puck* 29, no. 749, July 15, 1891, 25 × 34 cm (9 ⅞ × 13 ⅜ in.).

object of the gaze at every level: that of the individuals around her and that of *Puck*'s readers, to whom the image is complacently offered. The advances of photography and the growing number of people who could see without being seen, concealed behind technological mediations, introduced an exacerbated form of voyeurism.

THE NOCTURNE AND THE AURA

In that environment, suddenly flooded with images created and circulated by technology, artists, even more than others at the time, felt obligated to reconsider their relationship to the visual. When daily life was perceived to be saturated with images, technology forced artists to explore a number of often-related questions: the nature of artistic representation, which was called into question by photographic "objectivity"; the artistic act, shunted aside by the mechanization of the image; and the place occupied by the various image producers in a rapidly changing market. The reaction of nocturne artists was in great part based on the "fetishistic, fundamentally anti-technical notion of art."[15] That entrenchment was identified by Walter Benjamin in "The Work of Art in the Age of Mechanical Reproduction": "With the advent of the first truly revolutionary means of reproduction, photography, simultaneously with the rise of socialism, art sensed the approaching crisis which has become evident a century later. At the time, art reacted with the doctrine of *l'art pour l'art,* that is, with a theology of art. This gave rise to what might be called a negative theology in the form of the idea of 'pure' art, which not only denied any social function of art but also any determination by a concrete subject."[16] Here Benjamin accurately identified the motivations for the negative redefinition of art advanced by Whistler and his imitators. The nocturne, in its rejection—including in its iconography—of "any determination by a concrete subject," typified that desire to defend the work of art's "aura," which was undermined by increasing pressure from the sheer volume of mechanically reproduced images.

Nocturne artists displayed an almost paranoid need to prevent the secularization of their works, cutting them off from any historical, political, or social referent and reaffirming the uniqueness of the artist's activity. In response to the multiplicity of images and the overabundance of content, they proposed a negative aesthetic, combined with an exclusionary set of social practices related to the image. Nocturnes, rarefied visions that were to be exhibited only infrequently, were very much at odds with the work of art's increasingly public nature, which Benjamin considered one of the factors leading to the loss of its aura: "In the past, a painting always had an excellent chance to be viewed by only one person or by a few. The simultaneous contemplation of paintings by a large public, such as developed in the nineteenth century, is an early symptom of the crisis of painting, a crisis which was by no means occasioned exclusively by photography but rather in a relatively independent manner by the appeal of art works to the masses."[17] The very form of the nocturnes, which were not readily reproducible, prevented them from being inserted into the most popular distribution circuits. Their dark tones, restricted palettes, and blurred outlines remained in great part inaccessible to the technologies of the time, despite the advances made. The nocturnes of Whistler's disciple Herman Dudley Murphy (see fig. 17) are a good example, if we are to believe one of his critics: "Mr. Murphy's pictures, even the portraits, in black and white, give but a poor idea of what his work really is. Much of it can not be reproduced by photography without losing the values."[18] Sometimes as well, nocturne artists refused to circulate their works, keeping them deliberately beyond the reach of the masses. In 1901 the painter Thomas Dewing chose not to send his paintings to the Pan-American Exposition in Buffalo, explaining to his client Charles Lang Freer that his paintings had no place there: "My pictures of this class are . . . above the heads of the public. My decorations belong to the poetic and imaginative world where a few choice spirits live."[19] Also in a letter to Freer, the artist Dwight Tryon expressed similar views, arguing that his painting *Rising Moon* was poorly suited to be exhibited before the general public: "Painting as I do without reference to public exhibition, I expect little in this line."[20] Nocturne artists, by keeping their works in short supply, justified both their aesthetic value and their exchange value. But the artists were thereby caught in the trap of their own contradictions: in positioning themselves outside commercial circuits, they inflated prices through the scarcity of their products. That amounted to nothing less than playing the market—in a rather sophisticated manner, to be sure—with methods close to speculation. This was archly pointed out in an illustration by Albert Sterner called *Quantity not Quality* (fig. 44).[21] A client visiting an artist's studio, presented with two paintings for which the artist is asking the same price, expresses her preference for the most animated composition—a scene depicting a flock of sheep—at the expense of a very Whistleresque seascape, all water and sky. Even as Sterner gently made fun of his female character, he seemed to display a certain sympathy for that

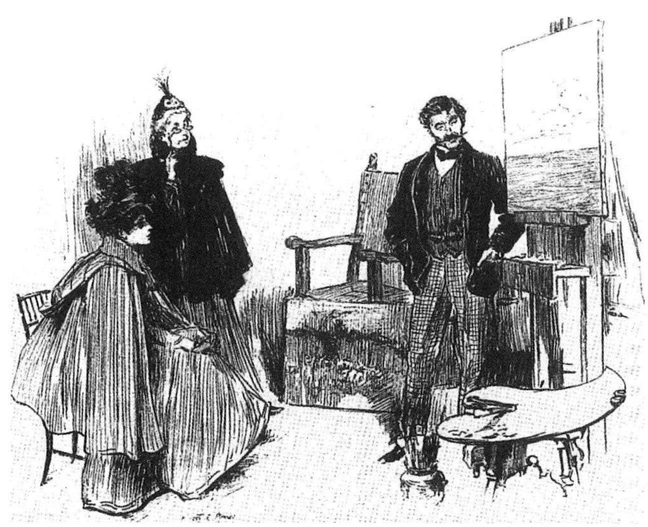

FIG. 44. Albert Sterner, "Quantity not Quality," *Harper's New Monthly Magazine* 94, no. 561, February 1, 1897.

commonsensical bourgeoise, who refuses to pay such a high price for "nothing more than water, horizons, and heavens."[22] The caricature indicates the irony of that new situation, where all distinctions were measured in quantitative—albeit negative—terms. Nocturne artists thus participated in an economy whose rules were ultimately the same for everyone.

As Sarah Burns has pointed out, Sterner's satire also evinces increasingly tense relations between the various image professionals. The new modes of creating and diffusing the image profoundly called into question the status of art and the artist. The commercial illustrator, who belonged to a category often held in contempt by easel artists, took his revenge. His situation sheds light on the divisions that were beginning to affect the world of image producers, where new categories were taking hold, and it was becoming important to define and hierarchize them. Nocturne artists and their critics, to distinguish themselves from their fellows, strove to impose a definition of "true" art. Their first gesture was to establish a rigid understanding of artistic vision. Faced with the growing domination of photography and of the notions of visual perception imported to the United States with impressionism, nocturne artists attempted to propose an alternative model of vision. The paradigm of a subjective, inward-looking gaze began to take shape, in opposition to the objective, externalized, and mechanized concept of photography. I will show later on how that discourse, particularly its engagement with the new psychology that developed in the late nineteenth century, contributed to conveying and shaping a new model of subjectivity. For the moment, I shall just indicate how artists and critics used this discourse to position the artists on the art market and, more generally, within the sphere of image production. Although it is true that nocturne artists were by no means the only ones to embrace that model, the nocturne serves as its systematic, even militant illustration.

Nocturne artists accepted photography as the instrument of an objective and scientific vision and defined their art as a reaction against it. Birge Harrison thus devoted a large portion of his reflections on painting to comparisons with photography. Adopting the conventional association of photography with objectivity and clarity, he contrasted it to art, which he placed on the side of an imperfect but human nature—superior, therefore, to the mechanics of photography. Even as Harrison conceded the scientific truth of photography, he developed the idea of a human and artistic truth, thus distinguishing the "factual," as recorded by scientific instruments, including photography, from the "visual," the result of an embodied and individualized vision. The "blur" and indetermination were not to be avoided: on the contrary, they were the forms closest to "nature," if by that word one understood the reality of human vision, including its limitations. In a chapter titled "The True Impressionism," Harrison discussed at length the repositioning of art vis-à-vis photography: "The human eye, and the human brain behind it, declined to accept as a symbol of motion anything which the eye had not been able to see for and by itself unaided. . . . The Kodak had revealed hitherto unsuspected facts and aspects of motion, but the eye would have none of them, and clung only to that which was visual. . . . Shortly also, it began to be seen that the impression, in fact, which the eye received from nature was not that which was rendered by the camera; and that, therefore, the human brain could never accept the photograph as a thoroughly satisfactory transcript of nature. It gives us scientific facts; and scientific facts are generally artistic lies."[23] Harrison reversed the terms of the opposition and reinstated human vision, with its known shortcomings, as the superior form of vision that art ought to approximate.

The chapter's title reveals that Harrison's remarks on the human eye's superiority over the Kodak camera were directed at least as much against impressionism, as it was understood in the United States at the time, as against photography. In that sense, they illustrate the keen competition among the various schools of painting and the different segments of the art market. Impressionism, because it shared the instantaneity of photography, was in fact often perceived as a mechanical art based on an automated vision. The painter Kenyon Cox, for example, described the impressionist painter William Merritt Chase as a "human camera, a seeing machine."[24] From the perspective of American critics, impressionism, by virtue of its formal characteristics, its choice of subjects, and its political commitments, was shocking, incapable of elevating the beholder's moral and aesthetic sensibility. The European impressionists' efforts were seen as mere tricks, an alienating mechanical method applied to the landscape from the outside. Alfred Trumble's description of impressionism as a violent and unnatural art, published in *The Collector* in 1891, is representative in that respect: "You are surrounded by explosions of paint—wild bombardments of the primary colors, hurled at your eye by brushes as brutal as the blows of slug-shots.... [Claude Monet] seizes on the mildest forms of nature... and tears all grace and beauty from it, covers it with furious splotches, rips it into iron lines and jigs it into saw edges, carves it with knives and mangles it with brush handles, smears it here, battles it there, and baptizes it with white lead and chrome yellow, which pass for light with him."[25] Contrary to the artist-prophet who revealed the truth of nature, the impressionist painter ripped and destroyed, in violent paintings where the tools (knives, brush handles) inflicted on the view represented the scars of a landscape ravaged by industry or railroad construction. A few paragraphs later, Trumble discussed the nature of "true impressionism": in his view, "all artists are impressionists, provided they are artists at all." To illustrate that "true" art, Trumble chose, significantly, a nocturne by Jean-Charles Cazin: "You enter the gallery in broad daylight and directly before you... the wall opens and you are looking out upon a moonlight and a midnight three thousand miles away. There is no trickery about it; it is only a picture; but it is painted with such extraordinary observance of nature and with such an extraordinary adherence to her, that certainly no mere words can convey more than a dim impression of the work they describe."[26] According to Trumble, Cazin's nocturne had the value of an authentic act of witnessing: it gave the beholder the perfect, magical illusion of looking at an actual night landscape, because the connection between nature and the work had not been broken by "trickery," a mechanical mediation and fragmentation, as practiced by photographers and impressionists.

ART FOR ART'S SAKE IN PHOTOGRAPHY

As it happens, these questions also arose among photographers themselves, who in the late nineteenth century strove to promote photography, or rather, a certain kind of photography, as an art. The British photographer Henry Peter Emerson's *Naturalistic Photography for Students of the Art,* one of the founding texts of the pictorialist movement in Europe and the United States, promoted photography as a pictorial art in its own right, reaffirming the separation between an artistic vision faithful to what the human eye perceived and a mechanical and scientific vision.[27] Significantly, a first article by Emerson, preceding and anticipating that book, appeared in a Philadelphia newspaper at the same time that Eadweard Muybridge was displaying in that city the spectacular images of his research on motion in photography—a discipline that, though it contributed to revitalizing the fine arts, was conceived as a scientific investigation.[28] The ambition of Emerson's book was as vast as its subject matter: the author began by elaborating a history of art, from ancient Egypt to modern Europe, in which photography would have its place. Then Emerson lavished advice on young photographers: he recommended to his readers that, as far as possible, they should avoid artifice (painted studio sets, props), stay away from urban views, and instead favor landscapes preserved from the traces of modernity. The aesthetic that Emerson embraced was beholden to two models: first, the physiology of vision as described by Hermann von Helmholtz; and second, Whistler's practice as a painter. Emerson, a physician who abandoned his profession to devote himself to photography, based his definition of artistic truth in photography on Helmholtz's discoveries regarding the physiology of visual perception, and especially, optical focalization. For example, he put forward the idea of a "mental focus" that would complement and adjust technical focus, which he linked to sight with the naked eye. Michel Poivert construes that return to an imperfect vision on the part of photographic technique as an antimimetic impulse, which, for the pictorialist photographers, led to an "aesthetic of aberrations" with the camera imitating the astigmatism or distortions that can affect the human eye.[29] In a paradoxical movement, then, photographic technique was manipulated by photographers in a bow to the limitations of visual human perception and its imperfections. The second aspect of that reformulation of photography was aesthetic: art photography, in reproducing human visual perception as Emerson suggested, adhered to formal principles fairly close to those of the nocturne. The influence of Whistler, who was also a friend of Emerson's, is evident in the photographer's writings. Although Emerson's early photographs usually consisted of rural genre scenes inspired by Jean-Baptiste Corot, John Constable, and the Barbizon School, by the 1890s he had dedicated himself to photographing deserted, misty, or snowy landscapes similar to those favored by Whistler. He was at odds with those who expected a hyperdetailed image with well-determined outlines: one of the pieces of advice that he dispensed to his readers was that they not confuse "accuracy and truth."[30] "The chief merit of most photographs is their diagrammatic accuracy, as it is their chief vice," he remarked with Whistleresque sarcasm.[31] Pictorialist photography, placed under Whistler's authority, also emerged as a form of militant and elitist antivision.

The views formulated by Emerson received a great deal of attention from a handful of American photographers, who wished to distinguish themselves from the "button-pushers" and other fans of Kodak prints. As amateur clubs centered on a photographic practice more recreational than creative spread, the New Yorker Alfred Stieglitz set out to outline an American art of photography. Stieglitz, the son of wealthy industrialists and himself an amateur photographer, took up the defense of the photographic avant-garde. He would ultimately become one of the foremost promoters of modern art in the United States. Between 1890 and 1902, he published *American Amateur Photographer*, then *Camera Notes*, in which he championed an aesthetic elitism, in contrast to the democratic approach of amateur photography clubs. *Camera Notes*, the official organ of the Camera Club of New York, sought to define that elitism, particularly through the selection of photographs published in the review. Stieglitz insisted on including in each issue, in addition to halftone illustrations, two photogravures chosen for their aesthetic quality: "In the case of the photogravures the utmost care will be exercised to publish nothing but what is the development of an organic idea, the evolution of an inward principle; a picture rather than a photograph, though photography must be the method of graphic representation."[32] Formal quality thus took precedence over technique, a distinction that was not without its contradictions, as the end of the passage quoted indicates: in spite of everything, that nonphotographic picture had to be produced through the medium of photography. Stieglitz's commitment to aestheticization ultimately led him to establish his own movement outside the Camera Club. In a tribute to the Munich and Vienna Secessions, he called it the "Photo-Secession." Stieglitz, surrounded by critics such as Charles Caffin and Sadakichi Hartmann and by photographers such as Edward Steichen and Jerome Kerfoot (all contributors to *Camera Work*, the journal associated with the Photo-Secession), set out to establish the legitimacy of the art of photography in the United States. The status of art photography became a familiar subject in the columns of *Camera Work*, but it was Steichen who pushed the aesthetic claims of the Photo-Secession the farthest. Comparing art and photography, Steichen brazenly acknowledged that photography was "a flagrant imitation of the technique of inferior media."[33] Himself a practicing painter as well as a photographer, Steichen constantly blurred the line between the two arts. In his photographic *Self-Portrait* conspicuously retouched with a brush, the artist imitated the great masters as well as Whistler's portraits, emerging from the darkness with brush and palette in hand. The picture was obviously something of a manifesto (fig. 45). And Steichen went even further: in the first issue of *Camera Work*, he responded to those who would criticize him for distorting the photograph through his manipulations, saying that all photographers were fakers. He thus upended the myth of an "objective" photography faithful to nature.[34] There is never anything natural in photography, said Steichen, and every shot, every print, is already a manipulation that introduces a gap between the photograph and its supposed truth.[35] In that sense, Steichen turned on their head the reproaches that the fine arts were making against photography and, in sum, pushed artifice to its logical conclusion.

Even so, several historians have noted that, behind the rhetoric of these definitions, the secession advocated by Stieglitz and Steichen was an aesthetic revival at least as much as an institutional rift.[36] Above all, it entailed emancipating oneself from the amateur clubs and their democratic practices to set in place an exclusive caste of art photographers. Like the nocturne artists, the pictorialists strove to define a socially distinguished taste: the Photo-Secession movement was spearheaded by a small elite of New York artists. True, it took shape at the same time as other photographers' societies abroad, which were motivated by similar intentions, including, notably, the Brotherhood of the Linked Ring in England. But the cosmopolitan exchanges that occurred among these various groups simply add to their social elitism. For example, *Camera Work* regularly reprinted articles published in the *Amateur Photographer*, the review of the Linked Ring, and Stieglitz and several of his American companions were members of that group even before they founded the Photo-Secession.

What distinguished the pictorialist photographers from other amateur photographers? Strictly in terms of technical considerations, the differences between the two groups were altogether relative. In practice, the pictorialists used the same tools as ordinary amateurs, and though

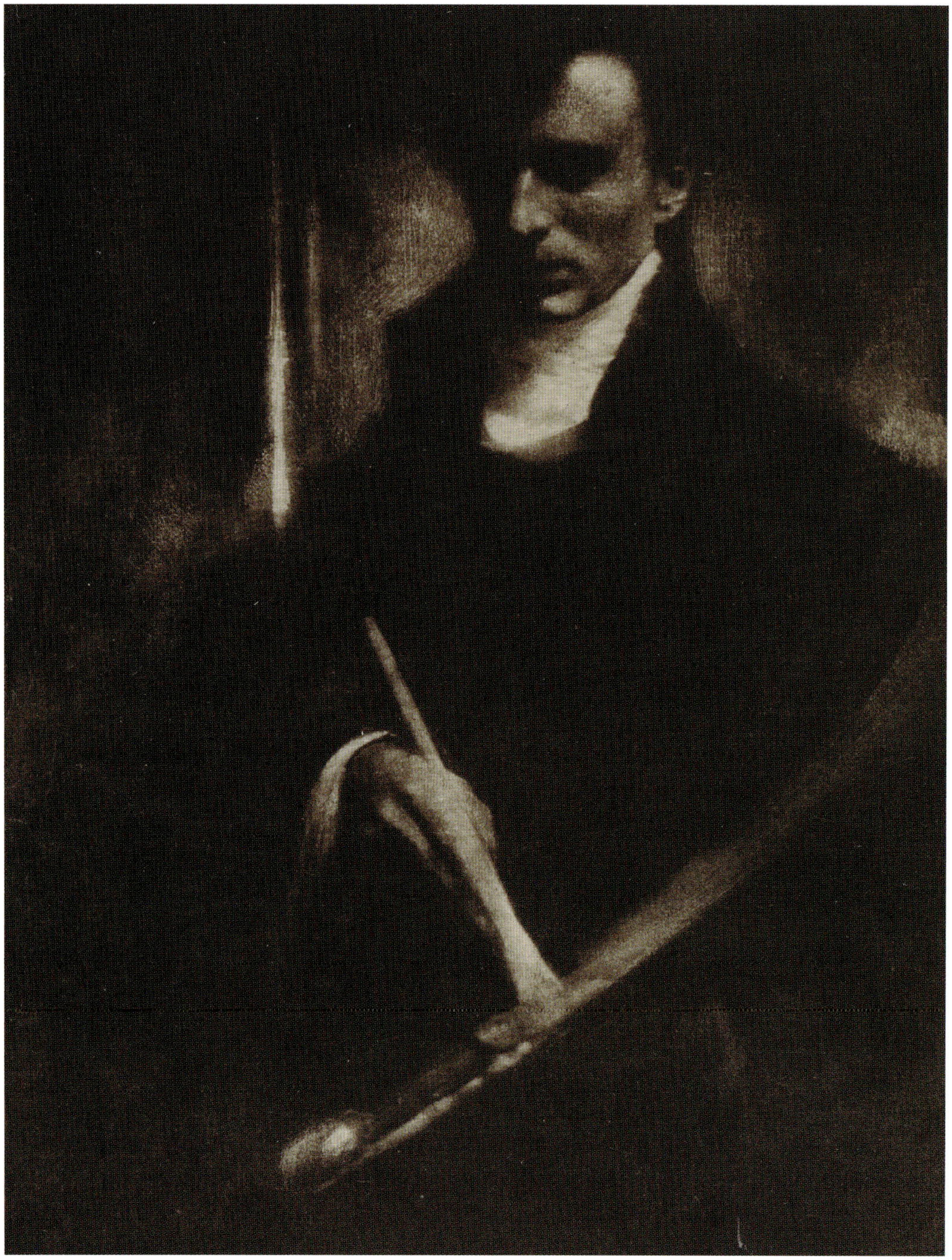

FIG. 45. Edward Jean Steichen, *Self-Portrait*, 1903. Photogravure, 20.3 × 25.4 cm (8 × 10 in.). Yale University Art Gallery, New Haven, Connecticut. Gift of Susan and Arthur Fleischer, Jr., B.A. 1953, LL.B. 1958 (2011.129.24).

they disavowed the simplified practices introduced by Kodak, a large part of their aesthetic remained indebted to them. In 1897, for example, Alfred Stieglitz published a piece praising the portable camera, admitting he had wrongly disparaged the light, handheld devices with which Eastman (who went unnamed in the article) had "flooded the market."[37] Stieglitz acknowledged the merit of these cameras, which restored the photographer's mobility and freed him from the constraints imposed by the clumsier mechanisms of older cameras. The Eastman firm also provided Sunday photographers with increasingly sophisticated development tools. In particular, it popularized enlargement and cropping, methods that the pictorialists regularly employed. Furthermore, Eastman's technical simplifications played a role in redefining the art of photography: it would allow the photographer to make adjustments "without a conscious thought" and to develop a practice of photography as a "second nature."[38] The organic and the unconscious took precedence over the mechanical and the rational, freeing up the artist's

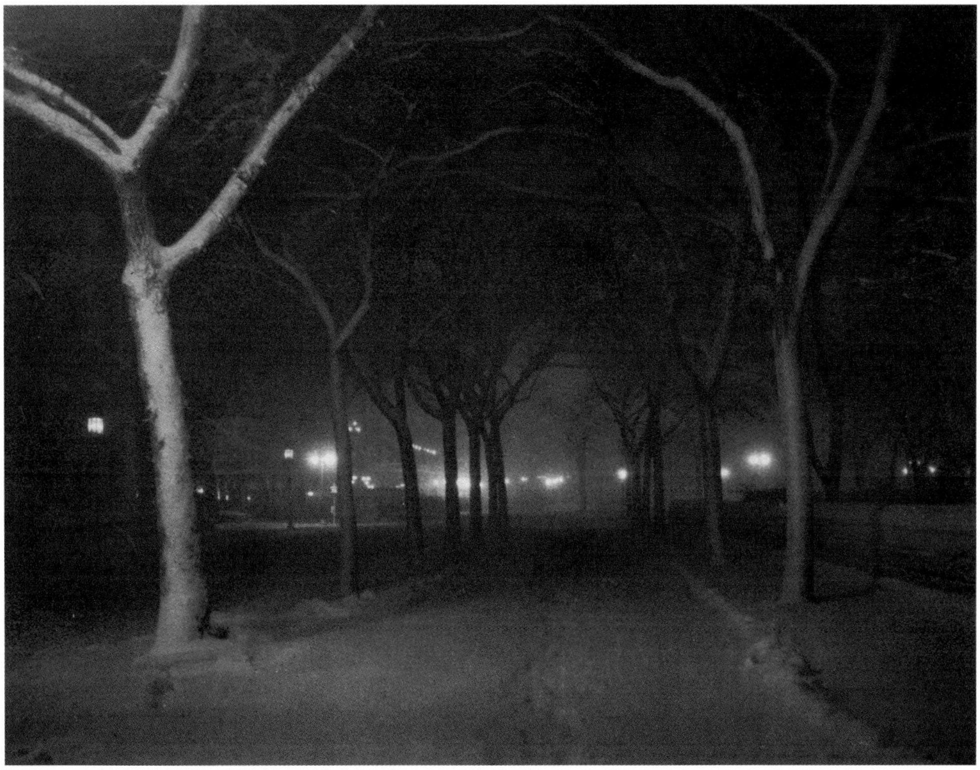

FIG. 46. Alfred Stieglitz, *Icy Night, New York*, 1898. Photogravure, 12.7 × 16.2 cm (5 × 6 ⅜ in.). Museum of Modern Art, New York. Transferred from the Museum Library.

subjectivity. The photographer's eyes and mind now determined the photographic object and, paradoxically, it was through this technical progress that eye and mind prevailed over mechanics, reaffirming the figure of the artist as an individual and independent genius. The innovations introduced by the Eastman firm thus contributed indirectly to the strategy of advancing photography as an art.

That strategic revision of the relation to technology was accompanied by aesthetic choices that were also clearly intended to restore to the photographic image an aura that mechanization had supposedly placed in peril. The artists of the Photo-Secession, having inverted the definition of photography to make it a nonmechanical art, proceeded to a second reversal, endeavoring to deny the traditional association between photography and light. The very first descriptions of photography as an art of light (also attested in the etymology of the word, "*photo*graphy") could still be found in the advertising of the Kodak firm. It announced the elimination of the darkroom, thanks to a simplified developing machine, and vaunted products "as plain as daylight." In contrast to the sunny photographs of tourists and amateurs, who followed to the letter the advice of the user's manuals provided by Kodak, Steichen and his Photo-Secessionist partners, like Emerson, demonstrated a marked preference for cloudy or foggy landscapes (fig. 46). That tendency culminated in the night photographs produced by the pictorialists, veritable technical feats antithetical to Kodak photography.

The pictorialists' repurposing of the technology is apparent, for example, in Stieglitz's *Hand of Man,* his *Glow of Night—New York,* and also his *Reflections: Night—New York.* The first of these photographs relies on atmospheric effects created by the plume of a steam locomotive, the other two on the gleam of electric lights reflected on the wet pavement (figs. 47–49). Ironically, the three photographs place technology at the center of the image, only to take their distance immediately and to concentrate on its aesthetic effects. The wording *The Hand of Man* sounds like a provocation on Stieglitz's part: it not only points to the technical progress achieved by human beings by means of the railroad but also suggests a second transformation of reality, this time by the artist's "hand." The sophisticated manipulations practiced by the pictorialists, and the care given to printing, reveal a desire to superimpose an artistic technique onto the pure mechanics of photography. The pictorialists made wide use of soft-focus techniques, filters, and special lenses: they deliberately underexposed or overexposed

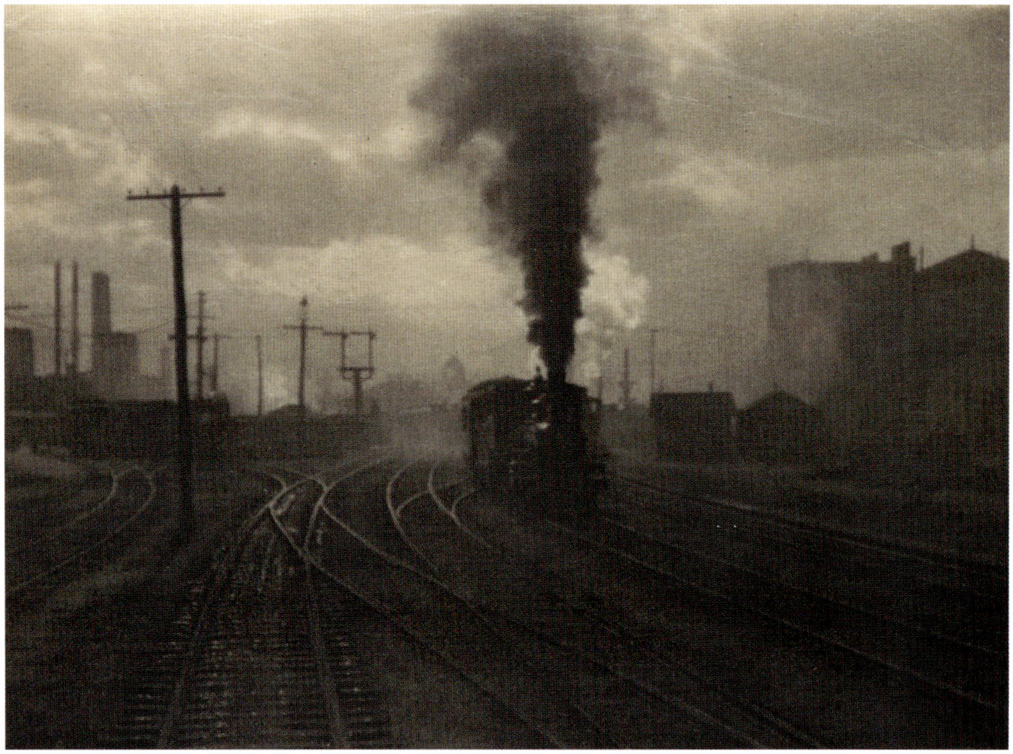

FIG. 47. Alfred Stieglitz, *The Hand of Man*, 1902. Photogravure, image: 21.3 × 15.6 cm (8 3/8 × 6 1/8 in.). Inv. PHO1981-22-7, Musée d'Orsay, Paris.

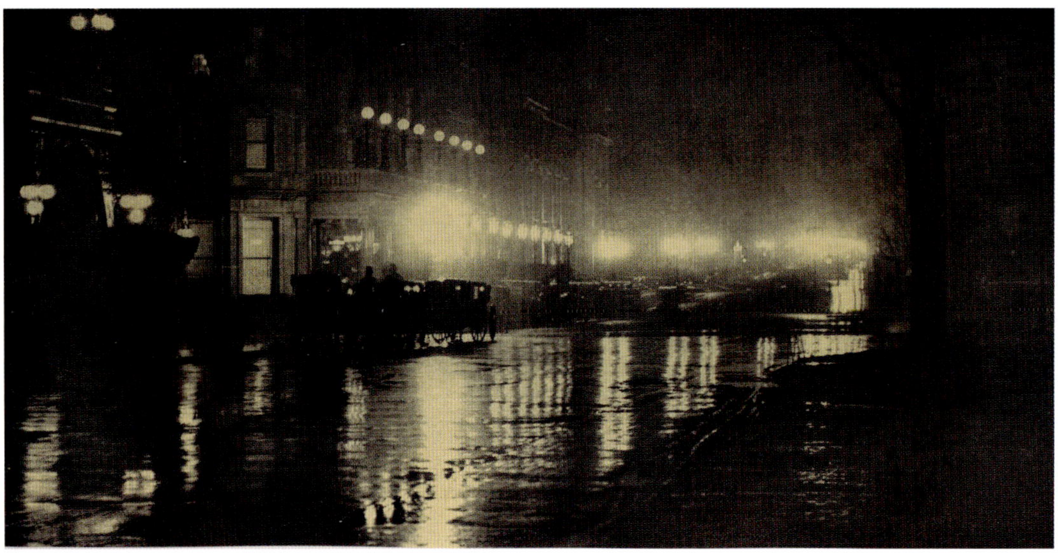

FIG. 48. Alfred Stieglitz, *The Glow of Night—New York*, 1897. Photogravure, image: 12 × 23.4 cm (4 3/4 × 9 3/16 in.); overall: 40.4 × 50.7 cm (15 7/8 × 20 in.). George Eastman Museum, Rochester, New York. Museum accession (1974.0054.0007).

their negatives, constantly cropped their shots, and used refined printing techniques, such as photogravure, sepia toning, or gum bichromate. A good number of these manipulations, such as the use of filters or the addition of transparent layers of pigment through the gum bichromate process, mimicked at the technical level the filtering effect of night. The photographic practice was thus congruent with the aesthetic content of the subject matter. The strategies developed by the pictorialists—blurry outlines, haloes of light suffused in a misty or clouded atmosphere—tended to reestablish almost literally a certain aura of the image. Jay Bochner shows, however, that the question of the aura in Stieglitz's art of photography and in that of his circle was inseparable from the artists' financial concerns. The pictorialists thus reintroduced commercial value, even as they conspicuously rejected it. Stieglitz, for example, in limiting the number of prints or highlighting their technical quality, attempted to restore to photography a value both aesthetic and economic.[39] For the pictorialists, as for the painters caricatured by Sterner, quantity and quality were carefully calculated and indissociable factors.

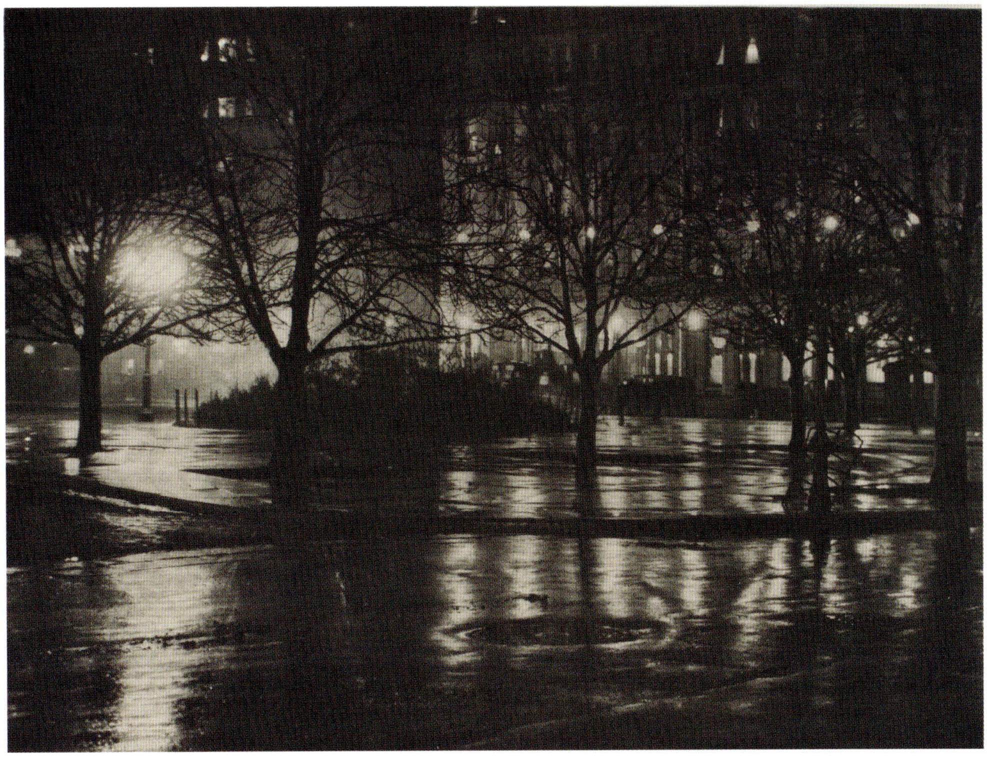

FIG. 49. Alfred Stieglitz, *Reflections: Night—New York*, 1897. Photogravure, image: 21 × 35.1 cm (8 1/4 × 13 7/8 in.). Philadelphia Museum of Art, From the Dorothy Norman Collection, 1968, 1968–68–4.

FROM COMMERCIAL ILLUSTRATION TO THE FINE ARTS: THE CASE OF FREDERIC REMINGTON

The pictorialists were not the only ones to make use of the night as a source of artistic aura. As the 2003 exhibition of Frederic Remington's nocturnes at the National Gallery in Washington has demonstrated, the illustrator proved that he fully understood the distinction that night could confer to his art and how it could advance his career as a "real artist."[40] Remington, bedeviled by his reputation as an energetic and virile but unrefined popular illustrator, managed to find his way into the most exclusive artistic circles by adapting his Western scenes to the nocturnal mode. Even today, Remington's nocturnes, the last phase in a career cut short by his early death in 1909, are viewed as the achievements of his artistic maturity, a surpassing of his limitations as a commercial illustrator. That radical turn in the artist's career exemplifies the tensions and contradictions that were rife in the world of image production around 1900—between the democratic art of illustration and an elitist taste expressed in nocturnes, between the illustrator's craft and art for art's sake as espoused by Whistler's disciples, and, above all, between competing or strictly hierarchical cultural institutions. Remington's fortunes illustrate not only these tensions but also a certain fluidity within the milieu of image producers in the broad sense, demonstrating that, though the differences were marked and somewhat stereotyped, it was still possible to move back and forth between the categories. Many artists in the American canon, Winslow Homer in the lead, began their careers as illustrators. Remington, however, is a particularly telling example: in an admirable about-face, he moved from one extreme to the other. His case illustrates the institutional impact of the nocturne form: in imposing the filter of night on his scenes of the American West, he completely transformed his identity as an artist.

Remington began his career by fashioning a professional persona based on technical competence and field experience. The image he constructed for himself was that of an illustrator who, though certainly rough around the edges, was authentic, patriotic, and virile, well versed in the "realities" he depicted. That image suggests, in negative outline as it were, the corresponding cliché of the academic artist, an effeminate, aristocratic, and cosmopolitan figure. Remington's biographers repeated over and over again that, though the illustrator had studied art at Yale, he quickly lost interest in copying classical models and preferred the company of his football teammates to that of his classmates, young women for the most part.[41] He then studied at the Art Students League, an institution where most professional illustrators trained but which did not have the prestige of the fine arts academies. Remington quickly turned to genre scenes of the West, and they became his trademark. After a brief stay in Kansas, he moved to Brooklyn in 1885 and thereafter only rarely left the east coast. Yet Remington did not hesitate to portray himself as an authentic Westerner. He showed up dressed as a cowboy to offer his illustrations to publishers, who often accepted his disguise at face value. Remington took advantage of the American public's infatuation with the mythology of the frontier. That cowboy image coincided almost naturally with that of an illustrator ready to capture the action on the spot, a faithful transcriber of a reality he himself had lived. One biographer described Remington rejecting the timorous conformism of the fine arts to live the life of a pioneer: "So young Mr. Lochinvar hurried out of the art schools, which were essaying to make a tidy mural decorator of his burning, blundering, unformulated gift, and sought the West, palette in hand. As far from the beaten track as possible he traveled on a broncho pony. He herded cattle with cowboys, shot antelope and buffalo on the trail for the provender necessary for his life."[42] Remington was successful enough in that vein to become one of the main targets of the journalist Emerson Hough in his pamphlet "Wild West Faking," which denounced and ridiculed the inconsistencies and lies of that supposedly authentic art.[43] The "Brooklyn cowboy," wearing his chaps backward and posing for the photographer next to a pedestal table, closely resembles the portrait of the young Remington decked out as a dashing pioneer, pretending to hold his wife at gunpoint, against an ornate decor (figs. 50, 51).

Nothing stands in starker contrast to that fabricated "cowboy" image than the refined art steeped in abstract sophistication produced by Whistler and his disciples. Remington portrayed himself as a truly "American" artist, whose work was marked through and through by an authenticity diametrically opposed to the artifice deliberately pursued by Whistler and, in general, to the elitism of art circles. Remington saw little place for himself there—or, rather, they made little place for him. From the start of his career, Remington maintained an ambivalent relationship with his profession, torn between his enthusiastic embrace of the figure of the cowboy and more conformist aspirations. Critics reproached him for offering an interpretation of reality that was too literal, too mechanically faithful for a true artist: "Some say that Remington, even in his most carefully thought-out pieces, is too illustrative, too photographic, less an artist than a reporter."[44] Remington himself seemed aware that he had not yet altogether achieved the status of an artist. He wrote to one of his friends in 1886, at a time when he was celebrating his first successes as an illustrator: "That's a pretty good break for an ex cow-puncher to come to New York with $30 and to catch on in 'art.'"[45] Remington's use of scare quotes demonstrates that he was aware that illustration was considered a minor art or merely a craft. His boasting was ambiguous: while claiming a background alien to the established art circles and embracing a career as a "self-made man," Remington also emphasized his desire to join the artistic class and his awareness of the distance that still separated him from it. Far from being satisfied with the status of illustrator, he tried his luck at the most exclusive fine arts institutions: every year, he submitted a painting to the National Academy of Design, where he was elected an associate in 1891 but was never awarded the status of an official member.

The turning point came in 1899, when Remington visited the California painter Charles Rollo Peters's exhibition *Paintings of the Night* at the Union League Club.[46] Peters had trained at the École des Beaux Arts in Paris, joining the hordes of American art students who arrived there in Whistler's wake. Peters even circulated the story that Whistler had said the California artist was the only one besides himself capable of painting the night.[47] After receiving a warm welcome from New York critics, Peters moved back to his native city of San Francisco, where his nocturnes became the latest fashion for the local elite.[48] It was through him that Remington came to accept Whistler's aesthetic codes. With increasing regularity after 1900, Remington adapted the nocturne "formula" to his paintings. Between 1900 and 1909, he produced about twenty nocturnes. His journals bear witness to his interest in Whistler: in 1908 he twice traveled from New Rochelle to New York City to see the artist's works at the Metropolitan Museum and at the Macbeth Gallery. Remington also owned a copy of Arthur Jerome Eddy's biography of Whistler, and his notebook of sculpture sketches included a reproduction of Victor D. Brenner's commemorative plaque for Whistler.[49] Even Remington's protestations, vehement as they were, are a sign of the attention he was paying to Whistler.

Above all, Remington's adoption of the nocturnal mode served to reposition him on the American art scene. In 1906 Remington exhibited a series of nocturnes at the prestigious Knoedler Gallery, which earned him a very positive critical reception: "It is a softened

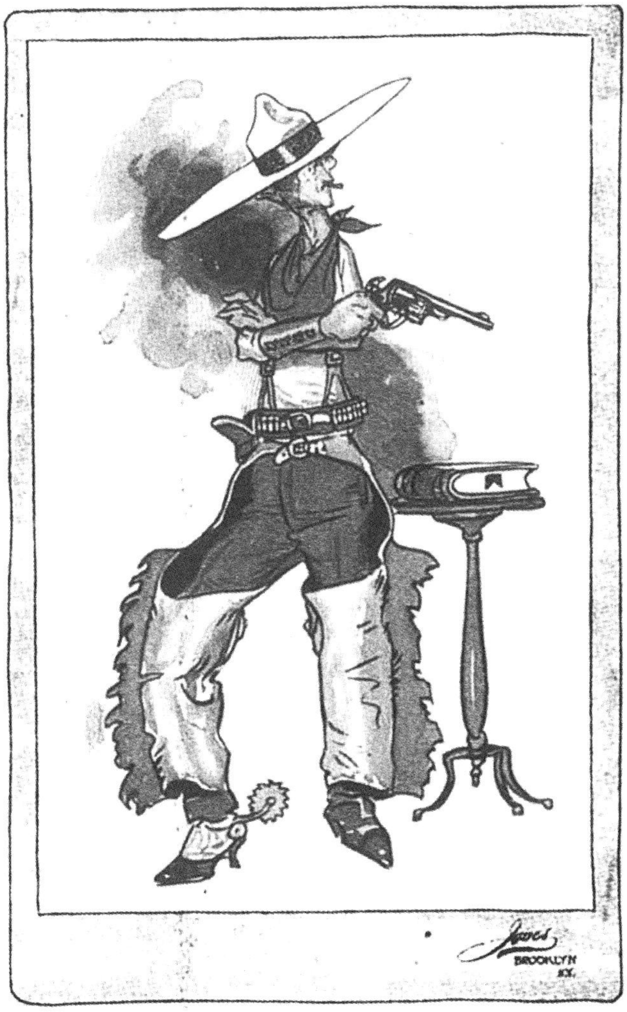

FIG. 50. "The Cowboy, as Created in Brooklyn," *Collier's* 42, no. 13, December 18, 1908.

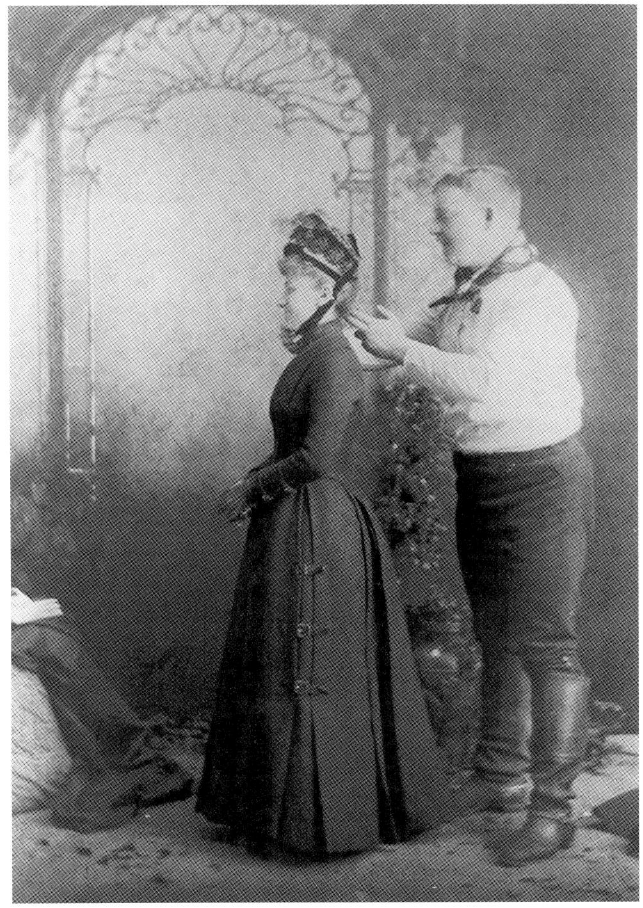

FIG. 51. Frederic Remington and his wife, c. 1885. Photograph. Courtesy Frederic Remington Art Museum, Ogdensburg, New York.

and harmonized Remington we find this year, his pictures having atmosphere. . . . It is sure that he takes the shades of night to help him to those tones of mystery which most of his previous pictures lacked."[50] The next year, Remington exhibited a second time at the Knoedler Gallery, and his nocturnes were once again a great success. The *New York Times* critic, after judging Remington's daylight scenes harshly, focused on the nocturnes: "The exhibition is not wholly without its new note, however, and this is in the most difficult and unexpected quarter: the painting of night, revealing genuine painter-like qualities. In these night scenes there is a marked forward stride in the rendering of atmosphere, the color is more expressive, and less painty, the brush work is looser, even the drawing is better and the whole has a breadth and freedom of execution that may presage great things for Mr. Remington if he chooses to follow this path seriously."[51]

In late 1909 the exhibition of Remington's nocturnal works received enough favorable reviews that the painter wrote triumphantly in his journal: "The art critics have all 'come down'—I have belated but splendid notices from all the papers. They ungrudgingly give me a high place as a 'mere painter.' . . . The 'Illustrator' phase has become background."[52] In an odd twist, Remington had left *Collier's* in January of the same year, after many months of tensions with Will Bradley, the magazine's new editor and a defender of art for art's sake, who found Remington too mundane for his tastes. Although Remington's death a few weeks after the journal entry put an unexpected end to that development, the genre he invented did not die with him: the artist Frank Tenney Johnson made the formula of the "Western nocturne" his own and exploited that niche market until the mid-1930s.[53]

But, as Nancy Anderson has shown, the transformation went even further: Remington not only adapted the

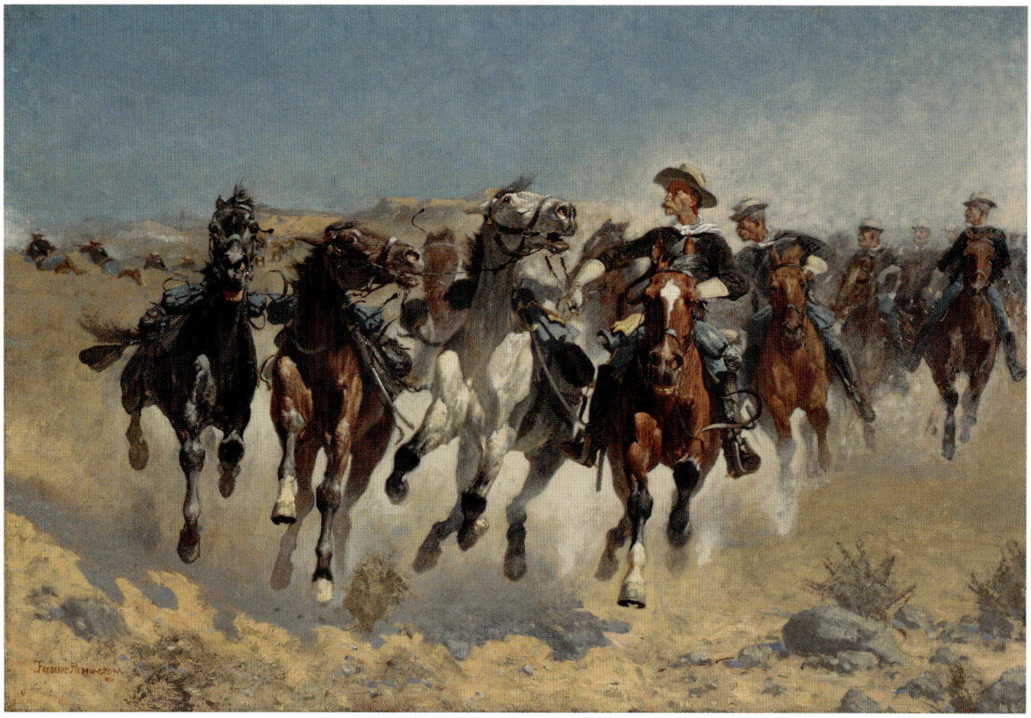

FIG. 52. Frederic Remington, *Dismounted: The Fourth Troopers Moving the Led Horses,* 1890. Oil on canvas, 86.5 × 124.3 cm (34 1/16 × 48 15/16 in.). Sterling and Francine Clark Art Institute, Williamstown, Massachusetts (1955.11).

nocturnal theme, he also adopted several of Whistler's aesthetic strategies.[54] He began by giving priority to color. Like Whistler, who placed tonal variations at the center of his process, even naming his compositions after the dominant colors, Remington displayed a special interest in tonal harmonies and shadings. In his early days as a painter, critics reproached him for his awkward use of color, which showed he was an illustrator more accustomed to creating black-and-white images intended for halftone reproduction than to handling subtle hues.[55] A *New York Times* critic wrote in 1890: "[Remington's] colors are so shrill and temperament so prone to violent movement that a collection of his pictures gives the impression of a thousand discordant noises, yells of battle, screams of dying horses, and the crudeness of existence between a pitiless sky and a pitiless earth, without the compensation of beautiful colors and noble forms. Mr. Remington . . . remains the illustrator in black and white who, with a magnificent but short-sighted audacity, has taken to color. He is not at home with oils and brushes; his paintings hurt."[56] Remington's journal attests to the growing attention he was paying to the question of color in the last years of his life. He noted, for example: "*Snow Trail* lacks color in figure and *Call for Help* is too green. I am looking to try and fix it up"; "low tones in the darks are fugitive."[57] And it was precisely color that Remington's critics applauded in his nocturnes, as in this review of *Night Halt of the Cavalry:* "It is in [Remington's] night scenes, however, that as mere art lovers we find the most satisfaction. . . . The general color of the picture is blue, and the tone dark. The indication of the figures of the men in the middle ground gathered around the fire is admirably done, and the whole effect is of sincere workmanship and a strong feeling for characteristic sentiment."[58] Critics felt that the harsh colors in certain scenes conveyed the reality of life on the frontier with journalistic fidelity; but when it came to pleasing "mere art lovers," the nocturnes prevailed. Color became feeling and gave rise to a truly aesthetic experience.

Remington also borrowed from Whistler's formula for the nocturne a sobriety of composition and a relative lack of narrative. Between his famous *Dismounted: The Fourth Troopers Moving the Led Horses* (1890) and *A Pack Train* (1909), a shift occurred: from full daylight to starry night; and from a tumultuous episode with a multitude of horses and men, who completely fill the frame with their gesticulations, to a restful scene in which the human figure, now an isolated silhouette, recedes in the middle ground, barely visible among the horses (figs. 52, 53). Remington also occasionally adopted the high horizon lines and visible texture of Whistler's canvases. As the figures retreated to the horizon and action gave way to immobility and silence, narrative, associated with his illustrations from the start of Remington's career, also disappeared. As the

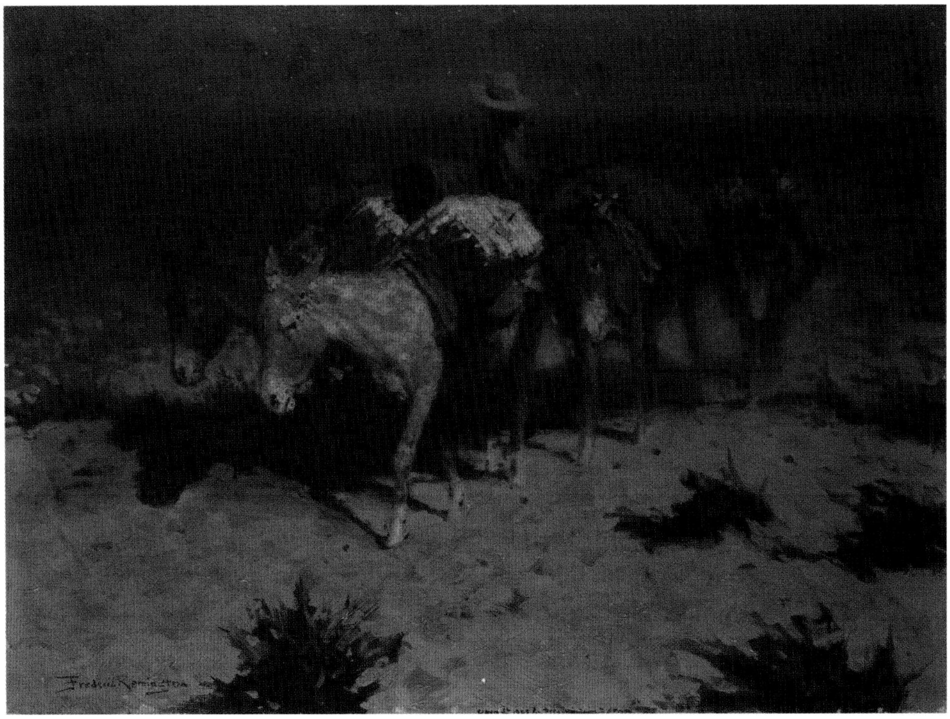

FIG. 53. Frederic Remington, *A Pack Train*, 1909. Oil on canvas, 68.6 × 101.6 cm (27 × 40 in.). Private collection.

years passed, for instance, he chose less and less detailed titles for his paintings. The illustration *Cheyenne Scouts Patrolling the Big Timber of the North Canadian* became simply *Indian Scouts in the Moonlight* in a 1902 nocturne that repeated the theme. Although he resisted on principle the doctrine of art for art's sake, Remington drifted toward an art of suggestion lacking any narrative thread. "Big art is a process of elimination," he explained in a 1903 interview for *Outing* magazine, advising young artists: "Cut down and out—do your hardest work outside the picture, and let your audience take away something to think about—to imagine."[59] Without espousing Whistler's contemplative abstraction, Remington relied on the imagination, turning away from an overly explicit narration and a fidelity to nature, which he understood were no longer in fashion. That movement was comparable to the one initiated by the pictorialists: they diverted the image from a too direct, too mechanical gaze, to make it a more inward-looking vision. Alexander Nemerov demonstrates that, for Remington, the shift to nighttime profoundly modified the content of his images. In that transition from animated scenes with a direct relationship to the reality they depicted to murky views that appealed to the beholder's imagination, Remington's West itself underwent a transformation. The images no longer aspired to convey the instantaneity and reality of lived events but simply suggested the memory of them.[60] Through that internalization and mediation of memory, the authenticity of lived experience made way for the truth of feeling. The Western nocturne thus turned the objective gaze back toward a subjective and abstract vision, dominated by the imagination and by memory. These "antivisions" did not merely constitute a rejection of direct vision; they also set forth an inverted form of sight.

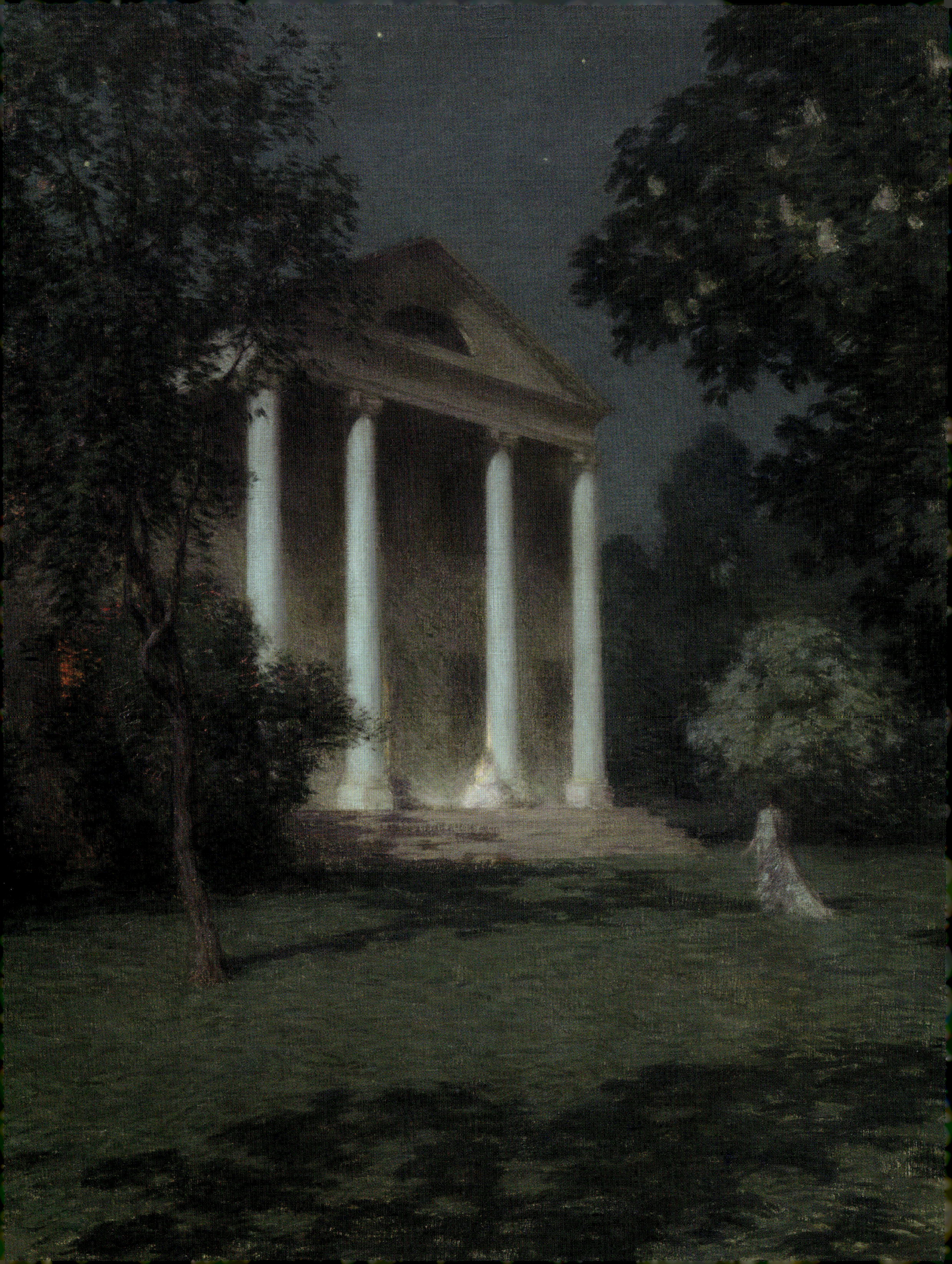

4 Visions of the Mind and Spirit

The "antivision" proposed by the nocturnes rested in reality on a threefold rejection of vision: first, formal abstraction; second, an effort to escape the domain of the visible, which was invaded by an aggressive proliferation of images; and third, a corresponding movement toward interiority. The discourse surrounding nocturnes abounded in reflections on the concordance between the nocturnal atmosphere and the "mood," "feeling," or "sentiment" they supposedly expressed. Nocturnes, exploiting the ancient poetic associations of nighttime, presented themselves as interior landscapes, highly subjective mental objects seen by the mind's eye.[1] In their formal strategies, they conformed to the description of the work of art that John Van Dyke developed in his *Art for Art's Sake.* Following Coleridge's formula, Van Dyke placed the work of art between "a thought and a thing": "It is not a statement of fact, but a suggestive impression; not a realization of absolute nature, but a hint of those deep meanings which will not bear realization—those meanings which a sensitive soul may know and feel, and yet be able to express only in part. For the idea in art is at the best not like a clear-cut intellectual thought, but rather like a sympathetic sensation or an emotional feeling."[2] According to Sadakichi Hartmann, the painters of his time opened new vistas, filling the need for "some spiritual support, some science of the soul" left by the increased secularization of Americans' lives.[3] What matters here is that the abstract realm toward which the nocturne was moving was not that of a clear rationality but that of a subjective interiority. A California critic detected in the paintings of "moonlight conjurer" Charles Rollo Peters "a reminiscent mood" and affirmed that these paintings were "first aids to reverie."[4] Darkness played a crucial role in the pursuit of that vision, turning the gaze away from material reality to allow the artist's inward vision to emerge. Thus, for instance, Whistler described how the actual subjects of his portraits were absorbed into the darkness: "As light fades and the shadows deepen, all petty and exacting details vanish, everything trivial disappears, and I see things as they are in great strong masses: the buttons are lost, but the sitter remains; the sitter is lost, but the shadow remains; the shadow is lost, but the picture remains. And that, night cannot efface from the painter's imagination."[5] The veil of night served as a projection screen for the artist's subjectivity and for the beholder's as well. It was an ambiguous space, since the opening that the

Fig. 55 detail

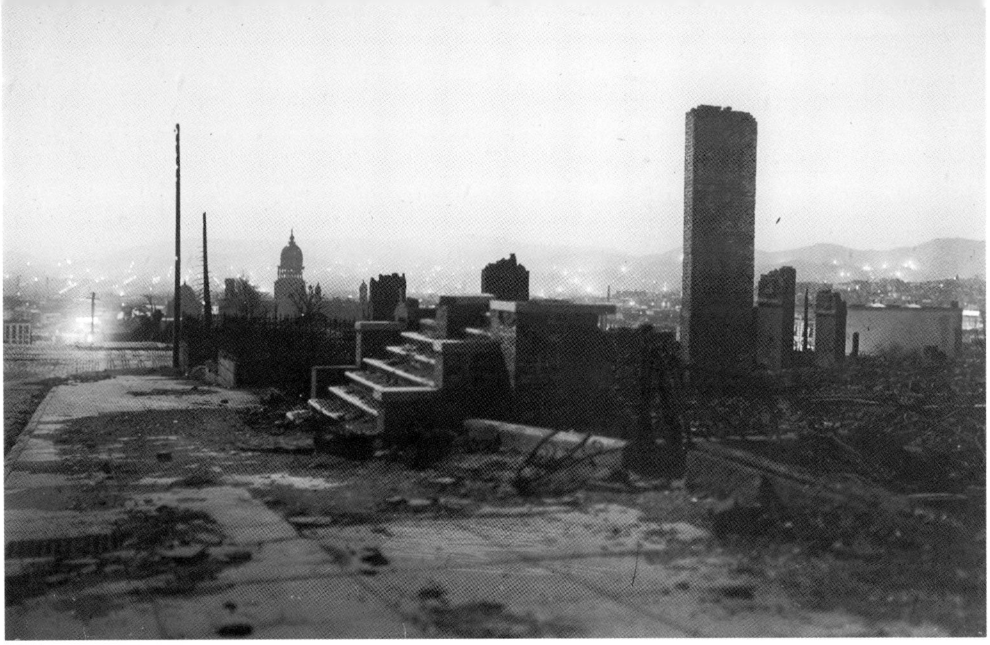

FIG. 54. Arnold Genthe, *Steps That Lead to Nowhere (After the Fire)*, 1906. Diapositive, 12.7 × 17.78 cm (5 × 7 in.). Library of Congress Prints and Photographs Division, Washington, D.C.

nocturne provided actually sent the beholder back to her own interiority: nocturnes often revealed a complex play between surface and depth, openness and closure. Critics of nocturnes, insisting on the genre's affinities with the imagination, memory, madness, and artistic genius, drew on the romantic imagery of the night. But they also incorporated nocturnes into concerns that were acquiring new urgency in the late nineteenth century, when psychology had attained the status of a science, and research on the supernatural and the unconscious was growing.

GATES OF THE NIGHT: AN INWARD MOVEMENT

Nocturnes reactivated the romantic correspondence between scenery and subjective interiority, with critics often reading them as "intimate landscapes."[6] One of Ralph Albert Blakelock's biographers, describing the artist as a "dreamer, a poet, a mystic," refused, for example, to classify him as a landscape painter, situating him instead in the realm of mental and formal abstraction: "To call him a landscape painter is incorrect. He made use of natural forms with which to express himself and through these we find his moods, inspirations, and his eccentricities expressed in an imaginative synthesis of rich color and harmonies."[7] In the nocturne, the process of abstraction distills the real landscape into a place within the mind: "[Whistler's landscapes] are places of dreamland, landscapes of the mind, summoned with closed eyes, and set free from everything coarse and material, breathed upon the picture and encompassed with mysteries. . . . This wonderful harmonist has the art of simplifying and rendering all things spiritual, whilst he retains the mere essence of forms, and of colours only what is transient, subtle, and musical."[8] A number of critics, such as Frederic Fairchild Sherman discussing Dwight Tryon, also emphasized the purely subjective character of the artistic vision: "His art is subjective and his interest is in the spiritual significance of the visible world as it is made intelligible in immaterial beauty."[9]

Nocturnes often play on the various levels of the beholder's engagement with the imaginary and pictorial space, using several types of strategies. First, on the level of iconography, the gate or portal motif appears repeatedly in nocturnes. These physical signs of passage often have a temporal dimension as well, suggesting a gradual transition toward contemplation. Peters's *San Fernando Mission* (see fig. 8) and the pictorialist photographer Arthur Genthe's *Steps That Lead to Nowhere* both provide nostalgic meditations, the first on California's Hispanic past, the second on the San Francisco earthquake of 1906 (fig. 54). The ruins indicate a lost past, whose darkness, by virtue of its formal abstraction (a "nowhere" expressing the conspicuous neutrality of the nocturnes), suggests recollection and introspection. These gates of the night are sometimes enlivened by female figures, allegories that feed the desire for a transcendence of the merely visual. Such is the case, for example, in Willard Metcalf's *May Night* (fig. 55), in which a young woman dressed in white approaches the portico of a house illuminated by moonlight. Similarly, Steichen's *Lady in the Doorway* (fig. 56) shows Lilian Steichen's silhouette detaching itself in the artificial light streaming from the street or the house, protected by the door. Arthur Mathews's *Eve* declares its allegorical character more overtly, aligning the nude figure of a woman with a sculpted female bust framed by foliage and surrounded in a halo of moonlight (fig. 57). The mediation of the young women is ambiguous, because their invitation also takes the form of an exclusion: the female figure in *May Night* has her back turned to the beholder; Lilian Steichen and the young woman in Mathews's picture are only dark silhouettes, their faces turned away, clearly absorbed in thoughts that remain inaccessible to the viewer.

That give-and-take between openness and closure can also be found in the materiality of the canvases, beginning with the sophisticated working of the surfaces. Most often, artists relied on a dialectic between opacity and transparency. Whistler, to give his paintings the aspect of "breath on the surface of a pane of glass,"[10] the translucence of a light and colored mist, developed a laborious process inspired by great masters such as Titian and Rembrandt. This practice consisted of accumulating multiple layers of paint, which drew the eye to the quality of the surface itself (in contrast to the illusion of transparency cultivated by French academicism, for example) in order to create the optical illusion of depth. Whistler also revived the technique of glazing;

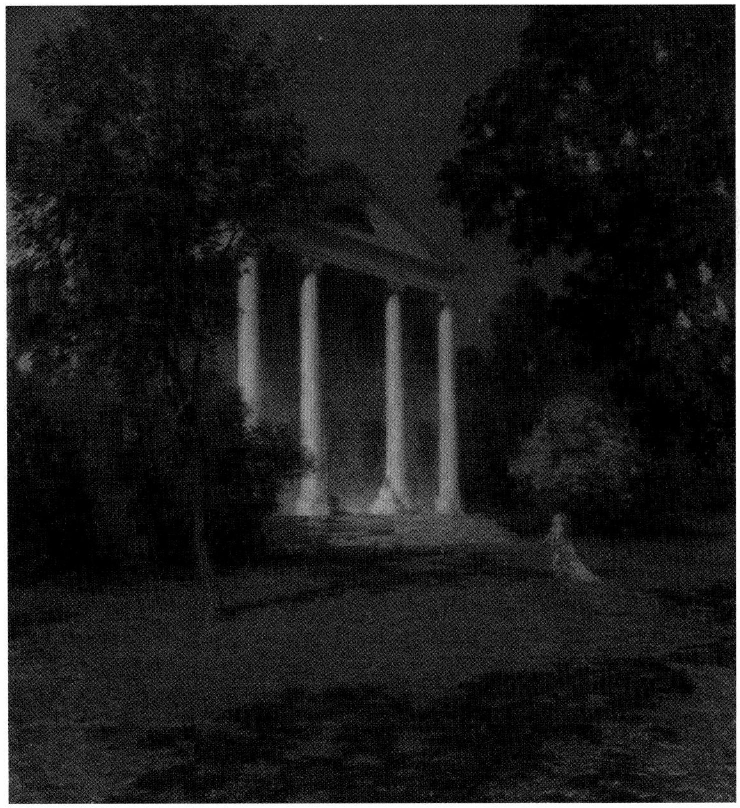

FIG. 55. Williard Leroy Metcalf, *May Night*, 1906. Oil on canvas, 99.5 × 91.8 cm (39 3/16 × 36 1/8 in.). National Gallery of Art, Washington, D.C. Corcoran Collection (Museum Purchase, Gallery Fund), 2014.136.6.

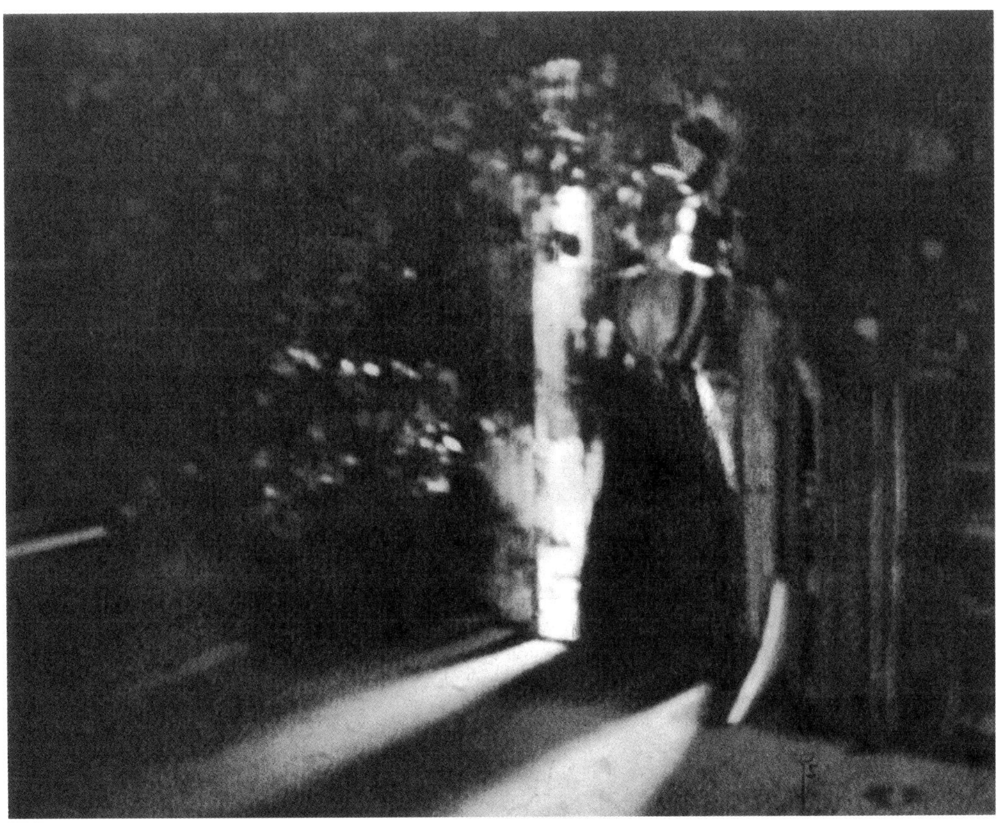

FIG. 56. Edward Steichen, *Lady in the Doorway*, 1897. Photogravure, 18 × 21.75 cm (7 1/8 × 8 1/2 in.). Collection of the author.

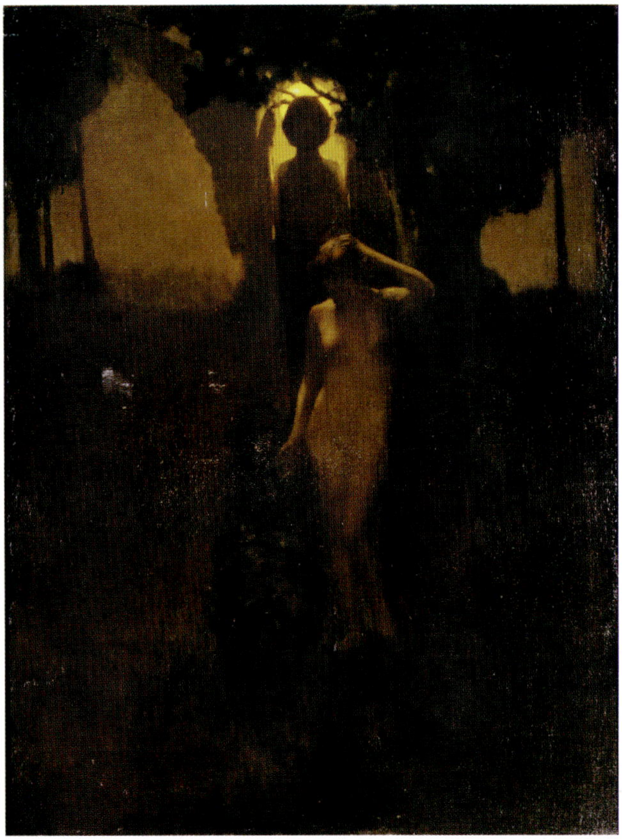

FIG. 57. Arthur Mathews, *Eve,* n.d. Oil on canvas, 167.64 × 135.89 cm (50.5 × 38 in.). Collection of the Oakland Museum of California, Gift of Concours d'Antiques, the Art Guild of the Oakland Museum of California (A66.196.9).

he superimposed countless layers of varnish, very lightly colored with pigment, to create a translucent effect. A number of his disciples adopted these techniques and, like him, used canvases prepared with imprimaturas, whose color filtered through the successive layers of paint—often extremely diluted—within a particularly fluid medium.[11] The resulting pictures stand halfway between materiality and immateriality, revealing themselves to the eye and evading it in turn. A critic cited by Whistler in his catalogue *Nocturnes, Marines and Chevalet Pieces* aptly translates the eerie impression produced by these subtle manipulations of paint: "His paintings seem like half-materialised ghosts at a spiritualistic séance. I cannot help wondering when they will gain substance and appear more clearly out of their environing fog, or when they will melt altogether from my attentive gaze."[12] The generally small format of the nocturnal landscapes further encourages an inward-looking gaze. Once again, openness and closure coexist in paradoxical fashion, creating an apparently contradictory movement: the expansion of space, produced by the elimination of visual landmarks and the undercutting of the traditional principles of landscape painting, is simultaneously counteracted by a contraction of the visual field, which is restricted to the surface of the canvas. In reality, if the space does expand, it does so only for an individual and isolated beholder. The landscapes, either deserted or with a single human figure to accentuate the void, foreground individual contemplation. The obscuring of spatial reference points and the reconfiguration of the relationship between the beholder and the work culminate in an internalization of vision.

Edward Steichen's nocturnes provide a particularly interesting example in that regard. His night landscapes appear to be ambiguous spaces, suspended between interiority and exteriority. In three of his paintings—*Nocturne, Yellow Moon,* and *Moonlit Landscape*—darkness, in blurring perspectives and disorienting the beholder, accentuates the sense of confinement already created by the narrow canyon of *Moonlit Landscape* and the horizons obstructed by groves of trees in *Nocturne* and *Yellow Moon* (figs. 58, 59). Their almost square format reinforces the impression of closure by underscoring how the landscape is framed, displayed in a box as it were. At the same time, within that limited space night creates a formless but uniform space, which seems to lend itself to mental projection. Steichen's famous photograph *The Pond—Moonrise,* constructed on the same model, produces what appears to be a form of antiphotograph entailing multiple inversions: not only does moonlight replace sunlight, but the moon itself is obscured and distanced behind a row of trees and within a hazy atmosphere (fig. 60). The alignment of the slender but close-set tree trunks obstructs the horizon of the landscape, circumscribing the view to the small body of water that gives the photograph its title. The pond furthers the effects of indirection, by reflecting the trees in their entirety, even though the actual treetops are cut out of the frame. The beholder's gaze, rather than occupying a dominant position and projecting itself into a landscape with well-lit vistas and sharply delimited contours, is cramped within a space that offers only an inverted reflection of the external world. The scene functions as a sort of natural camera obscura, in which the moon, the only point of light at eye level, is the aperture that gives a glimpse of a world beyond reach. Similarly, photographic techniques seem to serve as an optical paradigm for the three paintings, which all replicate that tiny aperture of the glowing

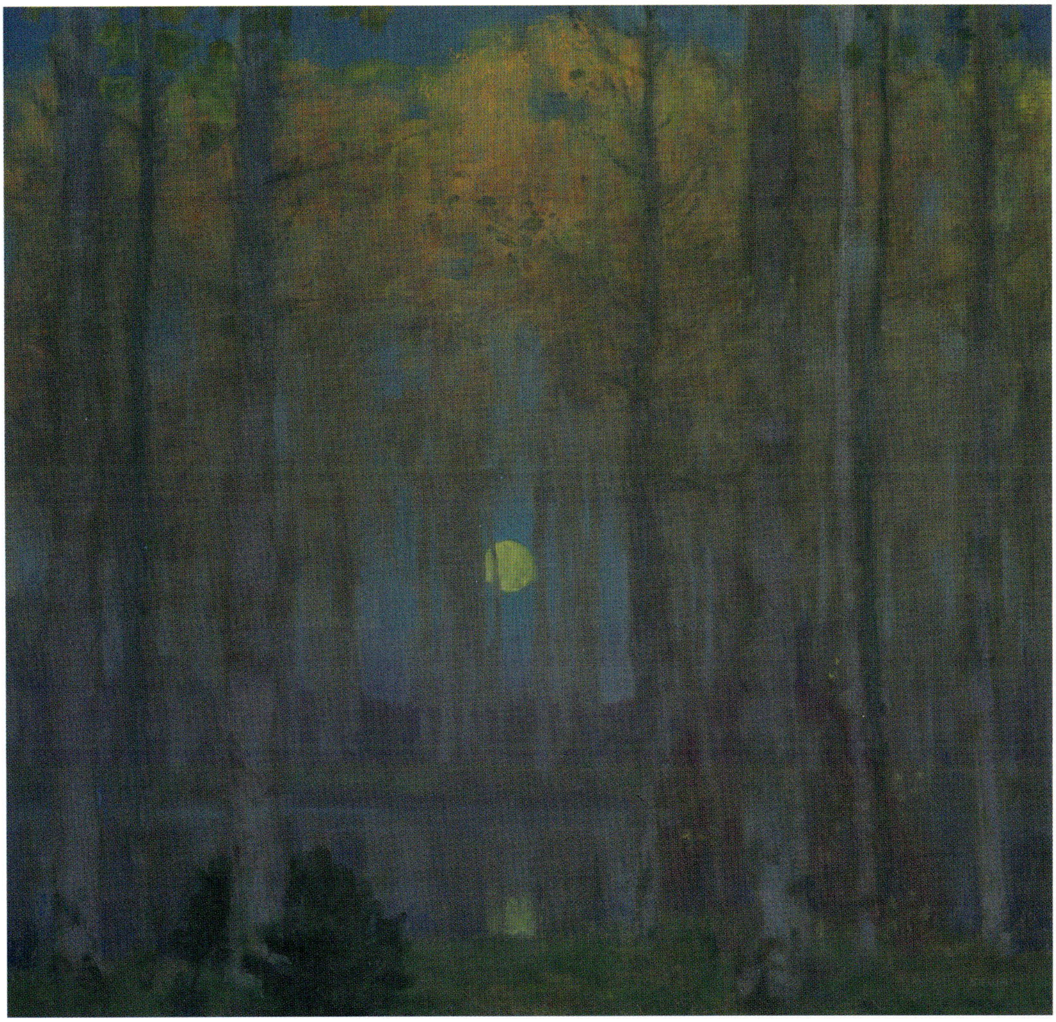

FIG. 58. Edward Steichen, *Nocturne*, 1900. Oil on canvas, 60.96 × 63.5 cm (24 × 25 in.). Snite Museum of Art, University of Notre Dame.

FIG. 59. Edward Steichen, *The Yellow Moon*, 1909. Oil on canvas, 61 × 64.1 cm (24 × 25 1/4 in.). Washington County Museum of Fine Arts.

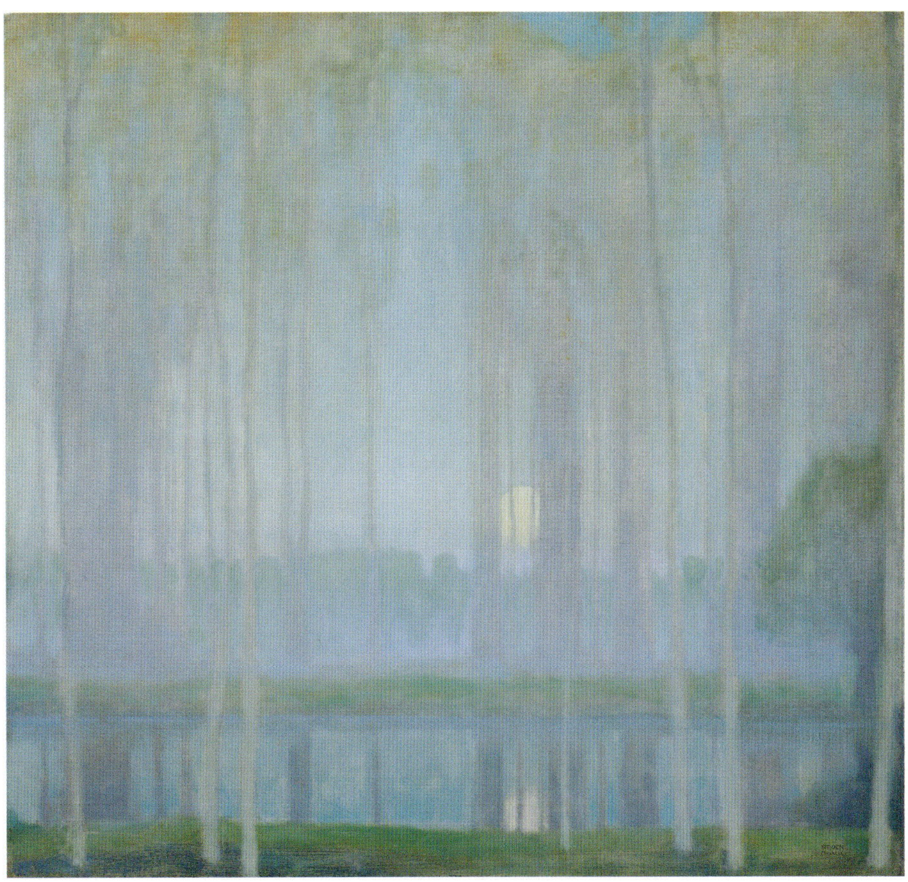

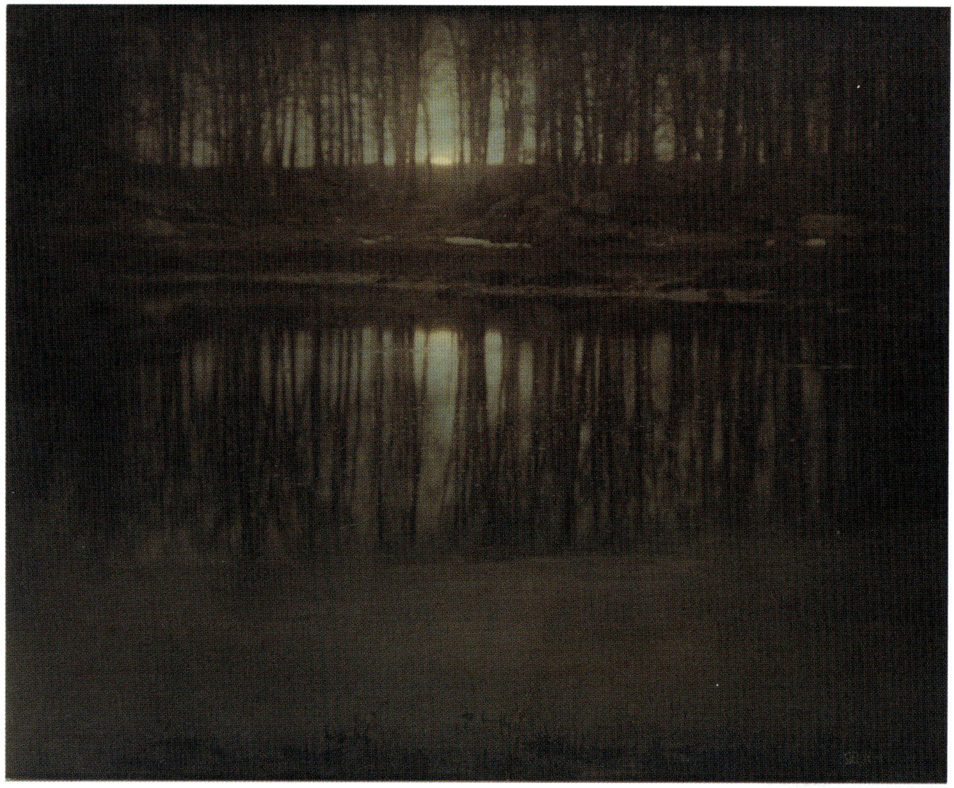

FIG. 60. Edward Steichen, *The Pond—Moonrise,* 1904. Platinum print with applied color, 39.7 × 48.2 cm (15 5⁄8 × 19 in.). Metropolitan Museum of Art, Alfred Stieglitz Collection, 1933 (33.43.40).

moon. In these as well as in *The Pond,* Steichen used the model of the photographic mechanism, but only to make it a space of vision in itself. No objective duplication of reality is implied by that model; rather, it suggests the possibility of a certain subjectivity. This landscape resembling a camera obscura stands as an intermediate field between the external world and consciousness, a field in which darkness would serve as the medium. The nocturnal landscape, like darkness, is neither altogether exterior nor wholly internalized and concealed. Presenting itself as an equivocal mode of visibility that combines dissimulation and unveiling, it constitutes the antechamber of an inverted vision.

By the turn of the twentieth century, the equivalence between the nocturne and interiority seems to have become self-evident. One journalist noted, for example, that "Alexander Harrison's seascapes grow more and more to be the product of his own inward vision."[13] Another understood Leonard Ochtman's nocturnes as "a seeing of the inward eye."[14] To Birge Harrison, the effects of nighttime, particularly the way it hampers direct vision, were used as the pretext for expressing a "mood," a subjective prism through which the landscape was envisioned: "The effect under which a subject is painted has come to mean more to them than the subject itself—the 'mood' more than the motive. . . . Thus the modern painter . . . has learned that the veiled and half-seen things make a stronger appeal to the human imagination. . . . Twilight and pearly dawn, moonlight and mist, the moments when things are glimpsed rather than seen, now grip him more forcefully than of old."[15] In what Harrison viewed as a modern gesture, landscape painting was reoriented toward a type of representation more concerned with psychology than with fidelity to external reality. In that respect, the American tonalist painters continued to explore a concealed interiority of the landscape, its fleeting, transitory, and hidden moods, where darkness itself provides enough substance for the picture.

NIGHT AND VAGUENESS: PSYCHOLOGY AND THE REVISION OF SUBJECTIVITY

Vagueness for Vagueness's Sake: The Nocturne, Parapsychology, and Psychology

The aesthetic return to a vague interiority corresponded to a scientific exploration of internal darkness or, to borrow William James's words, a "reinstatement" of the vague,[16] embraced as an object in itself and even as a scientific approach: "The boundary-line of the mental is certainly vague. It is better not to be pedantic, but to let the science be as vague as its subject."[17] In the last decades of the nineteenth century, a new scientific field opened up, one that made use of still-uncertain methods.

In fact, the field of psychology took shape in conjunction with a science of the occult that was still in its infancy. Although spiritualism had long had many followers in the United States, beginning in the 1880s its practices, previously empirical and popular, were augmented and even supplanted by more scientific research, through the American Society for Psychical Research in particular.[18] After the paranormal was incorporated into the scientific domain, it found a legitimate place in the discourse of art criticism. Nocturnes, in placing the emphasis on absence, encouraged their beholders to look for hidden presences as subtle as the shapes barely distinguishable on the canvas. In 1907 the critic and art historian Charles Caffin interpreted Whistler's *Nocturne: Blue and Silver—Bognor*[19] as a work that recorded a spiritual "presence" on the canvas and that also served as a medium for the beholder:[20] "The *Nocturne—Bognor* is penetrated with this quality of elusiveness; phantom shapes glimmering in misty, ethereal light, a spirit picture, rendering the impressions which such a scene in nature gently makes upon the imagination. So gently that, while we are filled with sensations, they are vague, unrealisable; our spirit is allured to infinite longings in the very unattainableness of which there is a poignancy of cleansing sadness. If you have come under the spell of this enchantment in the actual presence of Nature, you recognise it instantly in this picture; if you have not, the picture may lead you to find it."[21] According to Christian Brinton, Whistler's canvases reveal the artist's interest in parapsychology: "Reviewing in turn this succession of nocturnes, harmonies, symphonies, and arrangements, so full of suppressed color and almost audible melody, so intangible, so subliminal, it is difficult not to feel that Whistler enlisted qualities hitherto unknown to painting. . . . Spontaneously the mind travels back to those early London days, and to the tiny cottage in Walham Green where he used to busy himself with table-turning and spirit-rapping, or to sit up all night discussing with Rossetti things which lie just across the border-line of consciousness."[22]

The concurrent rise of psychology was characterized by a similar acceptance of vagueness and irrationality. This explains the almost equal interest William James showed in the two fields of investigation. It would be possible to read "spiritualist" interpretations of nocturnes as allegorical and metaphorical expressions of what in reality belongs to psychology.[23] The specters and supernatural presences haunting nocturnes would then be only a symbolic externalization of forces at work in the paintings that in reality can be traced back to the artist's inner life. In the late 1880s, psychology in the United States began to achieve the status of a scientific discipline. Simultaneously, it created new methods of investigation, acknowledging the obscurity of its object while conferring scientific legitimacy on it. The University of Pennsylvania, for example, established its department of psychology in 1887; it was followed by many other universities in the 1890s. The American Psychological Association was founded in 1892. Americans were increasingly interested in mental illnesses such as neurasthenia, a phenomenon that the neurologist George Beard described in 1881 as a national ailment.[24] In 1908 an article in the *North American Review* expressed concerns about its pervasive presence: "On every street, at every corner, we meet the neurasthenics," the author declared, citing statistics. Between 1880 and 1903, as the population of the United States grew by about a third, the number of patients in psychiatric hospitals nearly doubled each decade.[25] The increase, albeit real, also points to the greater attention being given to the question. Not only pathology but also mental life generally sparked ever more interest, which manifested itself in various cultural spheres. In 1907, for example, William Dean Howells published a series of "romances" under the title *Between the Dark and the Daylight,* which included short stories dealing with memory, forgetting, and telepathy.[26] These concerns also found expression in a playful mode, as, for example, in Winsor McCay's comic strip *Little Nemo in Slumberland,* published in the *New York Herald* from 1905 onward, which related the adventures of a little boy, known to the reader only through his dream life (fig. 61).[27]

The Nocturne as Reflection of the Soul and as Remedy for Its Afflictions

Nocturnes, in presenting themselves as the image of a reality seen through the filter of an imprecise individual aesthetic experience, became part of a profound revision of subjectivity. Psychology's inquiries into the nature of mental activity established a new foundation for the notions of individual identity, understood on the basis of deliberately imprecise models. The image of a distinct and almost unvarying self was gradually replaced by the idea that, on the contrary, the subject was vague and changeable. In Henry James's novel *Portrait of a Lady,* Madame Merle tells Isabelle Archer: "There's no such thing as an

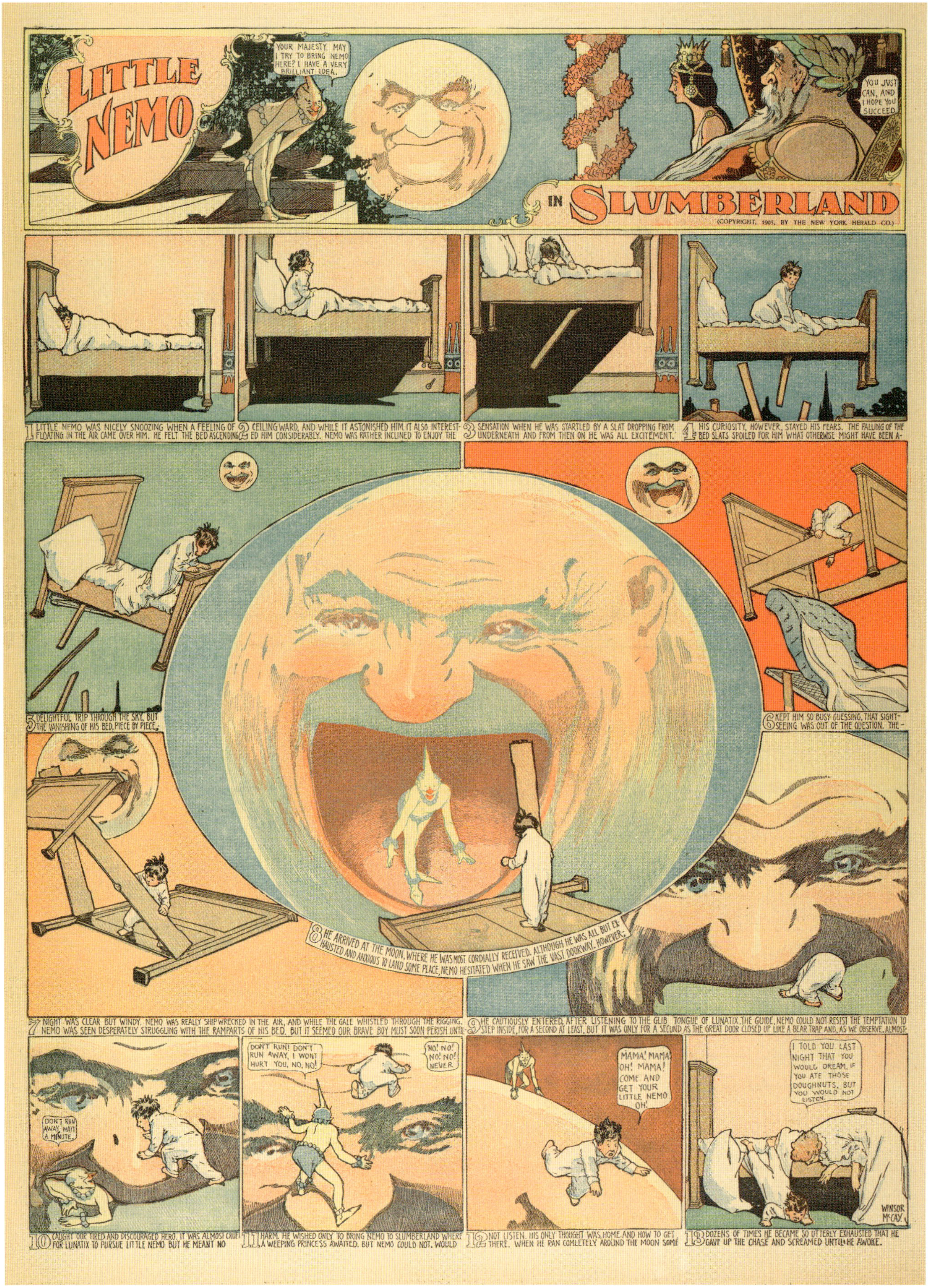

FIG. 61. Winsor McCay, "Little Nemo in Slumberland," *Los Angeles Times,* December 3, 1905. San Francisco Academy of Comic Art Collection, Ohio State University, Billy Ireland Cartoon Library and Museum.

isolated man or woman; we're each of us made up of some cluster of appurtenances." She goes on: "What shall we call our 'self'? Where does it begin? where does it end? It overflows into everything that belongs to us—and then it flows back again."[28] Madame Merle's questions, and her suggestion that one's only concrete identity is derived from the objects with which one surrounds oneself, point to the diffuse, shifting, pluralistic, and interactional character of modern subjectivity. And the radical empiricism of Henry James's brother William shifted the emphasis from the object itself to its perception by the subject, ultimately granting subjectivity the primacy of experience: "The inner state is our very experience itself; its reality and that of our experience are one."[29] The historian Nathan Hale describes the dawn of the twentieth century in the United States as a moment of intellectual ferment, when a vanguard of researchers, with William James, G. Stanley Hall, and John Dewey in the lead, were laying the groundwork for psychoanalysis. In particular, Hale explains the success of dynamic psychology, in contrast to the relative failure of two earlier models, "civilized morality" and the "somatic approach." "Civilized morality" placed the emphasis on the repression of drives, while the somatic method treated mental pathologies by focusing on the patient's physical condition. The forced rest cures and vigorous activity advocated by S. Weir Mitchell remain the most famous of these somatic treatments.[30] In opposition to these primarily external, moralistic, and rationalistic treatments, a much more flexible approach emerged, one that proposed to treat patients by focusing on their deepest inner life. The extremely hierarchical psychology of the faculties was replaced in the late nineteenth century by a much broader and more pluralistic science, one that no longer considered mental faculties such as memory or thought to be distinct processes.[31] William James refuted the static model of a sovereign consciousness in control of the body, a consciousness under the guidance of a rationality that exerted its mastery over the drives, and one occupied with discrete tasks performed in succession. In its place, he proposed a dynamic vision of consciousness—integrating the physiological and the psychic—whose activities conformed to the famous "stream of consciousness" model. In William James's view, though it may be possible to describe separately the various phases of the mental process, in reality they are superimposed, interwoven, intimately linked to one another.[32] The continuum of thought found a pictorial equivalent in tonalist painting: like the sensations and thoughts emerging from a single indistinct whole, in nocturnes the elements of the composition are not "joined together"; rather, they form a "fluid" harmony.[33] Dewing's human figures, for example, can be read as figurations of the psychic model William James articulated. Dewing's women, absorbed in the act of listening, singing, or performing music, visually immersed in a quasi-monochrome, vaguely delineated environment, are subjects who gradually emerge from the landscape in a "penumbral nascent way,"[34] like the fringe of consciousness as James described it: "Let us use the words psychic overtone, suffusion, or fringe, to designate the influence of a faint brain-process upon our thought, as it makes it aware of relations and objects but dimly perceived."[35] Even as the new psychology based its discourse on models dominated by vagueness and darkness, the nocturne laid claim to a psychological style of painting. Hartmann concluded his study of Whistler's oeuvre with a few reflections on the paintings of his heirs. What was distinctive about modern painting, he explained, was its engagement with mental activity: "This is more than a technical change, it is a new way of thinking. We concede a new attribute to these painters and call their achievements the psychological style of painting."[36]

This new model of painting, closely connected to the redefinition of subjectivity, is particularly apparent in the new relationship that nocturne artists intimated between their works and the people who contemplated them.[37] One of the strongest connections between nocturnes and the new psychology occurred through the therapeutic use of art: nocturnes were interpreted as images that offered beholders a salutary repose. The "American nervousness" described by Beard was of particular concern to William James, who described the habits of his compatriots as potentially detrimental to their health. An excess of energy and vitality, an unflagging pace of life, were supposedly turning Americans into "bottled lightning": "By the sensations that so incessantly pour in from the over-tense excited body the over-tense and excited habit of mind is kept up; and the sultry, threatening, exhausting, thunderous inner atmosphere never quite clears away."[38] In an environment that made too many demands on the individual, aesthetic contemplation was seen as one of the avenues toward the "relaxation" William James recommended. Several historians of American art have written about the therapeutic virtues attributed to that fin-de-siècle art, citing more particularly the reception of tonalist painting.[39] The notion of a therapeutic virtue of art flourished in the wealthiest social milieus of the Boston elite (white, Protestant, and male for the most part), to which Abbott Thayer, Thomas Dewing, William James, and the millionaire Charles Lang Freer belonged. That discourse, of course, had an undeniable socioeconomic value as it targeted members of the higher classes of society and conferred extra distinction to the artworks. Delicate paintings were reserved for elites, whose sensitivity was equaled only by their nervousness. Kenyon Cox, for example, praised Whistler's paintings as "an art of exquisite sensibilities and fine nerves."[40] In 1893 George Moore, in his *Modern Painting,* speculated that, if nature had endowed Whistler with a less nervous temperament, he could not have painted the *Nocturnes,* "which are clearly the outcome of a highly-strung,bloodless nature whetted on the whetstone of its own weakness to an exasperated sense of volatile colour and evanescent light."[41] The highly evolved sensibilities of artists and their most excellent patrons—best personified by Freer—were united in a refined aesthetic contemplation. Freer, a phenomenally successful businessman, abandoned the world of commerce to dedicate himself almost exclusively to his activities as a collector, where he found the peace of contemplation.[42] The works of the painters Freer particularly prized—Whistler, Dewing, Tryon, and John Twachtman—were a mediated response to worries about not only the individual's psychological equilibrium but also and more generally the health of American civilization and its capacity to overcome the challenges of modernity. Critics regularly interpreted the ethereal art of the nocturnes as the antithesis of modern hustle and bustle: "Tryon helps us by lifting [us] . . . out of the everyday scrambling vulgarity of the street. You . . . forget business and work looking at his pictures. They lure you away from worldly interests and cares."[43] Dewing provides a particularly significant example, in that his paintings function as a sort of mise en abyme of therapeutic contemplation: the young women engrossed in their aesthetic experience, visually dissolving into vague monochromatic environments, are emblematic of the "oceanic feeling" that supposedly seizes hold of the beholder as well.[44] Nocturne paintings, too, offered a modern answer to the constraints of modern life and responded to the ambient nervousness with an increase in sensitivity: "The cherished traditions of former times have vanished as in the night. Painting has here ceased to depict the glories of the past or the insistent realities of the present. It plays directly upon the nerves, the chief possession, or affliction, of these restless modern days. [Whistler] with his sensitive, nervous fingers unlocked a new and secret chamber of the soul."[45] The nervousness, whether "possession" or "affliction," that governed the modern world was also the quality that gave access to the aesthetic experience. Paradoxically, the antimodern escape of the nocturnes relied on a sensitivity inherently linked to the conditions of modern life.

The principal medium for that therapeutic effect, exploited systematically in the nocturnes, was color. Critical writings and treatises on painting conveyed the idea that "vibrations" of color, in acting on the nerves, affected the beholder's mental state.[46] That notion rested, in fact, on the conviction that sound waves and light waves were of the same nature, and that there was a continuity between them, even if the human senses were unable to perceive it. In this theory, color vibrations were literally treated like waves of music: "Harmony in color, like harmony in music, may be defined as rates of two or more vibratory waves that enhance one another; and discords are the reverse."[47] What mattered most for mental repose was thus harmony, understood on the musical model: it is clear that the tonalists' night landscapes, in accentuating their affinities with music, could in that context aspire to a greater psychological effectiveness. "[Color] pleases by a subdued, yet pervading beauty. It neither vibrates nor wearies the nerves of the eye, but is restful, good to live with, cheering at times, and soothing always," wrote John Van Dyke.[48] And some colors, Harrison explained, were more restful than others: "Imagine a bright vermilion world under a brilliant sun, and tell me how long it would be before all the inhabitants would be raving maniacs. The cool colors blue, green, mauve, violet, and all the delicate intervening grays are, on the contrary, restful colors in the emotional sense; and the wisdom of the choice of these tones for the landscape scheme of the world is hardly open to question."[49] Hence the sober and "cool" colors of the night would be perfectly suited to that soothing use of art. But the insistence on the capacity of that aesthetic to provide a calming retreat toward a cultivated inner life reinforced, by way of contrast, the image of a violent or chaotic external environment. The discourse surrounding nocturnes, in repeating the claim that they allowed the beholder to extricate herself from her context, in reality spoke volumes about what the authors were projecting onto and relegating to that external world, which had to be fled. The dialectical dynamic between interior and exterior extended from the individual to the collective: what seems to have been at issue was the establishment of a "civilized landscape" in which the destabilizing forces apparently threatening American civilization would melt away.

DARK HARMONIES: THE NOCTURNE AS "CIVILIZED LANDSCAPE"

The nocturnal landscape, a space of mental projection, ultimately became the locus of a definition of "civilization," offering its beholders a (re)ordered vision of their environment. The insistence, on the part of nocturne artists and their critics, on the "spirituality" and "harmony" of nocturnes revealed their anxiety in a context where religion on one hand and scientific positivism on the other seemed to have become incapable of ensuring the idea of a world governed by a stable system. The refined art of the nocturnal landscape, a cure for the soul of the individual victim of modern ills, also served to reaffirm a set of values salutary for civilization as a whole. George Inness linked the individual spiritual value of art to its collective importance: "The true use of art is, first, to cultivate the artist's own spiritual nature, and, second, to enter as a factor in general civilization."[50] Landscape painting would thus function as an instrument that measured the state of American civilization: "A nation's art is its intellectual barometer. It shows with infallible finger the mental drift and tendencies of the race which gave it birth; and the same law applies to the art of any given age or epoch. This movement in modern art is therefore symptomatic. . . . The artist simply keeps pace with the spirit of his times; but in so doing he is, we like to think, learning to speak in new terms of beauty, a little finer, a little more spiritual than any hitherto known to the world."[51] Nocturnes, faithful to that definition of art, conveyed a malaise that was afflicting the entire culture. Kathleen Pyne interprets several examples of American painting dating to that period from the standpoint of theories of evolution, and especially, Americans' particular adherence to the theories of Herbert Spencer, who proposed an evolutionist model more optimistic and less violent than Darwin's.[52] According to Pyne, Dewing and Whistler inserted their paintings into that discourse by proposing harmonious and refined visions, reflections of a utopian civilization, to which the evolution process posited by Spencer would ultimately lead. Nocturnes were spiritualized and idealized landscapes that in fact functioned as "visions of the world." That is also how one ought to understand the fierce opposition to impressionism on the part of nocturne artists and their supporters. Impressionism, a "mechanical" painting, was also seen as a potentially dangerous artistic enterprise, in that it rested on a chaotic representation of the world. Impressionist painting, associated with the radical political engagement of the Paris avant-garde, gave rise to mistrust, even rejection in the United States. The "violence" the art critic Alfred Trumble read into the bright colors and fragmentary technique of the impressionists was partly the result of an implicit equivalence he established between these formal aspects and the Parisian artists' radicalism, even anarchism.[53]

In contrast to an impressionist disorder that relied solely on immediate sensation, nocturnes strove to establish a unified vision of an idealized landscape. Yet their very darkness tended simultaneously to introduce a modern "atmosphere of doubt." The nocturne, an art of repose, also reflected the late nineteenth-century American culture's obsession with extremely pessimistic discourses about the evolution of the physical world.[54] The American public was for instance familiar with the theory of entropy, which informed a series of metaphors applied to various subjects. The first law of thermodynamics, known as the law of conservation of energy, holds that energy (heat and work) can change form, but its quantity can never vary. From that law, Lord Kelvin (William Thompson) drew the scandalous conclusion that the energy from the sun will someday be used up.[55] The second law of thermodynamics states that energy spreads chaotically and irreversibly, leading to the ineluctable increase of "disorder" in any isolated system. Even an optimist such as Spencer, who used the vocabulary of thermodynamics in the service of his own theories about the evolution of civilizations, was overcome with doubt when confronted with the consequences of that model. In 1858 he had written to the Irish physicist John Tyndall: "Regarding, as I have done, equilibrium as the ultimate and highest state of society, I have assumed it to be not only the ultimate but also the highest state of the universe. And your assertion that when equilibrium was reached life must cease, staggered me."[56] The logical conclusion was that the idea of an "equilibrium" achieved by (American) civilization at its highest degree of refinement was potentially destabilizing.[57] The equilibrium and harmony so important to the nocturne's aesthetics could thus be reversed into negative values, a threat to civilization rather than a culmination of its most valuable aspects. One of the images most often used to describe that state of entropy was the dispersal of smoke inside a room: in appearance, the smoky atmosphere is uniform, but at the molecular level it is actually chaotic. Darkness metaphors were often used to signify this exhaustion of energies. A popular science article by Camille Flammarion that appeared in the *New York Tribune* painted a disheartening picture of the future of the universe: "This sun is not yet beginning to cool; but, whatever may happen, it will begin to do so one day. Darkness will gradually come on. . . . Then the world must inevitably become, as all the other worlds of the solar system, a frozen cemetery, continuing doubtless to turn as a dark ball around another dark ball and to follow its movements in the eternal night, carried along with the other planetary tombs in the infinite abyss."[58]

These speculations on the fate of the physical universe were openly transposed to every facet of culture. Henry Adams, for example, conceiving human history on the entropic model, expounded that view in a book he wrote for American teachers of history: "The department of history needs to concert with the departments of biology, sociology, and psychology some common formula or figure to serve their students as a working model of vital energies; and this figure must be brought into accord with the figures or formulas used in the departments of physics and mechanics to serve their students as models for the working of physico-chemical and mechanical energies."[59] The logic of entropy, applied to the human sciences, posited that culture was becoming extinct. So proclaimed Max Nordau, whose *Degeneration*, denouncing the tendency of the West toward "overcivilization," was translated into English in 1895.[60] Painting was not exempt from such considerations and, by virtue of its refinement, ran the risk of suffering the same fate as the civilization it reflected and of degenerating into a bland formula. Nocturnes lend themselves particularly well to that type of interpretation: these dark and hazy landscapes illustrate almost literally the phase of the exhaustion of forces, a universe whose energy level was dropping to zero. In the conclusion to Charles Caffin's *Story of American Art* (1907), the author examined all the works exhibited by American painters at the Exposition Universelle de Paris in 1900. Although the Americans displayed subtle and cosmopolitan tastes, they seemed dangerously attracted to an enervated art: "The general impression of the ensemble was of a moderation, grateful in comparison with the ostentation and vagaries that abounded elsewhere, but in itself open to the suggestion of being too negative a virtue, a little fibreless and lacking in marrow."[61] The "negative virtue" explicitly cultivated by the nocturnes revealed their fundamental ambivalence: the very equilibrium they called for seemed excessive and abnormal. Caffin denounced in particular the "paralyzing" influence of the doctrine of art for art's sake and the "preciosity" engendered by Whistler's example.[62] Like many of his contemporaries, Caffin interpreted nocturnes as an art "civilized" in the extreme, and he highlighted the anxieties of his contemporaries about the nature of that civilization and its possible excesses.

FEMALE SENSITIVITY AND LUNATIC GENIUSES

The scope of the discussions of the nature and evolution of their civilization often allowed commentators on the nocturnes to indulge in a series of revealing stereotypes. Critics revived the romantic associations between darkness and mental life, insisting in particular on two conventional models: the nocturne was said to be, first, an art in which a feminine sensibility manifested itself; and second, a "lunatic" form of genius. Behind the facile images, readily recycled by the artists and their public, a set of more destabilizing implications can be discerned. No doubt the clichés about nighttime being the realm of a disordered or feminine mind were especially appealing because they suggested the possibility of an outflowing, an excess. Once again, the darkness and vagueness of the canvas assumed a semantic dimension: what is peculiar to vagueness is an implicit potentiality whose dynamics, precisely, are not always controllable.

The commonplace of a feminine sensibility in harmony with the night could in fact prove problematic for the painters who created the "subtle" art of nocturnal landscapes.[63] It was acknowledged, for example, that artistic genius, in addition to its affinities with mental illness, was also akin to feminine intuition, itself very close to animal instinct: "From the very nature of her bodily organization, woman is emotionally more resonant than man. . . . She has a greater number of nervous reservoirs, as it were, whence stores of emotional energy can be drawn to meet occasion; and in moments that conspicuously call forth this energy, one can see her whole bodily form vibrating to the particular chord that happens for the time being to be touched by circumstances. But this emotional endowment is not, we may be sure, a small matter in the economy of the race. It is the basis on which are reared the whole vast superstructures of the artistic, the musical, and the imaginative faculties."[64] It became necessary to reassert masculine control over that feminine sensibility: "There is, indeed, in all genius, however virile, a certain undercurrent of the best feminine characteristics. [Geniuses] have in them something of the womanly, though not of the womanish. In one word, the man of genius is comprehensively human. As he always results from a convergence of many fine stocks upon a single point, so also, it seems to me, he often results from a convergence of male and female qualities."[65]

That feminine principle underlying any form of art seemed to be expressed more particularly in the nocturne, by virtue of the traditional associations between night (and the moon's cycles) and women, but also because of its aesthetic, which revealed a sensibility commonly understood to be feminine. In particular, the privilege granted to color over drawing was part of that gendered interpretation: color, associated with emotion and sensuality, was supposedly feminine, while drawing was vested with the supposedly virile virtues of rationality and discipline. The young Whistler thus wrote to his friend Henri Fantin-Latour: "Colour—it's really a vice! certainly it can be and has the right to be one of the most beautiful virtues—if directed by a strong hand—well guided by its master drawing—colour is then a splendid bride with a spouse worthy of her—her lover but also her master,—the most magnificent mistress possible!—and the result is to be seen in all the beautiful things produced by their union!—But coupled with indecision—feeble drawing—timid—vicious—easily satisfied, colour becomes a swanky tart! making spiteful fun of 'her little fellow,' she really does!"[66] Years later, when Whistler and his disciples almost entirely abandoned drawing, they made their nocturnes—in the very terms of these notions—a feminine painting. That may explain Charles Caffin's need to reaffirm Whistler's masculinity: "There are piquancy and virility in all his pictures, not of lively colour and rampageous brush work, but attained through subtle surprises of detail and decorative originality, qualities gleaned from the Japanese."[67] A *New York Times* critic pointed out that, in Dewing's paintings, color is contained by a "stiff" drawing: "The union of such sharply defined drawing with an envelope of such mysterious shadowy beauty gives an impression of dreaminess combined with power and decision—one of the rarest combinations."[68] But that rather awkward insistence only reveals the anxiety of the artists and of the critics who supported them. Another text by Caffin on American landscape painting reveals that preoccupation more explicitly. Having defined tonalism as a delicate and at the same time specifically American landscape form, Caffin singled out the case of Dwight Tryon: "His eminence is due to the fact that beneath his subtlety, which may easily run into a certain effeminacy of ultra-temperamental feeling, is an extremely masculine regard for the strength and solidity of the facts of nature."[69] In the introduction to his chapter on Tryon, Frederic Fairchild Sherman let himself be drawn into general considerations on the art of American landscape painting of that period: "American landscape of today is remarkable rather for fineness than for largeness of vision," he explained, adding, "there ensues a measurable diminution of virility, together with an appreciable increase in subtlety of expression."[70] Worth noting here is the ease with which the subtlety of the tonalist landscape could drift toward an art considered effeminate. Even as the tonalist landscape reflected the highest level of culture, which the artists and their critics believed they had achieved, the American civilization they represented was at risk of losing its strength and virility.

I have already identified a few examples of the fleeting presence of the female figure in the nocturnal landscapes of Homer, Metcalf, Steichen, and Mathews. The most prominent painters in the nocturne genre were almost all men, and women are often only present as anonymous figures, sometimes reduced to silhouettes, performing an allegorical function. These female presences, which are supposed to serve as intermediaries between the external landscape represented on the canvas and a suggested interiority, assume a role equivalent to that of spiritualist mediums, opening the way for an experience dominated by darkness.[71] In fact, the mediums of parapsychology did no more than manifest an extreme form of a sensibility quite simply considered feminine at the time. Rationality and knowledge, activity and light, fell to men; imagination, feeling, a passive life, and the mysteries of darkness to women. That assignment of gender roles was pervasive in American culture at the turn of the twentieth century, and the treatment of the female figure was one of the aspects that distinguished American art quite sharply from its European—and especially French—models. American artists and the American public preferred idealized figures of angelic purity, confined to the chaste roles of wife, sister, or mother, rather than the femme fatale of European symbolism.[72] The majority of female figures that appear in the nocturnes are thus placed in the service of a spiritual dimension of the work and suggest a special relationship to mental life.

Here, however, the cliché allowed for a return of the repressed: the transparency or transcendence with which women were vested was covertly paired with a rhetoric of opacity and darkness. At a time when, in Europe, Sigmund Freud was beginning to explore the "dark continent" of female sexuality, the association between night and femininity promised to reveal truths more disturbing than the sanitized ideas proposed, for instance, by Dewing's idealized women. In her novel *The Awakening,* Kate Chopin attacked precisely this ideal of the "woman-mother." The stream-of-consciousness narration depicts the slow emancipation of the heroine, Edna Pontellier, who discovers simultaneously her sexual desire and the social impossibility of satisfying it. One of the central scenes in the novel shows Edna speaking up in public to express a fantasy so undetermined that reality and fiction are indistinguishable, in which darkness becomes a figure for sexual desire. The heroine invents for her listeners the story of a pair of lovers lost in a pirogue in Barataria Bay, and she takes enormous pleasure in describing the details of the moonlight on the still water, as the lovers vanish into the unknown and oblivion.[73] Significantly, the stages of Edna's "awakening" unfold in landscapes dominated by the vagueness of night and the ocean.

In about 1900 Henry Ossawa Tanner, whose works ordinarily did not breach the most chaste of proprieties, produced a painting that suggested another aspect of dark feminine desire. *Salomé* depicts a woman whose curves are shown off by her transparent clothing and whose body, bathed in light, contrasts with a face veiled in shadow (fig. 62). Alongside the young woman, a dark mass can be made out; a few drops of bright red paint indicate it could be the bleeding head of John the Baptist. Salomé herself seems to be beheaded by the darkness. Her face is obscured, but her gleaming eyes and teeth stand out threateningly against the black background. This Salomé resembles the symbolists' disquieting women more than the innocent figures of American painting (it is possible that Tanner was inspired by Franz von Stück's 1906 painting of Salomé, though there is no tangible link between the two artists). She suggests a different—equally stereotypical but more disturbing—association between women and the night. Female irrationality takes the monstrous form of a body both headless and potentially destructive, desirable and fearsome at once. Corresponding to the erotic overexposure of the body is the suggestion, equally intense, of castrating violence. The fate of Tanner's *Salomé* was also marked by repression: the artist never sold the painting, which rarely left his studio and was considered lost until it was rediscovered in the early 1980s, affixed to the back of another of the artist's works.

But as the expression "dark continent" suggests, the sexual connotations attached to the figure of Salomé in general and to this painting in particular must also be interpreted through the prism of racial difference. When Tanner's personal situation is taken into account—he was an African American who chose exile in France to escape discrimination—*Salomé* takes on a complex meaning. Paradoxically, the figure of Salomé, an emblem of Oriental sensuality, is distinguished by her whiteness. Atop the young woman's hypervisible, luminous body is a dark face, forming a kind of biracial hybrid. The symbolic split between the "low" and the "high" reverses racial clichés: the body, traditionally associated with sensuality, instinct, and often the supposed savagery of nonwhites, is here what brings light; conversely, her face, symbol of the soul and intellect—supposedly the privileged domain of white civilization—remains in shadow. Salomé thus stands as an equivocal, even subversive figure, suggesting that symbols can be turned on their head and extremes can merge. The painting allows us to see the opposite of what the slender young girls in evening gowns that adorn Dewing's decorative art were supposed to embody: in stark contrast to their refined civilization stands a powerful vision of femininity upsetting the norms of sexual and racial conventions.

Another particularly resonant cliché in the nocturnes is the association between creative genius and madness, already well established in romantic and gothic literature. As of the 1890s, the apologia for the half-mad artist was also greatly inspired by the views of the criminologist and psychologist Cesare Lombroso. In *The Man of Genius* (*Uomo di genio*), published in Italian in 1889 and translated into English in 1891, Lombroso portrayed a

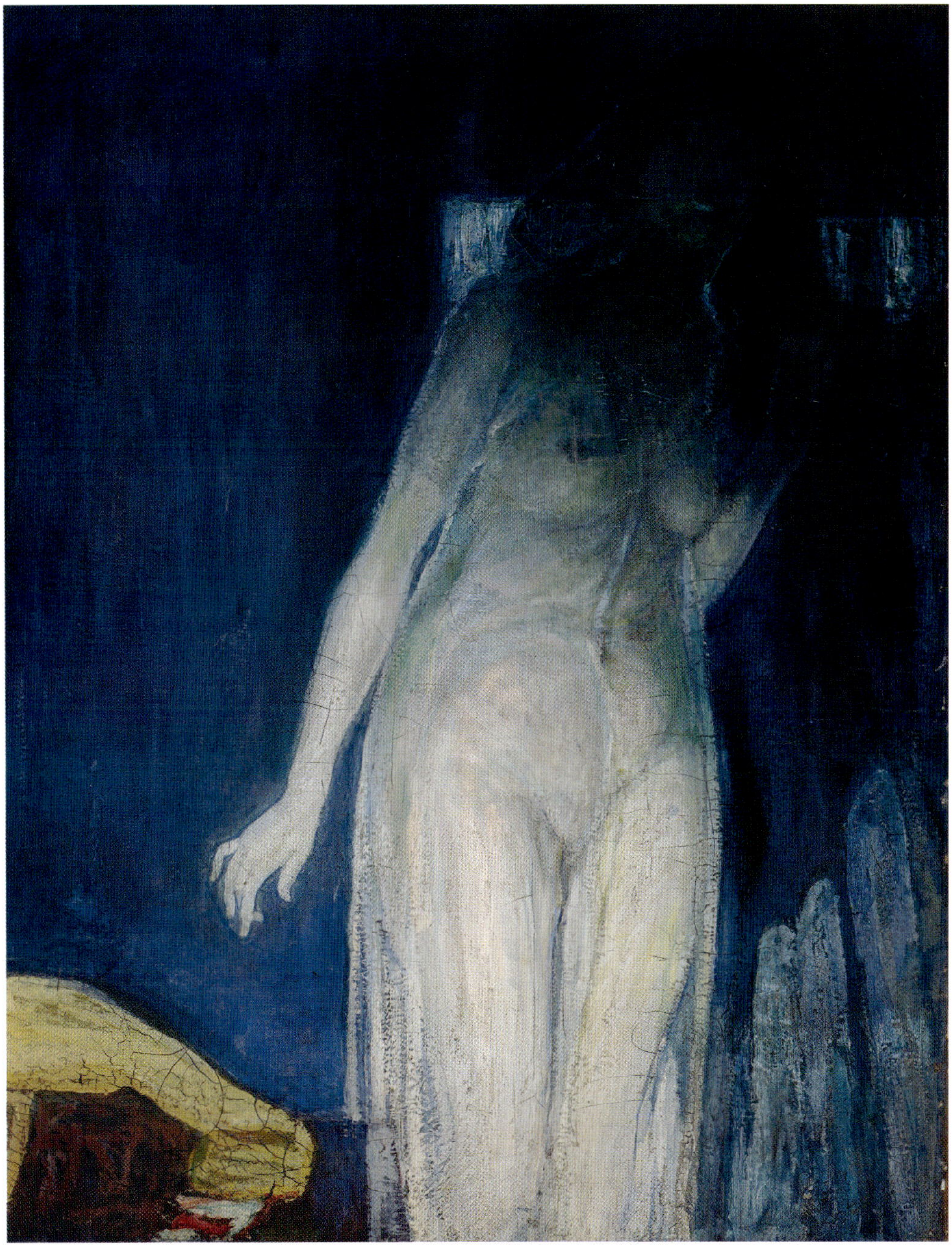

FIG. 62. Henry Ossawa Tanner, *Salomé*, c. 1900. Oil on canvas, 116.5 × 89.4 cm (45 7/8 × 35 1/4 in.). Smithsonian American Art Museum, Gift of Jesse O. Tanner (1983.95.207A).

pathological and deviant genius whose art was supposedly the result of "psychic epilepsy."[74] The book went through thirteen English-language editions between 1891 and 1917, and its views were commonly expounded in the daily press and in general interest magazines. The idea that artistic genius belongs to the same realm as mental pathology was widely discussed in the United States, as were the objections and responses made to that idea by Max Nordau.[75]

Two late nineteenth-century American painters conformed particularly well to that model of the mad artist. Unsurprisingly, these two artists also devoted themselves for the most part to nocturnes (see fig. 7; fig. 63). Albert Pinkham Ryder, who gained fame with his moonlit marines, drew from romantic literature and music in creating paintings such as *Siegfried and the Rhine Maidens* (1889–91; National Gallery of Art, Washington, D.C.) and *The Toilers of the Sea* (1880–85; Metropolitan Museum of Art, New York). What is important, in Ryder's case, is the way he was (mis)understood by his public. Sarah Burns, placing the reception of Ryder's paintings within the context of psychology and psychoanalysis as it developed in the early twentieth century, demonstrates that the emphasis Ryder's critics placed on the dreamlike

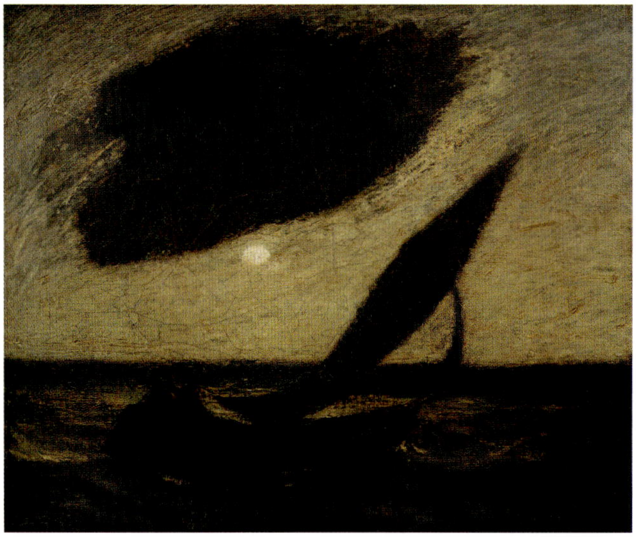

FIG. 63. Albert Pinkham Ryder, *Under a Cloud*, c. 1900. Oil on canvas, 50.8 × 61 cm (20 × 24 in.). Metropolitan Museum of Art, Gift of Alice E. Van Orden, in memory of her husband, Dr. T. Durland Van Orden, 1988 (1988.353).

quality of his paintings actually functioned as a form of censorship. Ryder, depicted as an innocently "lunatic" artist whose eccentricity only contributed to his genius, in reality also embodied a set of values unacceptable for the society that so lavishly praised him. For example, Burns describes Ryder's questionable hygiene and outlandish social behavior, and she shows that his critics, in persistently portraying the artist as contemplative and harmless, were attempting to repress a threatening deviance revealed in his works.[76]

The case of Ralph Albert Blakelock, though even more extreme, is consistent with that interpretation. In part, the figure of Ryder prepared the way for the reception given Blakelock, whose canvases were often compared to Ryder's. Critics noted in particular the habit the two artists shared of piling on the paint in thick layers interspersed with glaze and their sometimes disastrous experiments with various media, such as bitumen.[77] Interpretations of Blakelock's works, like those of Ryder's, drew from a set of preconceived images, channeling the artists' apparent eccentricity into commonplaces. Blakelock's biographers retraced the course of the accursed genius's mental illness, arguing that he was essentially unsuited to the prosaic constraints of life in society.[78] That emotional instability made him more vulnerable than other "mind-workers" to the pressures of modern life, especially its practical and financial demands. Almost all the stories about Blakelock's madness underscore the trauma that had triggered his pathology. On the very day that his eighth child was born, Blakelock, in dire straits, was forced to sell one of his paintings for an absurdly low price. The pathos of the artist as romantic figure grappling with a merciless environment thus took shape: "But our modern life imposes obligations in the mere business of keeping alive, which keeps this thought very prominently in mind, and no argument is needed in suggesting the value to any mind-worker of a mind at peace. This is one of the pitiful things in this man's career—that his advance toward that brilliancy which would have rewarded him and finally did honor his time, was so greatly impeded, if not measurably reduced, and the man himself broken upon the wheel of suffering. Of the shadowed mind which closed forever his labors, certainly the story is sad enough."[79] The story invariably repeats the conventional opposition between materialism and art so favored by the critics praising the nocturne's detachment from practical concerns.

Blakelock's personal life, combined with his predilection for night landscapes, made him the perfect illustration of the cliché of the lunatic genius. The moonlight landscapes that Blakelock painted from the mid-1880s onward often repeat the same formula: a composition centered on a radiant moon but framed by dark masses of trees, which, in a layout comparable to that in Steichen's paintings, establish an ambiguous space between interiority and exteriority. As Norman Geske has pointed out, at the beginning of his career Blakelock was relatively well integrated into New York art circles, well informed about the tendencies in vogue in that world, and intent on finding a style that would please the public.[80] Ironically, Blakelock's use of the nocturne genre, though promising, did not prove lucrative until he found himself excluded from the professional art scene. Shortly after his internment, the prices for his canvases spiked, which encouraged counterfeiters to flood the market with "fakelocks."[81] The fascination manifest in the accounts published at the end of his life, after his works had sold for record prices on the art market, lay in great part in the contrast between the figure of a martyred (and, above all, indigent) artist and the sums paid for his paintings. In 1916 *Moonlight* was purchased by the Toledo Museum of Art for twenty thousand dollars, which made it the most expensive work by a living American artist.[82] It was the very discrepancy between the two extremes that sealed Blakelock's fate as an accursed genius. All in all, Blakelock was never so well integrated into the capitalist economic system as when he was officially relegated to its margins. In a movement similar to the dreamwork, critics thus gave a central place to the artist's madness, the better to repress it: Blakelock was "institutionalized" in both senses of the term, becoming a fixture of the art scene even as he was locked up far from society.

Blakelock's misfortune is but an extreme example of a widespread concern for the roots of art in the deepest recesses of our psychology. Birge Harrison, in a chapter of his painting manual entited "The Sub-Conscious Servant," constructed a complex model of the psyche that combined temperament, character, and the "subconscious," whose particular importance in an artist's life was acknowledged by the author: "There is no man, probably, who has more need of the help of this faithful sub-conscious servant than the artist, for so many of the mental processes of art must be instinctive."[83] But the entire chapter consisted of reaffirming the hierarchy between that subconscious and reason. The former, characterized as a series of habits and a certain body memory, remained rather vague overall, without a specific content or independent motivations. Harrison refrained from attributing to that "servant" even a hint of rebelliousness, contrary to the Freudian theories imported to the United States only a few years before Harrison's book was published. The only danger lay in exhausting the subconscious: "If this ever-faithful helper fails to respond to the demands made upon him, it is through no unwillingness to serve the master but because of utter exhaustion and inability to react."[84] Ultimately, Harrison advised his students to cultivate a strict hierarchy, which, significantly, he modeled on a professional and social hierarchy: "The student's business is to learn all he can to train the subconscious servant to be the valuable helper that he must needs be later on; and this can be done day by day with as much adherence to regular hours as the business man demands of his assistants."[85] The aberrations of Blakelock's subconscious were ultimately placed in the service of the art market. According to Harrison, however, the subconscious had to be managed the way a manager treats his workforce: the irrational was acceptable only if, in one way or another, it could be reintegrated into the framework of a familiar rationality.

Once again, the discourse around the nocturnes seemed to maintain only a fragile balance between contradictory models, which threatened to escape control. In fact, in contrast to Harrison's disciplined model, the image of a subconscious or unconscious that was equal parts uncontrollable and invisible fascinated the public of the time. A whole series of fictional works exploited the theme, the best known by far being Robert Louis Stevenson's *Strange Case of Dr. Jekyll and Mr. Hyde.* While nocturne artists ostensibly looked for harmony and uniformity, their audiences, on the contrary, relished tales and images that allowed for the irruption of the Other. And they were prompt to associate that Other—psychological, sexual, racial—with night and darkness. In this view, Blakelock was understood to be more sensitive than others to the beauty of nature not only because he was especially sensitive, but also because he was still somewhat wild and outside of "civilization." Elliott Daingerfield thus portrayed Blakelock as an artist whose vocation arose in contact with the primitive culture of the American Indians he encountered in his travels to the West during his youth, "probably when he made his first journey to the West and began to study the Indians, when the barbaric depth of their color, the richness and plenitude of reds and yellows, the strength of shadow and brilliancy of light awakened his vision and set tingling those pulses of the brain which control the color emotions. His own soul an untamed one, responding to no conventional law, these children of forest and plain appealed to his deepest instincts."[86] Even as the nocturne artists insisted that art was a process of refining the primitive impulse, they ventured onto dangerous terrain by indicating their preference for darkness, given the number of equivocal associations night imagery elicited. At an individual level, the genius of the night could sink into madness, but, because he was primitive (even childlike), he could also lead civilization to regress to a less evolved stage. The artists and critics who made the nocturne the symbol of and means to achieve a civilized ideal, thus threatened by a loss of vitality, virility, and reason, seemed to hold a more than precarious position. The antivision in this case could be that of a past literally reverting to the mists—the darkness—of time. The universal and ideal night of civilization, having achieved its highest level, could thus fall back into the primitive formlessness of a nightmarish obscurity.

PART II

Heart of Darkness

The Nocturne as Metaphor for Racial Difference

When commentators equated civilization with the aesthetic refinement of the nocturne, they were proposing a political interpretation of landscape painting. In reality, the civilization they invoked was defined as an identity, one that was clearly local or national, but above all, ethnic. In the dominant discourse of American culture at the time, it was self-evident that the civilization under discussion was white. In sociocultural, geographical, and ethnic terms, nocturne artists formed a relatively homogeneous group: the vast majority were white men from the middle and upper classes living in the large urban centers of the east coast. Henry Ossawa Tanner was one of the very few black artists, and the California tonalists in Charles Rollo Peters's circle were not so much an exception geographically speaking as the reflection of a cosmopolitan and urban mode of life common to San Francisco, New York, and Boston.[1] Yet while the nocturne could be regarded as a form of landscape painting emblematic of white civilization, it also proved to be full of contradictions and ambiguities. Compared to the landscapes of the Hudson River School, it was a muted version of the triumphalist discourse of American imperialism.[2] The paintings of the Hudson River School offered the vision of a divine Providence protecting the enterprise of conquest by Anglo-American settlers;[3] the nocturne, by contrast, was a landscape that no longer promised anything. Whereas the works of the Hudson River School propelled their beholders toward an optimistic future, the nocturne indulged in nostalgia and melancholy.

That new point of view coincided with a change of direction in American foreign policy, which went through several major mutations between 1890 and 1917, particularly under the presidencies of William McKinley and Theodore Roosevelt. Abandoning the isolationist reserve of their predecessors, they set the country on the path of imperialism, guided by the rhetoric of the obligations that civilization bore toward the rest of the world. The United States, taking on the "white man's burden," to borrow Rudyard Kipling's expression,[4] "liberated" Cuba and Puerto Rico from the grip of the Spanish empire. After the U.S. victory in Cuba, McKinley proposed expanding "benevolent assimilation" to the Philippines.[5] But, bogged down in that enterprise, the government quickly found itself confronted with the contradictions of its own discourse. The fierce resistance of the Filipinos, under the leadership of General Emilio Aguinaldo, sowed doubt in the minds of the American public about the legitimacy of the colonial venture and the solidity of the proclaimed values of American civilization. In many cases, the roles of the warring parties—drawn from visual culture and assigned on the basis of stereotypes that contrasted the light of civilization to the darkness of savagery—quickly became blurred or even reversed themselves. Hence, in a context where light, whiteness, and civilization were conceived as equivalent terms, the preference for darkness expressed by the nocturne artists appeared paradoxical.

Imperialist designs were inextricably entangled with the definition of ethnic identities. The late nineteenth and early twentieth centuries witnessed the apogee of scientific racism in Europe and North America, with a proliferation of theories that classified various ethnic groups and justified political, legal, social, economic, and institutional inequalities on the basis of biological criteria, sometimes complemented by linguistic and geographical data.[6] This ideological hyperactivity evinces the dominant groups' deep need for stable and closed categories in a mutable environment. Herbert Spencer's evolutionist model was one of the first to transpose biological classifications to the realm of sociology. It elaborated a mythological hierarchy of civilizations to which the Western white middle and upper classes hastened to subscribe. Theodore Roosevelt, for example, delivered a speech at Oxford in 1910 in which, to justify his imperialist views, he drew a series of comparisons between biology and history: "We see strange analogies in the phenomena of life and death, of birth, growth, and change, between those physical groups of animal life which we designate as species, forms, races, and the highly complex and composite entities which rise before our minds when we speak of nations and civilizations."[7] Works of art, understood from the standpoint of that confusion between the biological and the cultural, were interpreted as symptoms or reflections of their creators' "race": in that regard, the nocturne was considered a "white" art. The world's fairs, in staging the imperialist competition between powers that grounded their superiority in racist notions, also served as showcases for these pseudoscientific theories.[8] From the anthropological sections exhibiting the customs of nonwhite peoples to the pavilions dedicated to the arts and technologies of Western countries, a single essentialist vision dominated, one that ranked the human "races" and "civilizations" in a hierarchical order.[9] Yet the genealogy invented by Frederick Jackson Turner, however epic, also gives us a glimpse of an uncertain and shaky American identity. As the phenomenon of the world's fairs attests, this was a time when exchanges at the global level were increasing and immigrants from ever more remote places and diverse backgrounds were arriving en masse on American soil. The American white middle and upper classes felt their identity threatened. That accounts for their anxieties, which a good number of them formulated in ethnic terms. For example, in 1916 Madison Grant published *The Passing of the Great Race,* in which he fantasized that whites were the heirs of a Nordic "race" in danger of extinction.[10] The nocturne's endless contradictions can be understood as expressing the worries and hesitations of white upper and middle classes that believed they were losing ground to its many "others."

The overseas imperialist venture was explicitly linked to the closing of the American frontier, and the nocturnal landscapes set in the West were both a nostalgic meditation on the completed conquest and an anxious reflection on the one beginning elsewhere. In 1890, when the American authorities declared the Wild West entirely conquered, the last confrontations between whites and Indians signaled what the American public saw as the death of the Indian "race." The tragedy at Wounded Knee at the end of that year was the most emblematic of these conflicts. White Americans, having arrived at continent's end, suddenly looked with new eyes at the Indians, who ceased to be enemies and assumed the role of ancestors of the American nation.[11] The declared end of the Wild West gave the historian Frederick Jackson Turner the opportunity to formulate, after the fact, his theory of the frontier, namely, that American identity was forged in that unique space of struggle and transition that separated two Americas, one savage and the other civilized. The pioneers, faced with the extraordinarily challenging circumstances of the natural environment, were said to have developed the spirit of enterprise, equality, and solidarity from which American democracy issued forth.[12] Simultaneously, and in view of that shift, popular culture revived the theme of the "vanishing Indian," supposedly destined for extinction. That topos was taken up by visual culture: Edward S. Curtis's magisterial work of documentary photography, *The North American Indian,* immortalized the Indian peoples and at the same time contributed toward their symbolic disappearance.[13] In the works of Curtis, Frederic Remington, and also Peters, a complex reflection about the nature of American identity took shape. That identity was vanishing in part along with the Indians, even as it symbolically reincorporated them into the national heritage. In these cases, night served as an ambiguous space, conveying the hesitations of Americans divided between conquest and loss.

The exotic climes of the Philippines and Cuba and the nostalgic past of the frontier indirectly tell a story about two peoples subjected to American domination. But a third group determined by racial difference—namely, African Americans—must also be considered in relation to the nocturnal landscape. For American artists and their public, the question of African Americans had an urgency and a proximity even more troubling than that of Indians or Filipinos, which might explain why the issue was only rarely raised. The living conditions of blacks deteriorated sharply in the last decades of the nineteenth century; a generation after the end of the Civil War, African Americans were stripped of their civil rights. Violence between whites and blacks reached a fever pitch at the turn of the twentieth century: in 1901 the *Appeal,* a black daily newspaper published in both St. Louis and Minneapolis, listed more than three thousand cases of lynching in the twenty previous years, noting that most of the victims were black and that almost all the crimes took place in the Southern states. It is significant that the filmmaker D. W. Griffith chose to give his film adaptation of Thomas Dixon's racist novel *The Clansman* the title *Birth of a Nation:* that choice shows that the definition of American identity entailed the exclusion of African Americans.[14] The visual dimension of the difference is crucial here: views on ethnic identity—both in white racist discourse and in the writings of W.E.B. Du Bois—were in fact dominated by the vocabulary of brightness and darkness, but also of visibility and invisibility. In that play of meanings, paradoxes and displacements abounded. Nothing, or almost nothing, in the nocturnes referred explicitly to relations between whites and blacks in America. Given the context, however, it is difficult to imagine that this art concerned wholly with darkness made no reference, however indirect, to race relations.

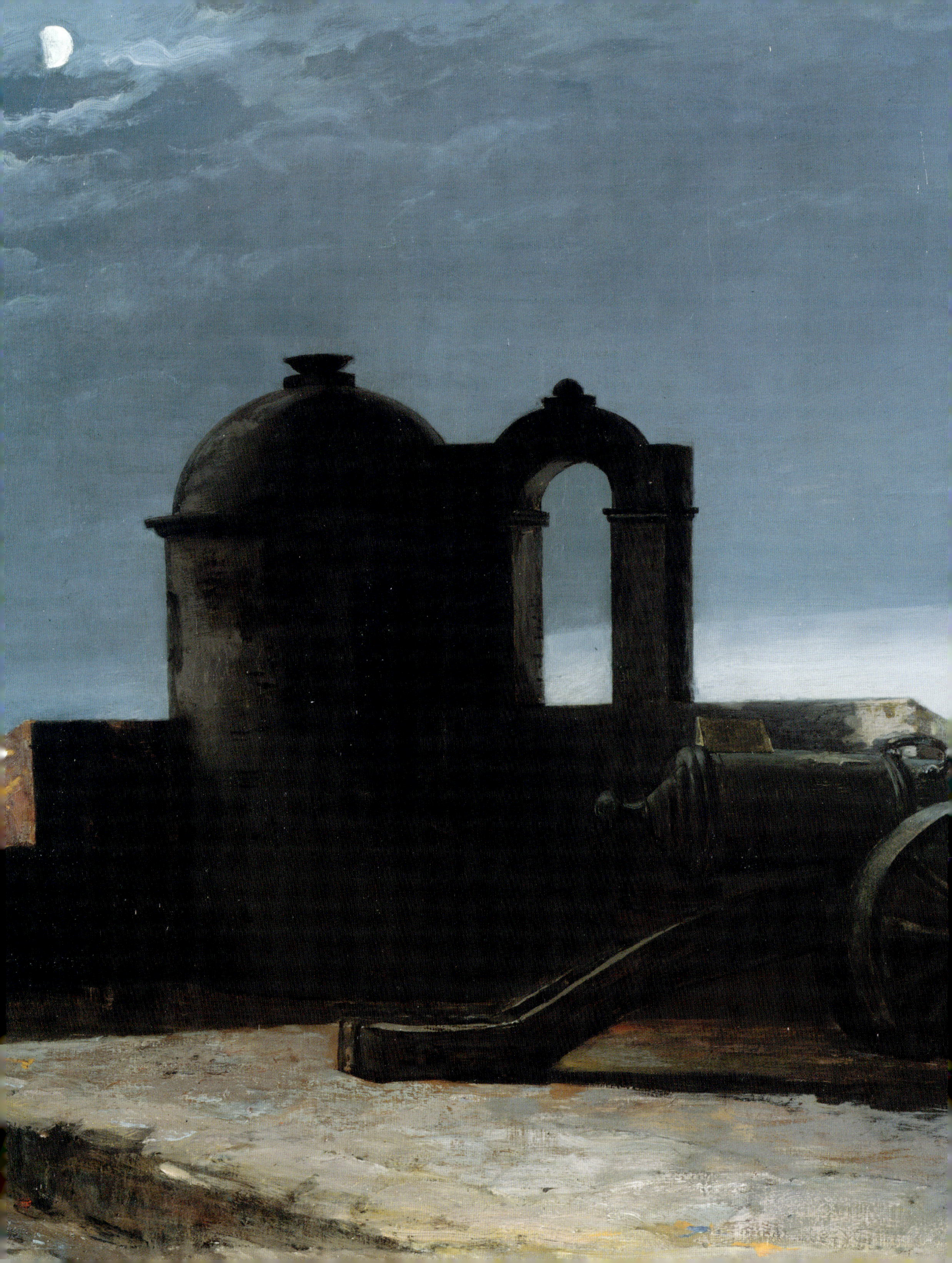

5 Inverted Light

The Nocturne in the Age of Imperialism

I would first like to address the methodological problems raised by a "racial" interpretation of the nocturnes. How is it possible to read into these landscapes, usually devoid of any human presence, a discourse on the political relations between various ethnic groups? What status should be assigned to darkness from that standpoint? Even as the United States was launching the imperialist conquest of Cuba and then of the Philippines, nocturnes for the most part remained silent, conspicuously detached from the international events of the time. The night as Whistler and his disciples represented it, supposedly universal and eternal, was generally interpreted as a "transparent" object. Nocturnes, indeterminate landscapes devoid of picturesque markers and defined solely by their atmosphere, almost never laid claim to local attachments or signs of identity. The titles the artists chose for their paintings often reflected atmospheric conditions (Alexander Wyant's *Moonlight and Frost,* Birge Harrison's *Soaring Clouds*), the season (Winslow Homer's *Summer Night,* Charles Warren Eaton's *Winter Night*), or a generic location (Tryon's *Sea: Night* and *Night: A Harbor,* Léon Dabo's *River*), without referring explicitly to a local communality, let alone an ethnic one. The very limited presence of human figures and the near absence of characters who could be clearly identified as nonwhite mean that, if a racial discourse can be attributed to the nocturnes, it is usually allusive.

I shall draw my inspiration from the methods developed by the field of white studies,[1] which sets out to reconstruct the ethnically oriented meanings behind the dominant vision. In following that example, I shall endeavor to present the more or less "invisible" discourses that provided the context in which the nocturnes were created and evaluated, and to uncover the ideological commitments concealed behind their apparent silence. The nocturne, which was defined by its declared neutrality, in fact participated in white "invisibility": critics' insistence on its formal sobriety (verging on vacantness), its immateriality, and its spiritual dimension would indicate that it belonged symbolically to the sphere Richard Dyer designates as "socially white."[2] And like the other products of white culture, its very "whiteness," in the sense of belonging to that ethnic group, was obscured by the fallacious self-evidence of a supposedly universal truth. In reality, the more the nocturne professed its detachment from racial and political concerns,

Fig. 65 detail

the more it manifested a white attitude. And though it may have evaded the direct representation of ethnic questions, I will show that the formal darkness it continually explored cannot be divested of racial meanings.[3]

To bring to the surface the implicit discourse underlying the nocturnes, it is necessary to correlate it with other discourses more explicitly focused on the ambient racial questions. I shall therefore compare the nocturnes to other visual products, for example, racist images in advertisements, attractions at the world's fairs, colonial postcards, and photographs of lynchings. Furthermore, I shall broaden the notion of image to include verbal images: in fact, the discourse on ethnic identity is largely governed by the metaphorical connection established between image and discourse. Metaphor, because it constantly shifts the content of urgent or delicate political questions onto apparently trivial objects, would appear to be one of the privileged modes of racist discourse. That is the hypothesis put forward by Toni Morrison in an essay entitled *Playing in the Dark: Whiteness and the Literary Imagination,* which demonstrates American literature's propensity for treating ethnic identity in figurative rather than literal terms.[4] For the purposes of my argument, I shall concern myself with the slippage between verbal and pictorial images, and with the dynamic interaction that places metaphor halfway between language and image.[5]

THE NOCTURNE AS THE LANDSCAPE OF WHITE CIVILIZATION

Beyond these methodological considerations, I shall situate the art of the nocturne within a historical and cultural context that, through the notion of civilization, granted art a national and racial representativeness. The absolute autonomy of art to which Whistler and the defenders of art for art's sake laid claim was not unanimously accepted by American nocturne painters. A certain tension persisted between the ostensible aloofness of Whistler and his followers and the need to define nocturnal landscape painting as a specifically American art, style, and tradition. Many critics sought to repatriate landscape painting, and the nocturne along with it, to the sphere of Western, even explicitly American, civilization: "In spite of present practice, and quite apart from [Whistler's] *Ten O'Clock* . . . , art is still believed to be in some way an expression of a time, a place, and a people. The world has not yet grown so small that it does not continue to exhibit race characteristics in its art manifestations. . . . The all-the-world-as-one idea may be farther-reaching, more universal in its scope, and therefore loftier in its art expression. . . . Still, even then, with cosmopolitanism in the saddle, there will be the need and the use of tradition."[6] Here, John Van Dyke was expressing an anxiety shared by many American commentators vis-à-vis recent developments of their art. Critics strove to reconcile the cosmopolitan careers of American artists with the definition of an art that would represent the United States on the international scene, but without lapsing into provincialism.

An "American" Art in the Global Age

The world's fairs, cosmopolitan sites par excellence, reflected the ambitions tinged with apprehension perceptible in Van Dyke's words. They were the occasion for the various Western countries to define themselves in the eyes of the world and to justify their claims of cultural, commercial, and political hegemony. In his review of the American works displayed at the fine arts pavilion of the World's Columbian Exposition in Chicago in 1893, Van Dyke lamented the effect of European influences on young American painters, handicapped by the "Gallicisms" and "world-isms" of international art.[7] Charles Caffin wondered whether it was even possible to speak of an American school of painting in a context where American artists, though they had no doubt reached artistic maturity, had done so only by means of an apprenticeship abroad: "Is there yet a distinctly American school of painting; and, if so, how does it compare with other schools? But, strictly speaking, there are no longer distinct schools anywhere. . . . The whole trend of modern art has been toward a free-trade in motives and methods, the clearing-house of which for all the world has been Paris. Yet, while the age of close communities of artists, following some distinct tradition or influenced by some one leader, and producing work which bears the stamp of a common sentiment and manner of expression, is past, it is unquestionably true that the local conditions of race temperament and natural environment do still stamp with a certain general distinction the work of each country."[8] The terms "free-trade" and "clearing-house" are far from insignificant. They indicate the close association at the global level between artistic and commercial exchanges, and suggest that uniformization and standardization affected works of art just like all other products of exchange. The works of Whistler, Dewing, and Tryon were part of a vast network of influences and distribution that ran parallel to that of commercial exchanges, a system of economic and symbolic transfers in which their patron Charles Lang Freer played a pivotal role.[9] In that respect, Dewing's and Tryon's art were more "global" than universal, like the world's fairs, which were in reality dominated by the great Western powers. From that standpoint, the views of Caffin, who tried to anchor painting in the natural order, appear incongruous. The dissonance between the evocation of free trade and "race temperament and natural environment" reveals his hesitations. But the less pertinent and the more arbitrary that notion of art is in terms of race, the more significant it becomes.

Race and Landscape

The ethnic question can almost always be discerned behind efforts to define a civilization or national identity as it is expressed in the arts. According to Harrison, for example, every work of art reflected not only the artist's individual vision but, atavistically, that of an entire human group: "Each artist is, first of all, a unit of some specified human group or race. Therefore, if he truly and conscientiously records his own impressions, he will also record the accumulated impressions of the race to which he belongs. That he does this is amply proved by the fact that any reasonably expert judge will tell you whether a picture belongs to the French or the Dutch or the Scandinavian school, without knowing the name of the painter, or anything more of the picture than the canvas itself discloses. It is impossible, therefore, to avoid the conclusion that racial individuality in art is fact, and a very real and solid fact at that."[10] That is why commentators on nocturnes were able to interpret them as landscapes characteristic of the white, Western "race": the "civilized landscape" was also the landscape of a particular civilization. None of them disputed the fact that Western civilization happened to be the one that they thought had achieved the most advanced level of civilization, in the absolute sense of the word. Van Dyke, reviewing the artworks of the various national sections represented at the World's Columbian Exposition, established a hierarchy both geographical and artistic: he began with the countries of southern Europe (Italy, Spain), before considering the case of France, then discrediting German and British painting,[11] which had the "racial" flaw of being too literary, and finally turning to the Scandinavian and American schools, which, in Van Dyke's view, had the brightest future. "Following the track of civilization, painting writes the color history of the people and when the land and the people are young, the record is full of aspiration, hope, and energy. Fortunately for the Scandinavians and ourselves, the period is that of youth."[12] According to Royal Cortissoz, painting was primarily the doing of the northern countries: "The genius of mere paint . . . appears to have been very largely a Northern prerogative."[13] Birge Harrison, in the first pages of his treatise on landscape painting, asserted the racial nature of the particular link between Nordic Western civilization and its natural environment, and therefore its superiority in the art of landscape: "For some occult reason in which the two factors of race and psychology are intimately blended, landscape art in its best expression is and ever has been confined within the narrow geographical limits of Northern and Western Europe. . . . The simple existence of our Aryan ancestors ([who] lived close to nature in the constant companionship of elemental things) has found expression in the landscape art of their remote descendants."[14] The landscape "instinct," woven into the fabric from which Westerners had been made for millenniums, could also be found—naturally, as it were—on the painter's canvas, reflecting a shared temperament on the part of the Western artist and the nature he depicted. Harrison, having traced the long history of that developing taste for landscape, reaffirmed more clearly the association between landscape painting and Western civilization, showing that the genre was a product specific to American modernity: "The fact is that the open has claimed us as a people! We devote ourselves with ever-increasing enthusiasm to out-of-door pleasures and out-of-door pursuits; we have learned to love out-of-door nature and out-of-door beauty. It is our best achievement as a nation; and our artists in this are, therefore, simply keeping step with the march of modern civilization."[15] Here Harrison borrowed the already-old theme of landscape painting as an American "heritage," the American democratic equivalent of European history painting.[16] But he adapted the theme to the spirit of his time, when leisure culture was emerging, eminent personalities such as Theodore Roosevelt were championing an active lifestyle in the open air, and the naturalist John Muir was popularizing the cause of preserving the wilderness.[17] If we are to believe Harrison, because the natural landscape was one of the privileged sites where modern American civilization developed, its representation in painting became the perfect emblem for national (white) identity.

The subdued tones of the nocturne encouraged that interpretation, in that they conformed to a widespread discourse on the racial connotations of colors. In 1901, for example, the organizers of the Pan-American Exposition in Buffalo assigned the muralist Charles Yardley Turner the task of elaborating a color scheme that staged the progress of civilization. "The color scheme will represent in epitome the growth of the color sense of the race," the newspapers announced, explaining the hierarchical arrangement of colors within the exhibition space, from the brightest tones to the most subtle nuances of civilization at its apogee: "All the savage races have manifested a great fondness for strong, crude colors, and these will be found in the buildings nearest the main entrance. The advancement of man in intelligence and civilization has been marked by a desire for mere refined color combinations, with the culminating point of subtlety and grace of color being in the Electric Tower, which, representing the highest advance in material civilization and occupying the leading position architecturally and sculpturally of the whole Exposition, naturally enough has come in for the finest color notes."[18] Color, in both the literal and symbolic sense, was directly projected onto the exposition's artificial landscape. On canvas, the subtlety of the tonal transitions deployed in the nocturne was in keeping with that racist understanding of vision. The capacity to distinguish colors was perceived as a factor in racial but also social "evolution," a physical aptitude as much as a class marker. "Evolved" or "civilized" taste favored the subtlety of "refined color combinations": the model of a colored environment invented by Turner repeated Whistler's rhetoric and adapted it to the political field.

That refinement of colors was combined with the notion of a range of "temperaments" characteristic of each race, which corresponded to the full spectrum of colors, from the warmest shades to the coolest. Cool colors, a cool climate, and a cool individual temperament could supposedly be found in the nocturne. Like Van Dyke, the critic Haywood Laudendale made landscape art a prerogative of the Scandinavian schools, which he gathered together into a single "Gothic stock": "In impulse, what is most characteristically Gothic in the life of all peoples of the Gothic stock belongs to the open air, so that landscape painting in modern art is as much indebted to the Gothic mind for its development as the painting of the human figure is to the mind of Italy."[19] In this article, which, according to its title, was devoted to the art of northern Europe, none of the thirteen illustrations was European, and no such art was cited directly in the text. On the contrary, all the artists represented in these pages were American, and only two women were included, by way of genre scenes centered on a female figure. Apart from a sculpture titled *Solitude* and the portrait of an Indian, all the paintings chosen were landscapes, half of them nocturnes. Although the text did not explicitly point out the connection between that art of the (nocturnal) landscape and the art of the northern European schools, the layout indicated at the very least that the editors of *Brush and Pencil,* where the article was published, perceived an affinity between the works and these words. That link suggests that the American nocturne carried with it the values of a white identity, embodying on canvas its virility and Nordic character. This connection also motivated an article devoted to Henry Ossawa Tanner's oeuvre, in which the journalist Eunice Tietjens commented on his use of color in conjunction with his ethnic identity. Having noted that, when Tanner became a mature artist, he abandoned the brown and gold tones inherited from Rembrandt and Thomas Eakins for a palette dominated by blue, Tietjens speculated on the compatibility between colors and ethnicity: "[Tanner's cold palette] does not seem temperamentally suited to him. The cold end of the spectrum, the violets, blues and cold greens, belong naturally to the Anglo-Saxon and correspond with a certain hardness of disposition and outlook. But the more warm-blooded peoples, beginning with the Latins, are more at home in the warmer tonalities."[20] The racial distribution of colors Tietjens chose is very significant: rather than a gradation from bright to dark, she based her critique of Tanner on the idea of color temperature, which led her to consider the "disposition" of peoples by way of what she deemed a "natural" connection. Not without contradiction, but tellingly as well, the order of distinctions she chose to adopt here superseded the more obvious categories of light and darkness.

Japanism

In addition to that inconsistency, a major objection could be raised to those who claimed that the nocturne was a "white" and fundamentally American art: it actually

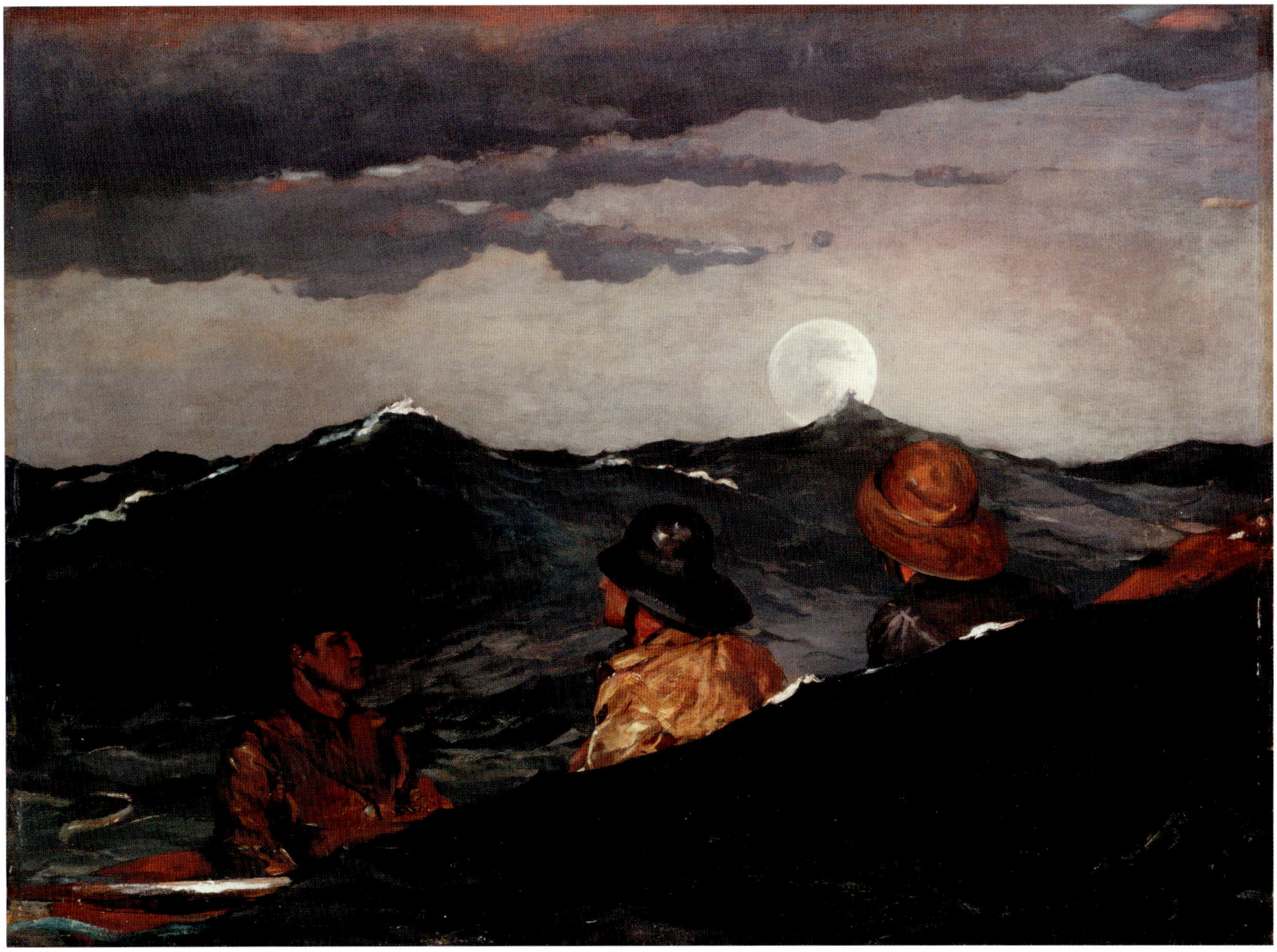

FIG. 64. Winslow Homer, *Kissing the Moon*, 1904. Oil on canvas, 76.84 × 101.6 cm (30 ¼ × 40 in.). Addison Gallery of American Art, Phillips Academy, Andover, Massachusetts, bequest of Candace C. Stimson, 1946.19.

borrowed a large share of its aesthetic codes from Japanese art. Whistler and his disciples did not hide their attachment to Asian art (which they declared, for example, in the monograms they created to use as their signatures, like Whistler's famous butterfly). Even the painters most remote from Whistler's circle, when they adopted the nocturne, were also occasionally inspired by Japanese art, as was, for example, Winslow Homer with his *Kissing the Moon*, whose theme and flat surfaces are reminiscent of Hokusai's famous *Great Wave off Kanagawa* (fig. 64).[21] A journalist reporting on the content of the Japanese fine arts section at the World's Columbian Exposition in Chicago explained the fondness of the Japanese—strange for most Westerners—for monochrome works. His description of Japanese tastes suggests an affinity with the aesthetic preferences of nocturne painters in the United States: "The Japanese . . . discover more spiritual, or occult beauty, in what appears to be but a vapory suggestion of a picture, than one in which form and color are rendered in strong and decided work."[22]

Japanese culture was introduced to the United States by personalities such as Ernest Fenollosa, a historian of Japanese art. He was as influential in Tokyo, where he served as foreign adviser to the emperor and founded a university and a museum, as he was in Boston, where he was director of the Asian art collection at the Museum of Fine Arts, gave many lectures, and published popular works on the art of Japan.[23] At the 1893 Chicago exposition, the country received a remarkably favorable treatment: the landscape architect Frederick Law Olmsted set aside an entire island for the Japanese pavilion, a picturesque setting adorned with lanterns and groves of trees. But Japanism can also be seen as a cosmopolitan phenomenon, since it was often in Paris that American artists discovered Japanese art. The West's interest in Japanese culture, of course, was linked to the country's geopolitical situation. Following the American expedition conducted by Commodore Matthew Perry in 1851, Japan had opened up trade with foreigners, after two and a half centuries of being strictly closed to outsiders. The new arrival's rising power on the international scene did not fail to elicit some wariness, especially after Japan's victory over Russia in 1905. For the first time in over two centuries, a nonwhite people had inflicted a military defeat on a white power, giving rise to anxieties in the American public about the "Yellow Peril."[24] The ambiguous situation of Japan, a nonwhite civilization whose cultural and political legitimacy was nonetheless acknowledged by Westerners, was particularly visible during the world's fairs: while Japan was one of the rare civilizations at the expositions to appear in the industrial and artistic sections of the developed countries, it was also present in the anthropological sections, where nonwhites were exhibited to curiosity seekers.[25]

Although most commentators on the nocturne acknowledged the Japanese influence on its aesthetic, they did so with a certain reticence, always taking care to maintain the Japanese heritage in an inferior position. Van Dyke noted the incongruity of that art imported from the Orient to the banks of the Thames: "Toward 1870 another riddle was presented with the appearance of the nocturnes. They were things done along the Thames at dusk and were revelations of that blue-air envelope which forms when the shadow of the world begins to creep up the Eastern sky. The idea had perhaps been suggested to Whistler in the color prints of Hiroshige and he had afterward found its reality in English twilights."[26] Just as night "creeps up" the sky from the east, that art of the night came from the Orient. But Van Dyke was intent on distinguishing the suggestion from its final realization by Whistler. The writings of the critic Sadakichi Hartmann, an American born to a German father and a Japanese mother, displayed the same ambivalence about Japan. According to Hartmann, the imprint made by Japanese art on Whistler's oeuvre was essential but invisible: "The 'Nocturnes' . . . are imbued with the very essence of Hiroshige's art without resembling Japanese art in the least. Never have the elements of Eastern and Western art been so originally united as in these poems of night and space."[27] That merging occurred organically, according to Van Dyke, who employed a botanical metaphor: "[Whistler] strove to graft the Eastern shoot upon the Western stock, to take what was best of Japanese art and blend it with French art, thus harmonizing the two traditions."[28] In all these models, the union between the Japanese and Western arts, though harmonious, always culminated in an equilibrium where the West held the advantage and remained the "stock."

The views of Hartmann, Caffin, and Van Dyke conformed to the idea that Eastern culture, by virtue of its highly decorative nature, formed an inferior entity whose dominant counterpart was the West. The Eastern propensity for formalism was regularly interpreted in terms of gender, a displacement characteristic of racist discourse. Critics emphasized the abstract, extremely formal character of Japanese painting and read it as a sign of its femininity, situated at the opposite extreme from Western pictorial realism and reality. Van Dyke quite simply excluded Japanese and Chinese paintings from his *Textbook of the History of Painting:* "The arts of China and Japan . . . are so positively decorative that they should be treated under the head of Decoration,"[29] an art considered minor and domestic. Ernest Fenollosa embraced the same gendered distinction in the preface to his collection of poems titled *East and West:* "Eastern culture, slowly elaborated, has held to ideals whose refinement seems markedly feminine. . . . Western culture, on the contrary, has held to ideals whose strength seems markedly masculine."[30] That was also the scheme Van Dyke followed in predicting the decline of Japanese art: "The art of old Japan . . . did not run into formalism and never became trite until recent years. Its ruin lies straight ahead of it if it shall abandon its traditions and continue to coquette with Occidental art."[31] Japanese art, suddenly brought into contact with Western culture, ran the risk of following an irresistible decline, both aesthetic and moral, and of finding itself reduced to a role close to prostitution. Van Dyke's remarks suggest the Darwinian image of a civilization unable to resist the Western influence, necessarily the loser in an environment dominated by the latter. Fenollosa, Hartmann, and Van Dyke, in reasserting the masculinity, strength, and Americanness of the nocturnes in spite of what they borrowed from Japanese art, reflected the ambivalence of the United States toward Japan: even while acknowledging the value of that nonwhite civilization and granting it almost the status of an equal, could not help but reaffirm its difference and inferiority.

IMPERIAL LIGHT IN THE DARK NIGHT OF PRIMITIVE PEOPLES: METAPHOR AT WORK

The nocturne's contradictions become most apparent when considered in the context of the pervasive use of the metaphor of light and darkness at the time. This metaphor was strikingly potent in the displays of international expositions from the late nineteenth century to World War I. At the World's Columbian Exposition in Chicago in 1893, the heart of the fair, a group of giant neoclassical buildings painted entirely white and flooded with artificial lighting, was renamed the "White City" upon its opening. At the world's fairs held subsequently in the United States (Buffalo in 1901, St. Louis in 1904, San Francisco in 1915), light—and especially electric light—played a fundamental role in focusing attention on the architecture, even while imposing a series of conventional symbolic interpretations. In these nerve centers of imperialism, the use of artificial light offered a way to combine the demonstration of technological and commercial superiority with the assertion of political and cultural preeminence. The model that the American world's fairs were seeking to surpass was Paris, which in 1889 had capitalized on the conflation of light and Enlightenment: the organizers of the Exposition Universelle, which celebrated the centennial of the French Revolution, orchestrated a festival of light that embraced a highly metaphorical rhetoric. That rhetoric co-opted the discourse of the Enlightenment, in particular the notions of progress and freedom, to promote an imperialist ideology. At the foot of the Eiffel Tower, Jules Coutan's *Fountain of Progress,* one of the most remarked-upon attractions at the exposition, depicted an advancing ship laden with allegorical figures in an extravagant spectacle of spraying water animated by colored lights. Four years later, Chicago went a step further, with an output of electric light on an unprecedented scale. Every evening, it produced ten times as much artificial light as the Exposition Universelle de Paris.[32] From the flame of the Statue of Liberty to the allegorical figures powered by electricity that adorned the fairgrounds, the same image circulated: light, especially electric light, the emblem of technological modernity, symbolized the political progress which nations such as France and the United States considered their duty to bear to the least "enlightened" peoples. The increased output of artificial lighting on display at American fairs made visible the dynamic shift from the Enlightenment to imperial conquest. Light was to spread and spare no region of the globe. In particular, the figure of the light beam piercing the night represented this modern Enlightenment conquering the world. It appeared recurrently in literature, with titles such as *China under Searchlight* and *Searchlight on the Panama Canal, or America's Greatest Enterprise,*[33] and also in visual culture, with images in fields ranging from advertising to caricature to painting.

The association between light and Enlightenment had its dark counterpart, which was just as politically determined. The analogy between white Western civilization and light was correlated with its opposite, the equation between nonwhites and darkness. The racial metaphor transposed ethnic differences, marked visually by degree of skin pigmentation, onto an opposition between night and day. Examples abound in Western culture, from the late nineteenth to the early twentieth century, of that metaphorical use of light and darkness to address questions of racial difference. The metaphor constituted the guiding thread of Joseph Conrad's *Heart of Darkness* and reappeared, laden with biblical connotations, in Rudyard Kipling's poem about the "white man's burden": "Take up the White Man's burden / And reap his old reward / . . . The cry of hosts ye humour /(Ah, slowly!) toward the light: / 'Why brought he us from bondage, / Our loved Egyptian night?'"[34] Countless examples of the same metaphor can be found in American culture, from the attraction called "Darkest Africa" at the Pan-American Exposition of Buffalo in 1901 showing African villages "in their primitive state"[35] to the book *Benighted Mexico,* published in 1916 by Randolph Wellford Smith, who describes a country in such a crisis that "either the faces of its people must be turned to the sun or else they must forever pass over into the Land of Shadow."[36]

Winslow Homer's *Searchlight:* Questioning American Imperialism

While the racist metaphor of light and darkness was one of the most hackneyed images circulating at the time, nocturne artists raised a discordant voice in that otherwise almost unanimous concert, adopting a nostalgic and ambivalent attitude. Their approach stood in contrast to an optimistic imperialist discourse, which without qualms associated colonial conquest with the supposedly universal and humanistic values of the Enlightenment. The nocturnal landscape, viewed within that context, provides a different perspective on the

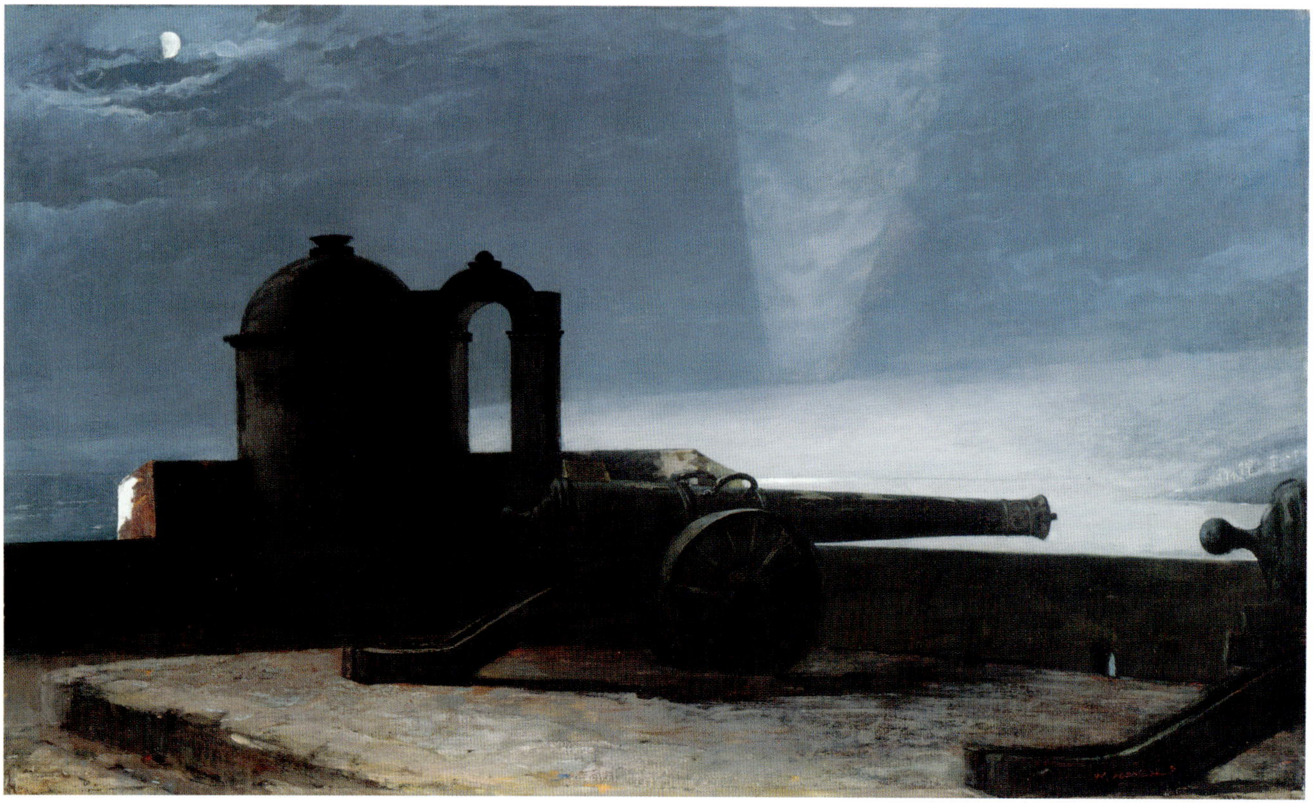

FIG. 65. Winslow Homer, *Searchlight on Harbor Entrance, Santiago de Cuba,* 1901. Oil on canvas, 77.5 × 128.3 cm (30 ½ × 50 ½ in.). Metropolitan Museum of Art, Gift of George A. Hearn, 1906 (06.1282).

American imperialist venture. Rather than show civilized light flooding into the conquered lands, it inverted the familiar rhetoric of bright and dark. The example of Winslow Homer's *Searchlight on Harbor Entrance, Santiago de Cuba* (fig. 65) illustrates the confusions, contradictions, and ambiguities between the image and its metaphorical import that the night landscape allowed artists to develop.

First, the painting offers a good example of the neutrality imputed to the nocturne. It was interpreted by critics as a work "created out of nothing"[37] and "precious near . . . a great affair of form, light, and air."[38] "The picture is grandly impressive. How is this impressiveness secured? It can be by nothing but composition, and by composition at its simplest. The perfect balancing of two or three masses, the perfect coordination of a few straight lines and a few segments of circles, and the thing is done—a great picture is created out of nothing and with almost no aid from any other element of the art of painting than this all important one of design."[39] In other words, *Searchlight* was considered an extremely formal work, abstracted from its material and historical context. Nonetheless, the painting retraces a crucial episode of the Spanish-American War of 1898–1901, namely, the American fleet's blockade of the port of Santiago. Night after night for several months, American cruisers kept the Spanish fleet trapped in the harbor with the aid of powerful electric searchlights trained on the harbor entrance.[40] *Searchlight* evokes the spectacle of lights sweeping the sky, observed from inside the harbor in El Morro, a fortress in Spanish hands at the time. But though the center of the canvas is occupied by large beams of electric light, their origin remains invisible. Of the American warships stationed offshore, the beholder, confined within the fortress's shadow, sees only the brightness they project against the cloudy sky. That distance from the electric lights and the attention given to the melancholic setting of the fallen Spanish colonial empire, along with the spare composition and the dark tones of the nocturne, often resulted in the painting being interpreted as a meditative work, at a remove from the historical event. A monograph on Homer, for example, interpreted it as a "unique and sobering view" of the war, one that was "content to show the conflict in the most understated manner." The view of El Morro stands apart from its geographical and historical reality, becoming a sort of inner vision: *Searchlight*, if we are to believe the author, "leaves almost everything to the viewer's imagination."[41] This interpretation was combined with a formalist discourse that tended to consider the work as evidence of the artist's evolution toward a modernist style. One of Homer's biographers compared the composition of the painting to Mondrian's oeuvre, and the art historian Nicolai Cikovsky Jr. went so far as to link the painting to "Picasso's erotic surrealist constructions."[42] That formal reading of *Searchlight* would profit from being incorporated into an analysis that takes into consideration the tensions between surface and depth, between the painting's overt sobriety and its ideological content. *Searchlight* does stand at a remove from the historical event, but in spite of everything the painting is pervaded by the political questions that were rife during that era. And though *Searchlight* replies to these questions with a circumspect silence, it is the responsibility of art historians to decipher the meaning of the shadows cast in the painting and to refuse to overlook the work's deliberate ambiguity.

Searchlight in the Context of Its Visual Culture: Politics of the Image and Racial Stereotypes

Although *Searchlight* does no more than allude to the Spanish-American War, by naming the strategic site of Santiago harbor and the technology used by the American fleet, the artist contradicted the idea that it was a painting detached from its historical moment. The inclusion, albeit indirect, of electric lights plays an important role in underlining the painting's historical dimension. As in *Summer Night*, the relation to electric technology is paradoxical: although, in a certain sense, electricity constitutes the raw material for the painting, Homer made it a diffuse, atmospheric element, whose source remains concealed. A distant half-moon, relegated to the margins of the painting, underscores the magnitude of the change: its glow, dimmed by the electric light, has become as obsolete as the fortress's antique cannons and turrets. And *Searchlight*, in addition to evoking the very recent history of the Spanish-American War, makes reference to events immediately contemporary to it. In 1901 Admiral Winfield Scott Schley and Admiral William T. Sampson appeared before a military tribunal charged with determining which of the two men was to be credited with the American victory against the Spanish fleet in Santiago de Cuba in 1898. The controversy kept the American public riveted throughout the year: it regularly made the headlines, spurred a series of publications on the war, and was even immortalized in one of the first films by Edison Studios.[43] Homer, in seizing on the subject at that precise moment, clearly set out to join the debate.

More generally, *Searchlight* appeared at a time when the link between the news event and its visual representation was conceived in political and strategic terms. The Spanish-American War was waged first by the press and the image. It served as a springboard for the newspaper magnate William Randolph Hearst, whose *New York World* introduced an innovative journalistic style at that time. "Yellow journalism," as it was called, frequently resorted to sensational photographs and illustrations.[44] A famous anecdote about Hearst reveals he had some awareness of how to manipulate public opinion through the image. He supposedly exclaimed to the illustrator Frederic Remington, sent to Cuba with a group of reporters: "You furnish the pictures and I'll furnish the war."[45] Homer's painting thus belongs to a context in which political and military events were, to an ever greater degree, intimately connected to their construction by the media.

Within that web of visual meanings, night supplied the central motif of a political and social discourse as implicit as it was omnipresent. In addition to the immediate historical context of *Searchlight*, that of technological development and the American imperialist venture, there was a preoccupation with race, transposed through images into a contrast between darkness and light. The question of ethnic difference, though not in the foreground of the Spanish-American War, did play an essential role, in the first place within the ranks of the U.S. army. African American troops had only recently been allowed to bear arms. This change sparked heated debates and created tensions at military bases in the South, where African American soldiers awaited transfer to Cuba with the rest of the U.S. troops.[46] The historian Amy Kaplan has shown that ethnic difference formed a link between the Spanish-American War and looming racial questions related to American domestic policy: "The representation of empire at the turn of the century could function both as an external catalyst and as a medium for resolution of domestic racial conflict."[47]

Kaplan comments in particular on another central and controversial episode of the Spanish-American War, the Battle of San Juan Hill, in which race became a major ideological issue. As in the Battle of Santiago, the question was who had truly contributed to the victory. Historians now agree that the role of the 24th and 25th infantry regiments, composed of African Americans, was to a great extent minimized in favor of that of the Rough Riders, the white battalion commanded by Theodore Roosevelt.

Kaplan has demonstrated that representations of the Spanish-American War emphasized a strict division of labor along racial lines, contrasting whites, seen as agents in the "liberation" of Cuba, and nonwhites, who were portrayed as its passive, cowardly, and lazy beneficiaries. The tensions between black and white Americans were thus displaced and extended to the imperialist venture, and were conveyed in great part through the imagery relating to it. For example, Theodore Roosevelt, in his account of the conflict, acknowledged the courage of African American soldiers but observed that they were completely disoriented when their white officers were killed: "No troops could have behaved better than the colored soldiers had behaved so far; but they are, of course, peculiarly dependent upon their white officers."[48] He suggested several times that the Cubans refused to fight: "General Castillo promised Young the aid of eight hundred Cubans. . . . This promised Cuban aid did not, however, materialize, the Cubans, who had been beaten back by the Spaniards the day before, not appearing on the firing-line until the fight was over."[49] The Rough Riders regiment, half of it made up of young men from the major east coast universities, the other half of men from the West (cowboys, gold prospectors, and hunters), also included a few Indians. Roosevelt, who made mention of the recent Indian Wars, took care to note that the men he had enlisted in his regiment were from the highest echelons of their tribe. He also minimized ethnic difference and emphasized the integration of the Indian soldiers into white civilization. For example, he related an episode in which one of the Indians had asked the barber to cut off his hair, saying: "Don't want to wear my hair long like a wild Indian when I'm in civilized warfare."[50] In that sense, the Spanish-American War provided a prototype for the many variants of the relations between American whites and nonwhites: Indians were assimilated into the corps; Cubans were considered the unworthy beneficiaries of the civilizing mission; and African Americans remained inexorably marginalized. Yet these differences, apparent in Roosevelt's text, had a tendency to become blurred in the visual order, where nonwhites performed interchangeable roles. A journalist from the *New York Times* explained to his readers that in Cuba, blacks, Creoles, quadroons, and octoroons coexisted without distinction in every class of society: "In benighted Cuba the shade of a man has never been greatly considered, and one finds dusky Othellos in every walk of life. . . . The color line has never been thought of, for the reason that African blood may be found, in greater or less degree, in some of the richest and influential families of the island."[51] But from the Americans' point of view, the colonial Other was an individual whose political, intellectual, and moral backwardness could be conveyed visually by a generalized blackness. Amy Kaplan comments on several examples from visual culture—films and photographs in particular—that indiscriminately used various nonwhite types to represent, depending on the case, Filipinos, Cubans, and even Spaniards.[52] Although commentators of the time were aware of the existence of real ethnic variations, visual relationships became polarized around the two categories—whites and nonwhites—in an often simplistic contrast, with nonwhites relegated to an indeterminate darkness.

The simple setting of *Searchlight* does not allude directly to the racist violence of colonization. But if Homer's painting is considered within the mass of images that formed the everyday visual environment at the dawn of the twentieth century, the metaphor of night takes on a more evident signification. An advertising card for the Fairbank Company dating to 1899, obviously also inspired by the nocturnal blockade of Santiago, displays striking similarities to *Searchlight* (fig. 66). The visual rhetoric, thematizing the American ship's beam of light, is very close to that used by Homer. In a nocturnal landscape dominated by dark blue tones, the searchlight of a military ship traverses almost the entire length of the image. In the distance, the moon shines on an American flag conveniently placed in its halo of clouds. The text printed on the back contains formulations that speak volumes. Under the name "FAIRY SOAP" (in addition to its fanciful meaning, the name reactivates a series of positive connotations associated with the word "fair," which suggests justice, beauty, purity, and clarity, as well as light complexion), the words "PURE—WHITE—FLOATING" are inscribed, followed by a text vaunting the soap's white color as a sign of its purity and pointing out that it contains "no coloring matter." On the front, the inscription in gold letters of "FAIRY SOAP" in the beam of the ship's electric searchlight associates the soap and its purity with the visible whiteness produced by electric technology and emitted by the U.S. Navy. Physical cleanliness, military might, and technological mastery are thus summed up visually by light and whiteness.

The ethnic dimension of that whiteness remained tacit in this advertisement, but many other examples formulated it explicitly. Fairbank's was not the only brand of soap to refer to U.S. foreign policy in its advertising.[53] Sapolio, for example, repeated the amalgam of cleanliness and light in an advertisement that depicts Columbia, an allegorical figure for the United States, dressed in white and brandishing a bar of soap placed over a globe of the world (fig. 67). Rays of light emanate from the soap, located directly above the map of the United States: they reach out to touch Cuba, Puerto Rico, and the Philippines, simultaneously dispersing the clouds that cover the southern hemisphere. The text declares that American might will travel "to darker lands beyond the seas and light them with SAPOLIO." Electric lights are here associated with the Enlightenment: Columbia's Phrygian cap, recalling the struggle for emancipation from slavery, and the antique draping of her gown, which evokes the Statue of Liberty (since 1886 the statue had dominated the entrance to New York harbor), confirm that "the use of Sapolio is a distinguishing mark of enlightened people." The Pears Company, for its part, appropriated the figure of Admiral George Dewey, elevated to the rank of national hero after the victory of Manila Bay in 1898 (fig. 68), and whose triumph was immediately expressed

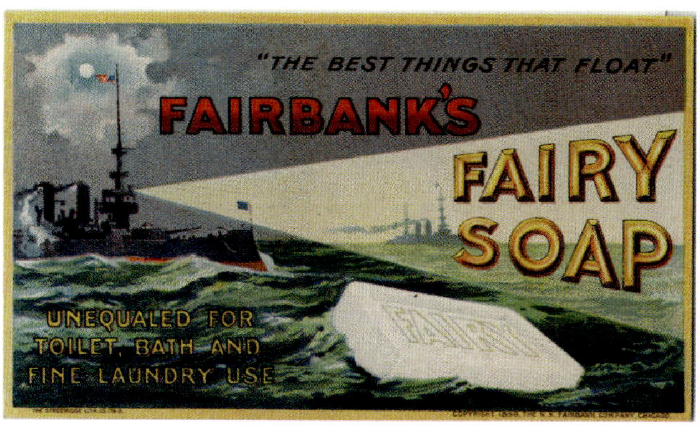

"THE BEST THINGS THAT FLOAT"
FAIRBANK'S
FAIRY SOAP
UNEQUALED FOR TOILET, BATH AND FINE LAUNDRY USE

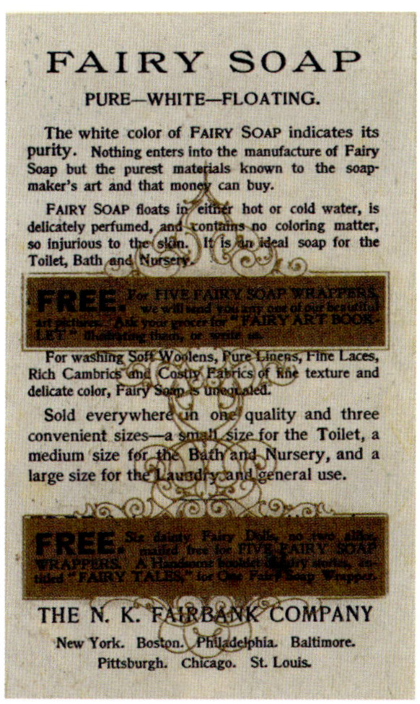

FAIRY SOAP
PURE—WHITE—FLOATING.
The white color of FAIRY SOAP indicates its purity. Nothing enters into the manufacture of Fairy Soap but the purest materials known to the soap-maker's art and that money can buy.
FAIRY SOAP floats in either hot or cold water, is delicately perfumed, and contains no coloring matter, so injurious to the skin. It is an ideal soap for the Toilet, Bath and Nursery.
For washing Soft Woolens, Pure Linens, Fine Laces, Rich Cambrics and Costly Fabrics of fine texture and delicate color, Fairy Soap is unequaled.
Sold everywhere in one quality and three convenient sizes—a small size for the Toilet, a medium size for the Bath and Nursery, and a large size for the Laundry and general use.
THE N. K. FAIRBANK COMPANY
New York. Boston. Philadelphia. Baltimore.
Pittsburgh. Chicago. St. Louis.

FIG. 66. "'The Best Things that Float': Fairbank's Fairy Soap," c. 1898. Advertising card, 9 × 15 cm (3½ × 5⅞ in.). Warshaw Collection of Business Americana, Archives Center, National Museum of American History, Smithsonian Institution, Washington, D.C.

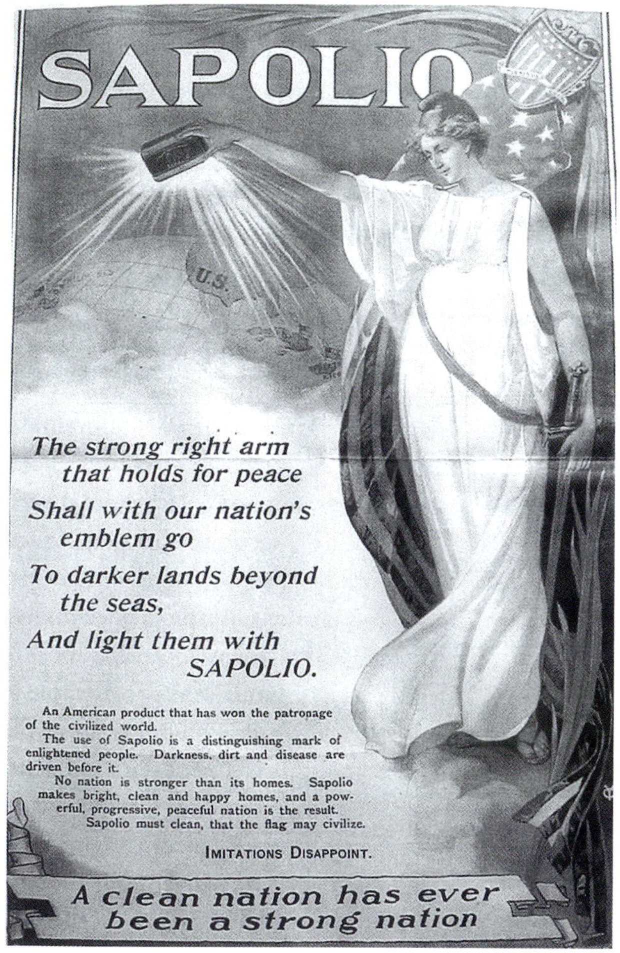

SAPOLIO
U.S.
The strong right arm
that holds for peace
Shall with our nation's
emblem go
To darker lands beyond
the seas,
And light them with
SAPOLIO.
An American product that has won the patronage of the civilized world.
The use of Sapolio is a distinguishing mark of enlightened people. Darkness, dirt and disease are driven before it.
No nation is stronger than its homes. Sapolio makes bright, clean and happy homes, and a powerful, progressive, peaceful nation is the result.
Sapolio must clean, that the flag may civilize.
IMITATIONS DISAPPOINT.
A clean nation has ever
been a strong nation

FIG. 67. Sapolio, "A Clean Nation Has Ever Been a Strong Nation," *Ladies' Home Journal* 16, no. 8, July 1899.

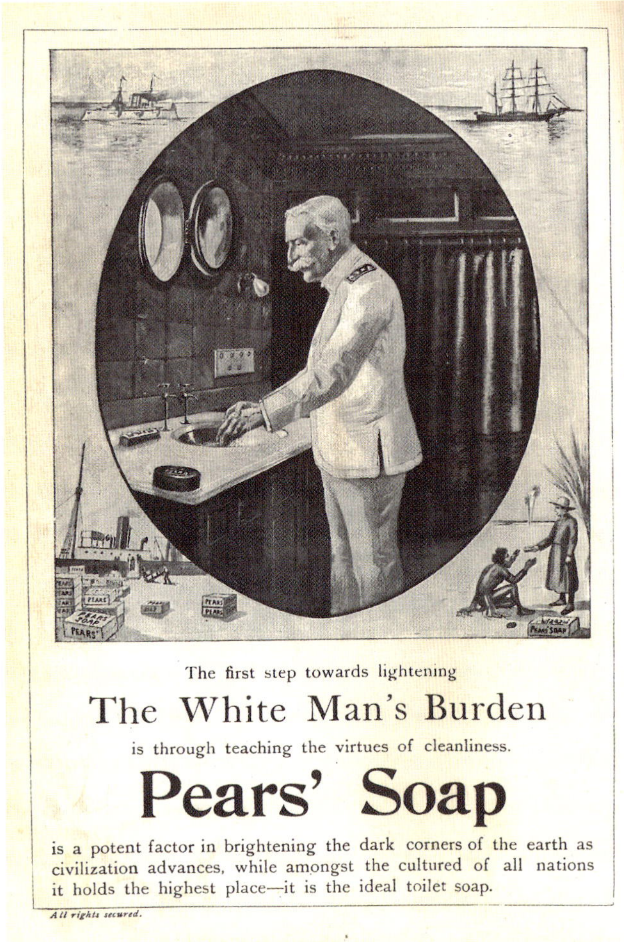
The first step towards lightening
The White Man's Burden
is through teaching the virtues of cleanliness.
Pears' Soap
is a potent factor in brightening the dark corners of the earth as civilization advances, while amongst the cultured of all nations it holds the highest place—it is the ideal toilet soap.
All rights secured.

FIG. 68. Pears Soap, "The White Man's Burden," *McClure's Magazine* October 12, 1899.

in terms of light. His return to New York after the Battle of Manila Bay was celebrated with an unprecedented illuminated display: for two days, an electric sign suspended from the Brooklyn Bridge spelled out the words "Welcome Dewey," as an array of spotlights, similar to the searchlights on military cruisers, formed an arc of light above the East River.[54] In the Pears illustration, Dewey, dressed in a uniform as white as his hair and mustache, is washing his hands in what is evidently a ship's cabin. At each of the four corners of the image, narrative vignettes complement the portrait: at the top, a merchant ship serves as a pendant to the military vessel, while, below, a white man dressed as a missionary offers the supposedly civilizing soap to a "native" seated at his feet. Under the central medallion, the words "white man's burden" stand out in imposing characters. The body of the text explains how Pears will be able to "brighten" (in the dual sense of "lighten" and "enlighten") the "dark corners of the earth as civilization advances."[55] These three illustrations, like Homer's painting, are striking for their almost total omission of the peoples about to fall under the United States' rule. The scenes depicted are deserted, or they feature white people, whom the beholder is encouraged to understand as ideal figures of whiteness. The only nonwhite presence is reduced to a minuscule silhouette in the lower right-hand corner of the Pears illustration, made even smaller by his position vis-à-vis the colonizer. The analogy between whiteness of skin and intellectual, military, and moral superiority, which the advertisements attempt to establish, cannot be sustained, however, unless that lightness is understood in opposition to darkness, which can only be conceived as a symbol for the ethnic Other. The nonwhite presence, both invisible and conspicuous, acts as a necessary negation, an indispensable foil, against which the white light shines. Nocturnal imagery thus entails a paradox: darkness serves to obscure the presence of the Other, even while granting it a metaphorical visibility. Critics who commented on the "strange impressiveness" of Homer's *Searchlight* may have perceived this tension.[56]

Considered against this dark background, electric technology acquired a different dimension: more than a factor of military might, it became the symbolic instrument of racist violence. Just as the territories coveted by the imperial powers were penetrated through the use of technology, electric light was also projected onto the bodies of the inhabitants, literally subjected to the power of the electric light. A souvenir book published for the Pan-American Exposition in Buffalo alternates between nocturnal views of the lights at the fair—directly powered by nearby Niagara Falls—and humorous illustrations featuring the various participants at the exposition. The ethnographic sections hold a prominent place, as they did at the fair itself, and further accentuate the intimate relationship between technical progress and imperialist conquest. The books published for the exposition, for example, revel in imagining the technological backwardness of the Filipinos, armed with wooden cannons, or the bewilderment of a "native" at the "Darkest Africa" attraction, stunned and blinded by the beam of an electric light.[57] Nonwhites, incompetent when confronted with technology, were necessarily subjugated by it. Electricity, the "white" weapon par excellence, was so intimately linked to the pale skin of those who had mastered it that, after the discovery of X-rays, some speculated

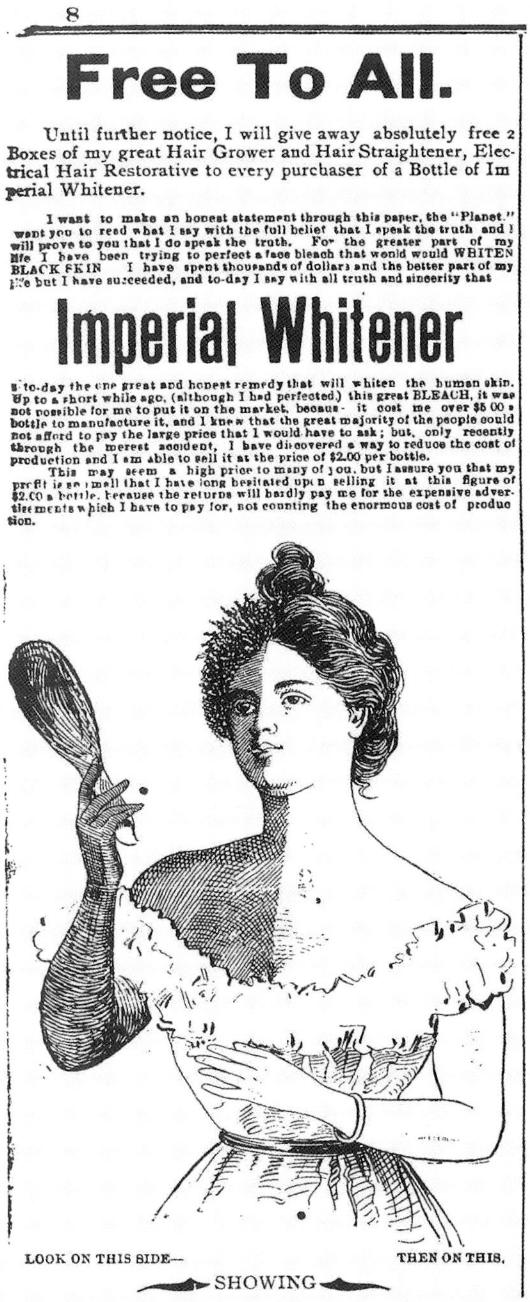

FIG. 69. "Imperial Whitener," *Richmond Planet*, June 9, 1900.

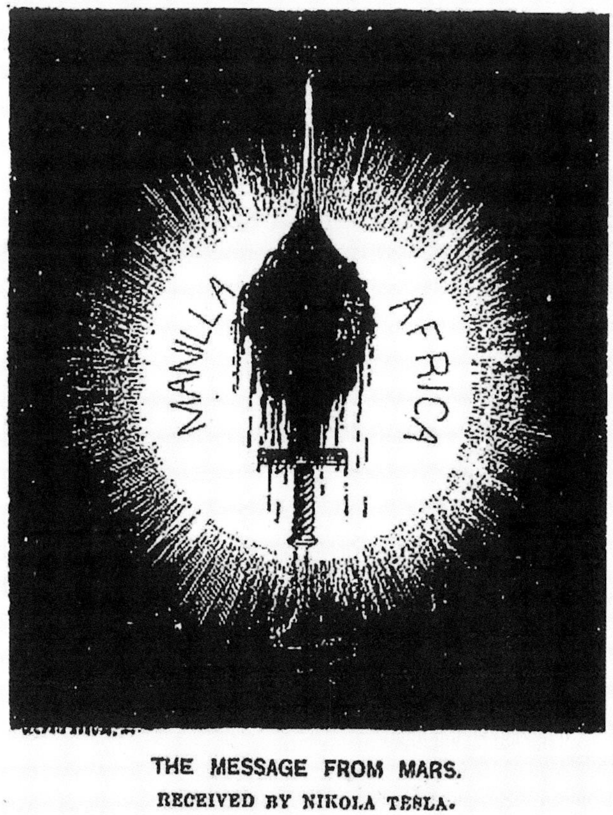

FIG. 70. "The Message from Mars Received by Nikola Tesla," *Life* 37, no. 955, February 17, 1901.

that electric technology could also whiten black skin.[58] Electricity and cosmetics also conspired under the sign of empire in advertisements such as the notice for the "Imperial Whitener," addressed to the female black readers of the *Richmond Planet* (fig. 69). One caricature published in *Life* magazine the same year Homer painted *Searchlight*, however, denounced the violence latent within these commercial and propaganda images. Called "The Message from Mars," the image works on two levels: technological or scientific research and imperialist conquest (fig. 70). The illustration shows a device emitting an intense light, which the caricaturist says was received by Nikola Tesla, famous both for his electric inventions and for his experiments in extraterrestrial communication. The "message from Mars" received by that device turns out to be more martial than Martian, however. On either side of the circle of electric light, the words "Manilla" and "Africa" are inscribed. It quickly becomes clear that the luminous focal point is composed of what is evidently a severed head stuck on a saber and from which the blood is still dripping. Coiled around the weapon's handle is a rope that, in an escalation of symbolic violence, brings to mind the sadly familiar ropes from which victims of lynching in the American South were hanged. The caricature radically reverses the rhetoric of shadow and light so often used by the defenders of imperialism. It suggests that the white light of technological progress, which the United States sought to dispense to the distant lands of Africa and the Philippines, emerges in reality from the heart of darkness.

Searchlight in Context

Where did Winslow Homer stand in relation to this visual context? To what extent did *Searchlight* adopt the racist metaphor of shadow and light? What position did Homer occupy within the discourse of his time on ethnic relationships? Although *Searchlight* plays on the same contrasts as those used in racist imagery, that play is complex and ambiguous. As Richard J. Powell notes, though Homer's "early links to the popular press certainly made him vulnerable to an undiscerning and mundane notion of Afro-Americans," he was one of the rare American artists who knew how to "paint blacks sympathetically."[59] Two years before *Searchlight,* he had painted *The Gulf Stream,* whose action is also set in the Caribbean Sea, but this time at noon (fig. 71). The painting depicts a black sailor alone in a small boat threatened by a school of sharks, in what seems to be a direct reference to a classic work of American art, John Singleton Copley's *Watson and the Shark.*[60] But though Homer chose a black hero for this painterly tour de force, the artist refused to give an epic interpretation to it. When his art dealer Roland Knoedler relayed to him questions from female visitors regarding the sailor's fate, Homer rejected any narrative explanation: "I regret very much that I have painted a picture that requires any description. The subject of this picture is comprised in its title and I will refer these inquisitive schoolma'ams to Lieut. Maury. . . . The boat and sharks are outside matters of very little consequence. They have been blown out to sea by a hurricane. You can tell these ladies that the unfortunate Negro who is now so dazed and parboiled,

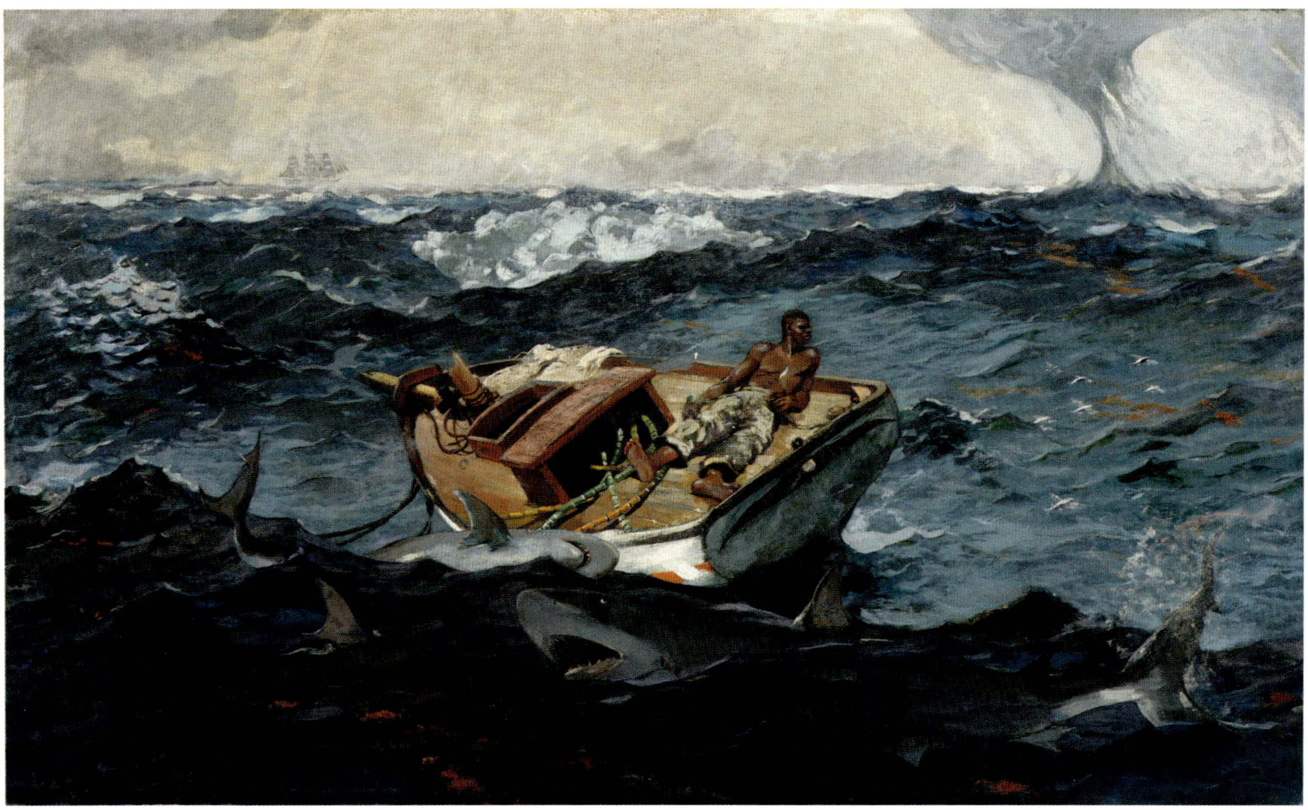

FIG. 71. Winslow Homer, *The Gulf Stream,* 1899. Oil on canvas, 71.4 × 124.8 cm (28 1/8 × 49 1/8 in.). Metropolitan Museum of Art, Catharine Lorillard Wolfe Collection, Wolfe Fund, 1906 (06.1234).

will be rescued and returned to his friends and home, and ever after live happily."[61] The artist's ideologically vague stance seems to be reflected in the equivocation that comes through in *Searchlight.* This position was strategic, in both the physical and ideological senses of the word. The painting's isolated point of view at the top of El Morro is extremely ambiguous, given that it is the perspective of the Spanish enemy. Homer, who reused a sketch for this composition he had made during his visit to the fort a few years before the conflict, likely chose that point of view for reasons both practical and aesthetic. But a second drawing, done in 1898, also places the painter and his beholder on the fortress side. In a letter sent to his brother Charles, Homer evoked in a humorous vein the anxieties of his neighbors and family members at Prout's Neck in Maine (fig. 72). The explosion of a U.S. Army ship—the USS *Maine,* in Santiago harbor—the first event in the escalation of the conflict, gave rise to all sorts of speculation about the impact of the war in the United States. Homer mentioned one of these rumors, namely, that an army battery had been set up in Prout's Neck. The illustration shows his neighbor Mrs. Putnam leaning out of the window of her house, protesting the presence of a piece of artillery pointed toward the ocean. Homer, who was fond of puns, was no doubt alluding to Cannon Rock, a geological curiosity on the shore just at the foot of the Putnams' house. But the sketch also evokes the obsolete cannons of El Morro. The illustration points to a convergence between the local and the global, both by the context to which it refers and by its formal similarities to *Searchlight.* A ship whose presence on the horizon is marked not by a beam of electric light, but by a trail of steam, brings to mind the invisible cruisers of *Searchlight.* In both cases, Homer placed himself as well as his beholder in a helpless position, far from the naval force undertaking that conquest—a warship disappearing on the horizon or concealed in the darkness, beyond the reach of the territory being conquered. The latter, invisible in the drawing of 1898, is barely discernible in *Searchlight.* The Cuban coast is reduced to a remote and marginal detail, yet starkly illuminated by the electric beam of the American ship (see fig. 65). The palm trees, under the pale electric light, look like a photo negative of the landscape. These quasi-human forms standing along the bank appear as a ghostly reminder of those whose presence has been concealed. They are, as it were, the luminous shadows of the island's residents. In

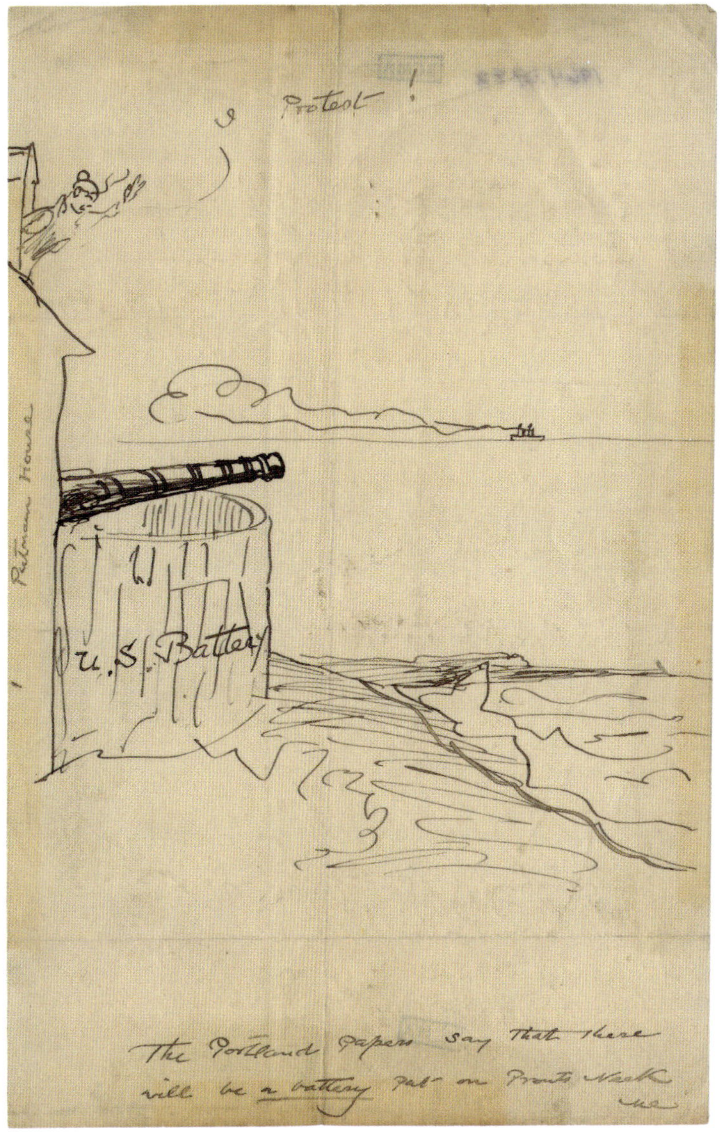

FIG. 72. Winslow Homer, *I Protest/Putnam House/The Portland papers say that there will be a battery put on Prout's Neck Maine,* 1898. Ink on paper, 22.5 × 14.1 cm (8 7/8 × 5 9/16 in.). Bowdoin College Museum of Art, Brunswick, Maine.

the foreground, an even more striking detail underlines that whitening of the landscape: the rays of light hit the outer wall of the fortress so hard that they visually whitewash it. Under the artist's brush, as in the searchlight of the American cruisers, "the Moor's fort" (for that is how "Castillo del Morro" could be translated) vanishes into whiteness.

PERVASIVE DARKNESS AND THE DECLINE OF THE EMPIRE

Incidentally, yet significantly, the name of the fortress, which is not included in the title of the painting, resurfaced in news reports after the second front of the Spanish-American War opened in the Philippines. I have already mentioned several examples of images that compared or associated Cuba and the Philippines, but I might point out as well the differences in status between the two conflicts. Although the United States wanted to transpose to the Philippines the Cuban model of a "splendid little war,"[62] and though Dewey's 1898 victory in Manila allowed the government to hope that, once again, it could wage a relatively quick fight—simplistically advertised as a battle in the name of freedom—the reality they encountered on the ground was completely different. The conflict in the Philippines very quickly bogged down. Once they had rid themselves of the Spaniards, the Filipinos led by General Emilio Aguinaldo turned against the Americans, organizing a fierce guerilla war against that new colonial occupation. The expansion of the Spanish-American War to the Philippines and the inglorious turn it took there contributed toward discrediting the emancipatory and humanist claims of the United States. Rather than bring the light of civilization and freedom to the Philippines, the Americans were drawn into a benighted colonialism.

In a way, the Filipino conflict was an extension of the conquest of Cuba, but it also uncovered the contradictions of American imperialism. Homer's El Morro alluded indirectly to that expansion of the conflict, by repeating the Spanish term that was used as a generic designation for nonwhites throughout Spain's overseas empire. In the Philippines, "Moro" designated more specifically Muslim tribes living on the Sulu and Mindanao islands, which had remained relatively independent from Spanish colonial authority. From 1902 on, these islands became some of the most solid bastions of the resistance. At the time Homer was painting *Searchlight,* however, they simply sparked a rather alarmed curiosity on the part of the American press:[63] "It is a queer and picturesque addition that has thus been made to our domains. The people are Musulmans and used to be pirates by occupation. Their swarthy features, bright-colored and fantastic costumes, primitive farming implements, strange manners, customs and rites, and whatever else seems odd to us, will be eagerly described and depicted, now that the Twenty-third Infantry is on the spot, and that the Islands are practically open to us."[64] An article in the *St. Louis Republic* reported the barbaric customs of this polygamous people who practiced human sacrifice, concluding with a few comic episodes in which individual Moros manifested surprise at American inventions, from the Colt revolver to electric lights to the telephone: "A few days ago one of our gunboats used its searchlight, sending long rays of electricity into one of the villages on the shore and lighting up the town. The next day a delegation was sent out to the ship asking that the people be permitted to submit, for they could not pretend to fight people who could turn night into day."[65] Yet these colorful descriptions raised questions that, in disturbing ways, echoed the history of ethnic relations within the United States proper. Indeed, the exotic customs of the Moros caused a certain uneasiness in Washington. In particular, a long debate ensued about slavery, which was still practiced by the Moros:[66] Was it the United States' responsibility to put an end to it? Or was slavery as practiced by a people considered half-civilized without importance? "We might, indeed, end the business at once by declaring the Moro slaves free, after the fashion of President Lincoln's emancipation proclamation, were it not that such a proclamation has never moved Mohammedan slaveholders elsewhere," explained Henry O. Dwight, a Civil War hero and missionary in Turkey.[67] In reality, the U.S. troops were apparently having too much trouble dealing with Aguinaldo's rebellion to concern themselves with justice and emancipation. Dwight used the argument of the Moros' irremediable religious fanaticism to justify the United States' inaction on that front: "Wherever it is found that Asiatic customs remain obstinately insoluble in the presence of the strong solvent of contact with Western civilization, we may be pretty sure that the great prophet of Mecca may be thanked for it."[68] (It is noteworthy that here again, Dwight envisages Western civilization as a cleaning—dissolving—agent.) Although some members of the public encouraged President William McKinley to keep his word and extend the "benefits of civilization" to the Filipinos, the U.S. administration confined itself to establishing an accord with the sultan of the Sulus that allowed him to continue governing his people, in exchange for his acknowledgment of U.S. sovereignty. That retreat says a great deal about the sincerity of U.S. humanist claims abroad. Slavery, barbaric among white people, became a secondary concern when practiced by nonwhites: in the end, the Moros were not considered civilized enough to receive all the benefits of civilization. Dwight concluded his article with a surprising proposal, which this time linked the Moros to the American Indians and renounced without compunction any possibility of "progress": "The Moros are a people apart, not as yet amenable to influences which will weigh with other inhabitants of the Philippines. Let them be treated as such. Let the Sulu Islands be classed in the same category as our Indian reservations, to be surrounded by a wall of steel for the safety of neighboring peoples, but to be managed internally by their own chiefs under existing laws and usages."[69] The news stories about the Moros are, of course, just an example among many other anecdotes and reports increasingly challenging their country's foreign ventures. The choice of point of view adopted in *Searchlight* also reflects this contradiction: Homer placed himself and his American beholders on the side of the Spanish colonizers' benightedness, which the American press regularly denounced, but of which the United States was also guilty.[70] Through that reversal of perspective, *Searchlight* seems to place in doubt the "Enlightenment" of American imperialism. Colonizers and colonized are indistinguishable in the symbolic darkness, and the civilizing light of the American searchlights crossing the Cuban sky compared to the clearly drawn beams of the Fairbank and Sapolio ads seems very hazy.

Although Homer's commentators confined themselves to reading the architectural landscape of *Searchlight* in formal terms, the attention drawn to the vestiges of the Spanish empire can be interpreted in a more political sense. JoAnne Mancini analyzes the interest taken in Spanish colonial architecture in the Philippines, a favorite subject for postcard manufacturers. She underlines the comparison implicitly made between these images and the relics of Spanish architecture in California and New Mexico, and demonstrates that such imagery, in emphasizing these comparable landmarks, established a continuity between geographically separate territories.[71] "Old Spanish empire" postcards thus invented a visual code that allowed the American public to conceive of the new territorial acquisitions as a coherent whole. Although Mancini focuses on the case of the Philippines, the elements that united the architecture of the California missions and that of the Spanish colonial buildings in the Philippines could also be found in Cuba, especially at El Morro. A journalist's enchanted description for *Outlook* magazine of the picturesque architecture of a Spanish Filipino fortress, viewed in the light of the rising sun, is thus somewhat reminiscent of the old-fashioned charm of the turrets of *Searchlight:* "Backed by this stage-like setting, at the very footlights, as it were, stood the romantic little citadel which Arolas raised against the warring Moros. Its white walls, pierced and turreted as in the days of mediaeval Spain, ran out into the placid waters of the open harbor, and in the center a heavy iron gate opened upon a white stone pier, cross-shaped at the end, and having on one arm a small castellated blockhouse."[72] Homer, in painting El Morro in Santiago de Cuba, thus created a picture that borrowed from that generic language and was part of a network of images circulating seamlessly from one geographical zone to another. This suggests that the ideological scope of the painting might extend beyond Cuba to embrace the entire American empire.

This fascination with the vestiges of a fallen empire displayed by Homer, his critics, and the American public (as consumers of colonial postcards) bears witness to a certain equivocation. In choosing the point of view of the former Spanish colonizer, in shrouding the painting in darkness, and in reducing electric power to the depiction of its effects on the landscape, Homer mitigated the optimistic, unilateral vision conveyed by the imagery of American progress enlightening the globe. Although his critics ordinarily read *Searchlight* as a nostalgic contemplation, that nostalgia must be revisited from a historical standpoint. It must be considered a possible meditation on the future of American imperial power, assessed in terms of the Spanish empire, whose successor it aspired to be. Seen from that angle, *Searchlight* may suggest that the United States, in embarking on the path of imperialism, also ran the risk of becoming the new upholders of the moral darkness for which the Spanish authorities were reproached.

Even before the Cuban conflict, the 1893 Columbian Exposition in Chicago formulated with naive confidence the idea that the nascent American empire was taking up the mantle of the former Spanish empire. A good part of its imagery centered on Christopher Columbus and Columbia. The organizers, to mark the four hundredth anniversary of Columbus's discovery of the American continent, ordered exact replicas made of the Convent of La Rábida, where the navigator had planned his journey, and of his expedition's three caravels.[73] Infanta Eulalia of Spain was invited for the occasion. After stopping in Cuba, she made a controversial appearance in Chicago, where the press took offense when representatives of American democracy bowed down to that inheritor of a reactionary regime.[74] The continuity, declared with some discomfort in 1893, turned to open conflict in 1898, when the United States supplanted Spain as the colonial power in Cuba and Puerto Rico, and a year later in the Philippines. The images of Spanish relics assumed a new significance at the time: the United States, in occupying the ruins of the fallen Spanish empire, symbolically imposed its authority over the territory. Mancini points out the violence of the transition, which sometimes entailed a destructive appropriation of the Spanish architectural landscape.[75] According to her, the facile nostalgia of colonial postcards concealed power relations that have been largely neglected by historians. *Searchlight* shows a pivotal moment in that transition, by means of the American occupation of the port of Santiago, which would culminate in El Morro falling into the hands of the United States. The nocturnal atmosphere attenuates and effaces the marks of violence: Homer refrained from directly representing American military and technological might, hence the invasion in and of itself; the view of the deserted fortress, in placing the focus on its architectural details, indicates that it had already passed over to the realm of the colorful architecture offered for consumption on postcards.

Because it participated in this visual culture of empire, *Searchlight* cannot be read without taking into account the far-reaching debate on the general direction of U.S. foreign policy. Several voices rose up against the expansion of the Spanish-American War to Asia. The most famous of these voices, and one of the most forceful, was William Jennings Bryan, who in 1900 waged a presidential campaign against Theodore Roosevelt on an anti-imperialist platform. An orator without peer, Bryan seized on the metaphor of light and darkness to oppose imperialism through the image of a country that championed true progress: "Behold . . . a republic which shakes thrones and dissolves aristocracies by its silent example and gives light and inspiration to those who sit in darkness. Behold a republic gradually but surely becoming the supreme moral factor in the world's progress and the accepted arbiter of the world's disputes—a republic whose history, like the path of the just, 'is as the shining light that shineth more and more unto the perfect day.'"[76] In 1901 Mark Twain took up the same reference—including the biblical quotation—in an ironic vein. In "To the Person Sitting in Darkness," Twain inverted the rhetoric of the Enlightenment by pushing it to the point of absurdity. In a tongue-in-cheek praise of imperialism, he revealed the inversion of values poorly concealed by flights of rhetoric: "Extending the Blessings of Civilization to our Brother who Sits in Darkness has been a good trade and has paid well, on the whole; and there is money in it yet, if carefully worked—but not enough, in my judgement, to make any considerable risk advisable. The People that Sit in Darkness are getting to be too scarce—too scarce and too shy. And such darkness as is now left is really of but an indifferent quality, and not dark enough for the game. The most of those People that Sit in Darkness have been furnished with more light than was good for them or profitable for us. . . . They have become suspicious of the Blessings of Civilization. More—they have begun to examine them. This is not well. The Blessings of Civilization are all right, and a good commercial property; there could not be a better, in a dim light."[77] Twain proposed, for example, that the proper functioning of commercial affairs should be reestablished in the empire by dealing honestly with the colonized peoples. He put words in the mouths of the promoters of imperialism that made the contradictions of white discourse apparent: "We have debauched America's honor and blackened her face before the world."[78] That symptomatic slippage is a good indication that, in Twain's words, the darkness was not so profound, nor the light so clear and bright, as the colonialist discourses made them out to be.

The nostalgic view that *Searchlight* gives of the conflict, without going so far as to invert light in such a radical manner, suggests that Homer had adopted an equivocal position. That ambiguity also stems from a temporal misalignment. Cuba, already conquered in 1901 when Homer was painting the picture, is represented as if it were yet to be conquered: the Spanish empire, still standing, is contemplated at the moment of its imminent fall. That oscillating, anachronistic movement prompts a dual reflection. *Searchlight,* an accommodating meditation on the defeat of the enemy and a moderate celebration of the American victory, can also be read as a prophecy in the form of a jeremiad. It announces, not the end of the Spanish empire but the future decline of the American one. Twain spoke ironically of the value of the American conquest in the Philippines, given that the Treaty of Paris of 1898 had already officially sold the territories of Cuba, Puerto Rico, Guam, and the Philippines to the United States: "We and the patriots having captured Manila, Spain's ownership of the Archipelago and her sovereignty over it were at an end—obliterated—annihilated—not a rag or shred of either remaining behind. It was then that we conceived the divinely humorous idea of *buying* both of these spectres from Spain."[79] The United States may have acquired only the ghost of an empire, a collection of useless ruins: the melancholic atmosphere of the deserted ramparts of Santiago depicted in *Searchlight* evokes that spectral vision of an already bygone empire. I cannot help but associate the painting with another pictorial reflection on the fate of the American empire, of which Homer could not have been unaware: Thomas Cole's series of paintings *The Course of Empire,* especially *Desolation,* the last work in the cycle.[80] *Searchlight* and *Desolation* both portray the vestiges of a fallen power, contemplated at night in a solitary setting. Cole's warning to the young, overly ambitious American republic, his prediction of a glorious but violent, and, in the last analysis, decadent future, seems to make itself heard in Homer's painting.

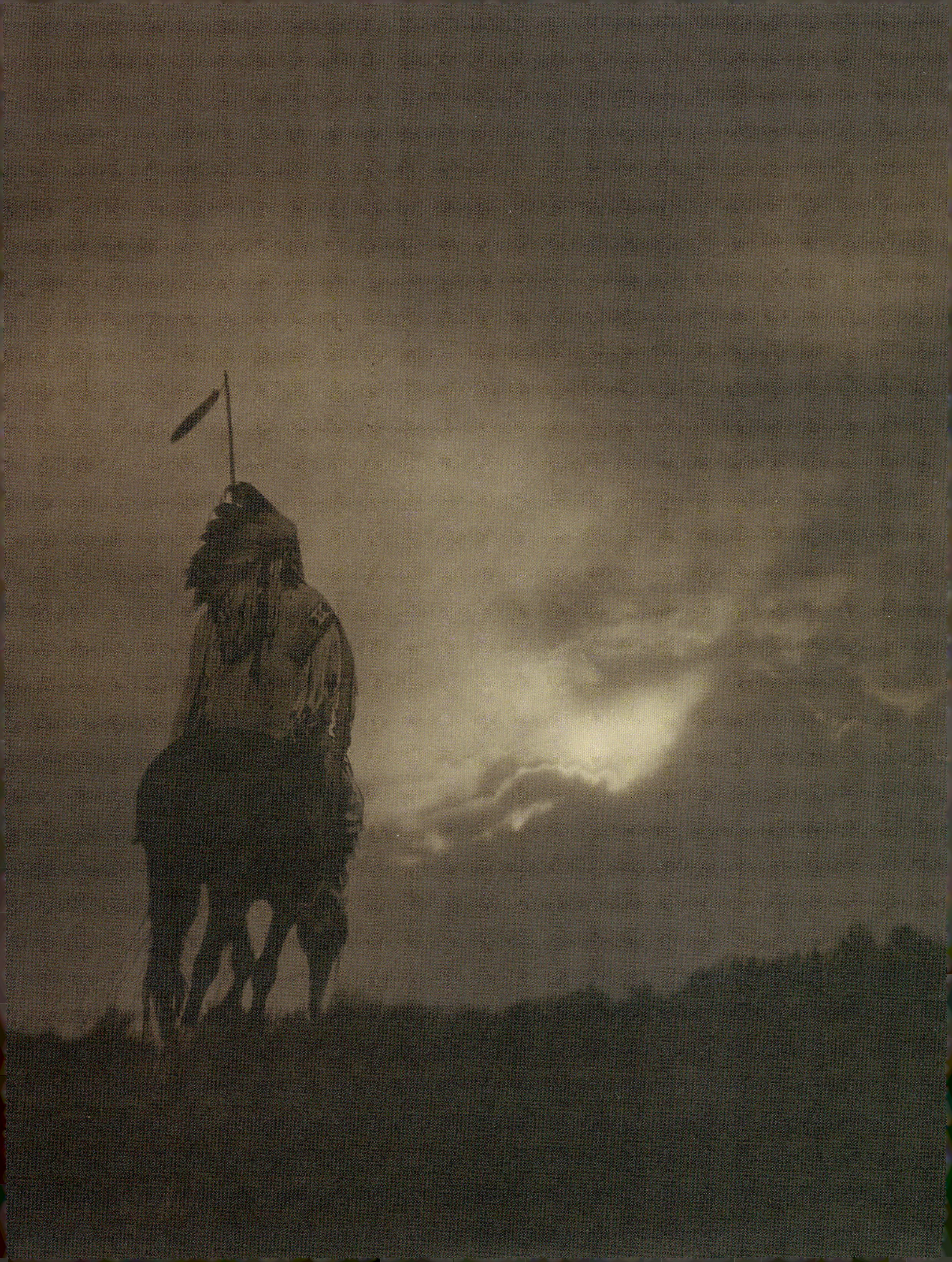

6 Vanishing Indians

Nostalgic Reminiscence and Haunting Presence

The anticipatory nostalgia of *Searchlight* mirrors the elegiac meditation conveyed by the nocturnal imagery of the West. Whereas Cuba and the Philippines symbolized the dawn of a global imperialism, the official closing of the frontier in 1890 marked the twilight of the conquest of North America. Here too, past and present conflated into an ambivalent discourse: it was precisely when the conquest of the West was ending that historian Frederick Jackson Turner anointed it the birthplace of Americanness. Night provided a visual outlet for this confused temporality. Painters Charles Rollo Peters and Frederic Remington, certainly one of the most celebrated image-makers of the West, and photographers Edward S. Curtis and Joseph K. Dixon repeatedly resorted to nocturnal settings. In the early twentieth century, such scenes accorded perfectly with the theme of the "vanishing Indian" that Curtis elaborated in photographs.[1] According to Patrick Brantlinger, that discourse belonged to a specific subgenre of imperialist discourse, which considered "primitive races" to be species destined for extinction as a result of contact with the white settler: "In art, in literature, journalism, science, and governmental rhetoric, extinction discourse often takes the form of proleptic elegy, sentimentally or mournfully expressing, even in its most humane versions, the confidence of self-fulfilling prophecy, according to which new, white colonies and nations arise as savagery and wilderness recede. Proleptic elegy is thus simultaneously funereal and epic's corollary—like epic, a nation-founding genre."[2] Alan Trachtenberg notes the particular fortunes of that language in visual culture. Paradoxically and "perversely,"[3] the more the Indians actually disappeared, the more visible their image became, through a profusion of representations in film, on postcards, and in photographs.[4] At the turn of the twentieth century, the figure of the Indian, vanishing but hypervisible, embodied a second paradox: in a radical reversal, that former enemy was now a figure onto which white Americans projected a mythic genealogy.[5] Even as the definition of Americanness became an increasingly sensitive subject for the class of white, English-speaking Americans (in the face of growth in immigration especially, as Trachtenberg shows), the Indian emerged as the symbolic source of that identity.

Night provided the ideal setting for that sentimental and nostalgic imagery. Through the frontier nocturne, artists lamented a lost West, metaphorically swallowed

Fig. 75 detail

up by the dark. But there again, darkness functioned as an ambiguous space of projection. The metaphor of night revealed the ambivalence inherent in the white mythology: white Americans, at the dawn of their empire, were able to contemplate the twilight of Indian civilization, but the temporal dimension of the nocturnal metaphor suggested that the cycle could continue. In a certain sense, it heralded the decline of white civilization itself. A cyclical vision thus competed with the optimistic image of linear progress, and the sharp contrast between Indians and whites coexisted with a more ambiguous model, in which their identities risked overlapping. These slippages were part of the nocturne's very form: the darkness of night, where it is difficult to distinguish the same from the other, served both to keep the vanishing Indian at a distance and to blur Indian and white identities. The nocturne thus contributed to a visual disembodiment of the figure of the Indian, even while incorporating him into the racist and nationalist mythology of whites.

THE NOCTURNE, ELEGY OF THE VANISHED FRONTIER

Just as Homer's *Searchlight,* whose prophetic echoes were revealed through the comparison with Cole's *Desolation,* can be read as a nocturnal meditation on the ruins of the Spanish empire, so too it can be linked to an image of the West contemporary to it, namely, Charles Rollo Peters's nocturne *San Fernando Mission* (see fig. 8). That painting also takes as its subject a relic of the Spanish occupation, this one located in California. Like *Searchlight, San Fernando Mission* meditates on the passing of the Spanish empire, supplanted by the American occupation.[6] The two works function as memento mori on the scale of American civilization as a whole, commemorating an act of destruction for which it was responsible, but which also threatened its own downfall. Although the two scenes are equally deserted, *San Fernando Mission* belongs to a visual discourse that more openly includes the presence—or thematized absence—of the nonwhite population that has implicitly fallen under American control. In Homer's painting, the residents of "benighted Cuba" and the overseas American empire remain a repressed and metaphorical presence. By contrast, Peters embraced a tradition of complacent contemplation of the "vanishing" Indian people. In Homer's work, the invisibility of nonwhites is contentious and paradoxical, whereas in the work of Peters, Remington, and Curtis, that invisibility constitutes the very subject of the image. The ruins of San Fernando were in fact emblematic of a global disappearance: they were the symbol of a bygone West, where Spanish missionaries, Indians, but also frontiersmen, had made way for urban and industrial expansion. The photographs capturing scenes of Indian life published by Joseph K. Dixon in his *Vanishing Race* exemplify that vision: explicitly aimed at demonstrating the "vanishing" of the Indian, the book grew out of an expedition financed by Rodman Wanamaker, the owner of department stores in Philadelphia and New York.[7] The image of the dying West, intended for consumption in the major urban centers of the east coast, owed its birth to the very thing that sealed the fate of the frontier: the advance of an urbanized society shaped by the capitalist system.

The Nocturne, Setting for the Myth of the Vanishing Indian

In the mythology of the West as recounted at the dawn of the twentieth century, the first to vanish was obviously the Indian. As Brian W. Dippie shows, that disappearance was announced by the early nineteenth century. Dippie's *Vanishing American* opens with a 1787 poem by Philip Freneau describing a ghostly Indian in a nocturnal setting: "By midnight moons, o'er moistering dews . . . / The hunter still the deer pursues / The hunter and the deer, a shade."[8] The association between the image of vanishing and the metaphor of night reappeared even in the speech that Chief Seattle is said to have delivered in 1854—according to the white journalist who published his remarks thirty years later—when he agreed to retreat with his tribe to the reservation offered by the U.S. government: "Day and night cannot dwell together. The Red Man has ever fled the approach of the White Man, as the morning mist flees before the morning sun. . . . It matters little where we pass the remnant of our days. They will not be many. The Indian's night promises to be dark. Not a single star of hope hovers above his horizon."[9]

The theme of the vanishing Indian, though already old and familiar by the late nineteenth century, took on broader scope after the official closing of the frontier and the end of the conflicts with the Indians, marked in particular by the massacre at Wounded Knee in December 1890.[10] Élise Marienstras points out the highly symbolic nature of that chapter, which left its stamp on the fin de siècle and the transition toward a political, economic, and cultural order dominated by capitalism: "The anonymous corpses [of the victims of the massacre] were endowed with a strong symbolic charge. They were the symbol of a past buried with the dawning century and of the anticipated victory of civilization over the savagery of men and in man, the triumph of Anglo-Saxon capitalism over the resistance of those left behind: the weak, the foreign."[11] Whites liked to dwell on the ineluctability of the Indians' extinction. In fact, their disappearance seemed to be confirmed by the census figures of 1890, the object of a special publication in 1894: the Indian population had dropped from more than 400,000 in 1850 to fewer than 250,000 in 1890.[12] At the time, the concept was endemic enough in American culture to resurface in a number of cultural products intended for a wide audience, beginning with new illustrated editions of James Fenimore Cooper's *Last of the Mohicans*,[13] Joseph K. Dixon's *Vanishing Race*, and Ella Higginson's collection of poems, also titled *The Vanishing Race*,[14] published in 1911 and dedicated to the photographer Edward S. Curtis, who published a series of articles explicitly devoted to that theme in *Scribner's Magazine* in 1906.[15] The notion of the vanishing of the Indian "race" was intimately linked to an aesthetic of darkness, which dominates Higginson's poems (the first in the collection set the tone: "Into the shadow . . . / Those last dark ones go drifting")[16] as well as Dixon's and Curtis's photographs. The first photogravure, called *The Vanishing Race* (fig. 73), in the first portfolio of Curtis's encyclopedic *North American Indian*, places the book as a whole within the register of the vanishing Indian: "The thought which this picture is meant to convey is that the Indians as a race, already shorn in their tribal strength and stripped of their primitive dress, are passing into the darkness of an unknown future. Feeling that the picture expresses so much of the thought that inspired the entire work, the author has chosen it as the first of the series."[17] The image shows a line of Indians on horseback, moving

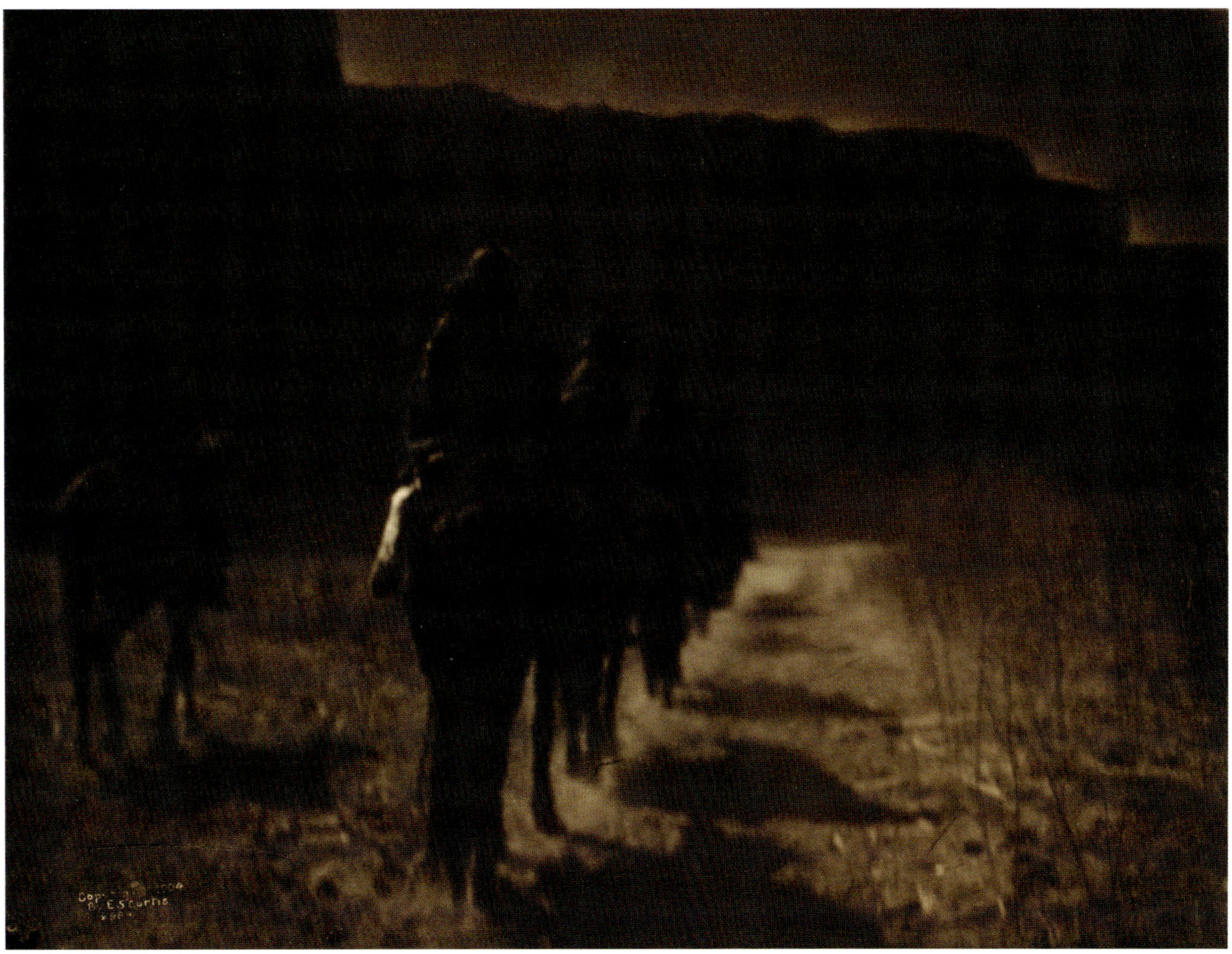

FIG. 73. Edward S. Curtis, *The Vanishing Race*, c. 1904. Photograph, 15.7 × 20.3 cm (6 ¼ × 8 in.). Library of Congress Prints and Photographs Division, Washington, D.C.

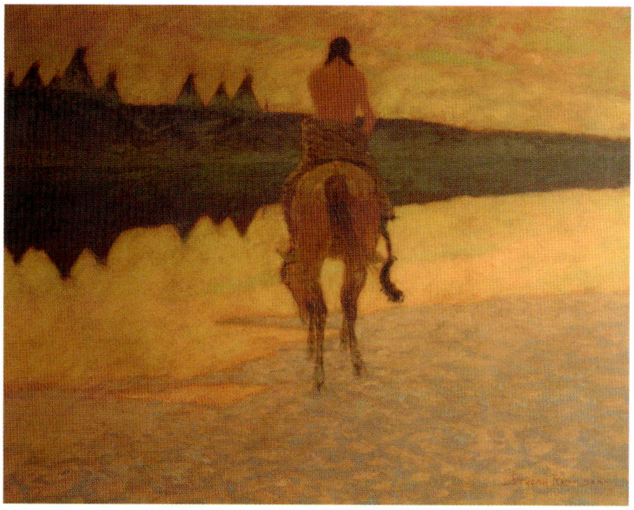

FIG. 74. Frederic Remington, *Sunset on the Plains*, 1905–6. Oil on canvas, 50.8 × 66 cm (20 × 26 in.). Courtesy of the West Point Museum Collection, United States Military Academy.

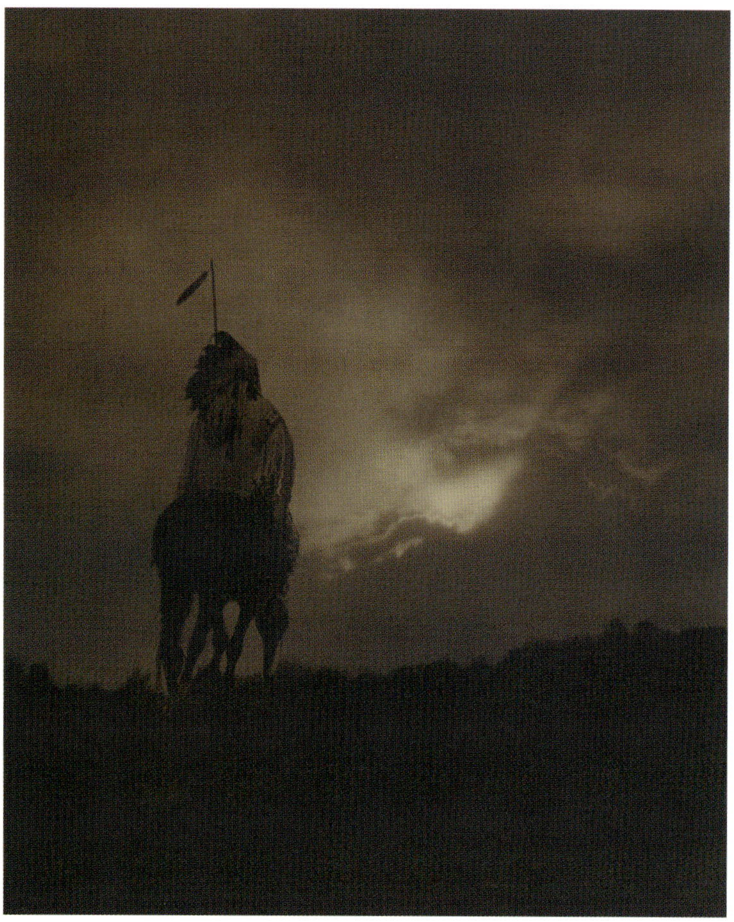

FIG. 75. Joseph K. Dixon, *The Sunset of a Dying Race*, 1913. Photogravure, 31 × 25 cm (13 3/8 × 9 13/16 in.). Collection of the Massachusetts Historical Society (137.7).

deeper into a vaguely defined landscape at twilight. Curtis treated romantically the Indians' presence in the landscape: swallowed up by the darkness that dominates the horizon, they are seen from the back, a position that indicates they are departing but that also evokes the romantic and solitary figures of the German painter Caspar David Friedrich. Curtis's silhouettes render their disappearance with pathos: their backs are hunched, or, like the next-to-last figure in the procession, they look regretfully at the beholder. Mathilde Arrivé, in her thesis on *The North American Indian,* compares Curtis's misty aesthetic to Stieglitz's and Steichen's pictorialism, showing it serves the discourse of the vanishing Indian: "[Some photographs of *The North American Indian*] seem motivated by the paradoxical desire *not to see* or, at the very least, not to see everything: concealing or masking reality might thus be a way of approaching it by having taken note of its inaccessibility. . . . Although, at the time the shot was taken, vanishing may have seemed an antiphotographic theme, Curtis succeeded in exploiting the resources of his medium, amplified by the expressive resources of pictorialism, to promote his own program."[18]

The same model was adopted by Remington in *Sunset on the Plains:* the isolated rider, also relatively downcast, is turned toward the setting sun, whose symbolism the painter fully exploited (fig. 74). The West is thus the vanishing point of daylight and the source of a symbolic discourse more than a real geographical space: space and time are emblematically united on the horizon of the Indian's fate. The painting underscores the ephemeral nature of the moment it captures, the crucial moment immediately preceding disappearance, and raises a dilemma: the Indian could be represented *vanishing,* but not vanished. Similarly conflicted vocabulary can be found in a large number of images,[19] beginning with the last chapter of Dixon's book, entitled "The Farewell of the Chiefs," whose words and images point insistently to loss and disappearance: "An Indian world revolves for the last time upon its axis. All the constellations which gave it light have burned out. The Indian cosmos sweeps a dead thing amid the growing lustre of the unfading stars of civilization and history. . . . In the deepening twilight all is silent—all speech is vulgar."[20] The photographs accompanying the text repeat the idea of a passing from view, with titles such as "The Final Trail," "Fading Sunset," or "Vanishing into the Mists."[21] *The Sunset of a Dying Race* (fig. 75) reproduces almost exactly Remington's

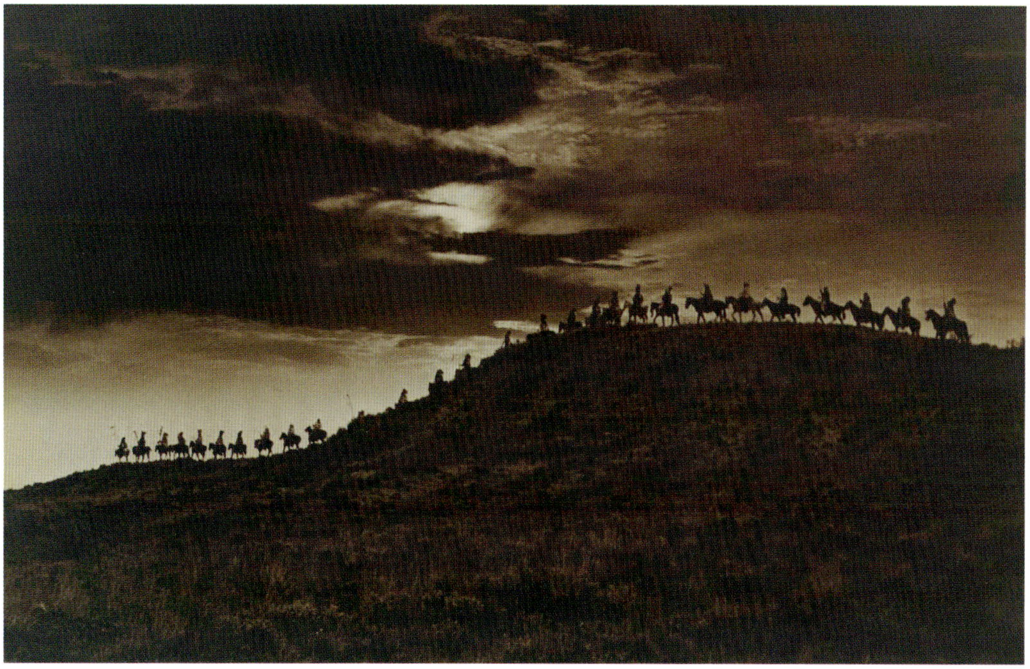

FIG. 76. Joseph K. Dixon, *Skirting the Sky Line*, c. 1908–13. Photogravure, 30 × 53 cm (12 × 21 in.). Denver Public Library, Western History Collection (Z-3167).

composition, while making its content more explicit. In Remington's painting, the figure's arched back might be explained by the posture of the horse taking a drink, but in Dixon's all ambiguity is dispelled: darkness envelops a stereotypical Indian, only his feathered headdress still visible. *Skirting the Sky Line* thematizes vanishing in an exemplary manner, even while showing the contradictions of that rhetoric (fig. 76). The outlined shadows of the Indians are eminently visible precisely because they are about to cross the horizon line, which they symbolically replicate. In this photograph, the horse riders, shadows of themselves, also personify their own vanishing horizon.

Night marks the logical culmination of that journey toward the setting sun: Remington's *Luckless Hunter* and *Hungry Moon* offer the pathetic spectacle of the Indian who has arrived at the end of the road, prostrate, his face turned away (figs. 77, 78). Royal Cortissoz gave a contradictory reading of the first picture, at first allowing himself to be carried away by pathos, then reducing the scene to a natural phenomenon: "I hardly know which is the more moving in his picture of 'The Luckless Hunter,' the stolidly resigned rider, huddling his blanket about him against the freezing night air, or the tired pony about which you would say there hung a hint of pathos if that were not to give, perhaps, too anecdotic an edge to an altogether natural episode."[22] As moving as it might be, this "episode" supposedly represents only the ultimate stage in the natural and inevitable process of the extinction of the Indian "race." Another critic considered this painting at some length in his review of the exhibition of Remington's nocturnes at the Knoedler Gallery in 1908: "In all of Remington's pictures the shadow of death seems not far away. If the actors in his vivid scenes are not threatened by death in terrible combat, they are menaced by it in the form of famine, thirst or cold."[23] Extinction is represented as literal exhaustion, both the physical fatigue perceptible in the figures' attitude and the exhaustion of vital resources, particularly the food supplied by bison hunts. *The Luckless Hunter* and *The Hungry Moon* are both implicitly about the environmental disaster caused by the destruction of herds of bison (often called buffalo), the main source of subsistence for many tribes. Whites were the principal agents of that extermination: Buffalo Bill Cody, for example, acquired his famous nickname by slaughtering entire herds.
In 1888 Albert Bierstadt depicted the last of the bison being killed by an Indian's spear rather than a white man's rifle, but this was a crude denial of historical reality (fig. 79). Beholders of Bierstadt's image were aware that the responsibility for that environmental tragedy fell on white settlers. The naturalist William Hornaday began his book on the extermination of wild animal species with these words: "I think that even the worst enemies of the plains Indians hardly will accuse them of killing large numbers of buffalo, elk or deer merely for the pleasure of seeing them fall, or taking only their

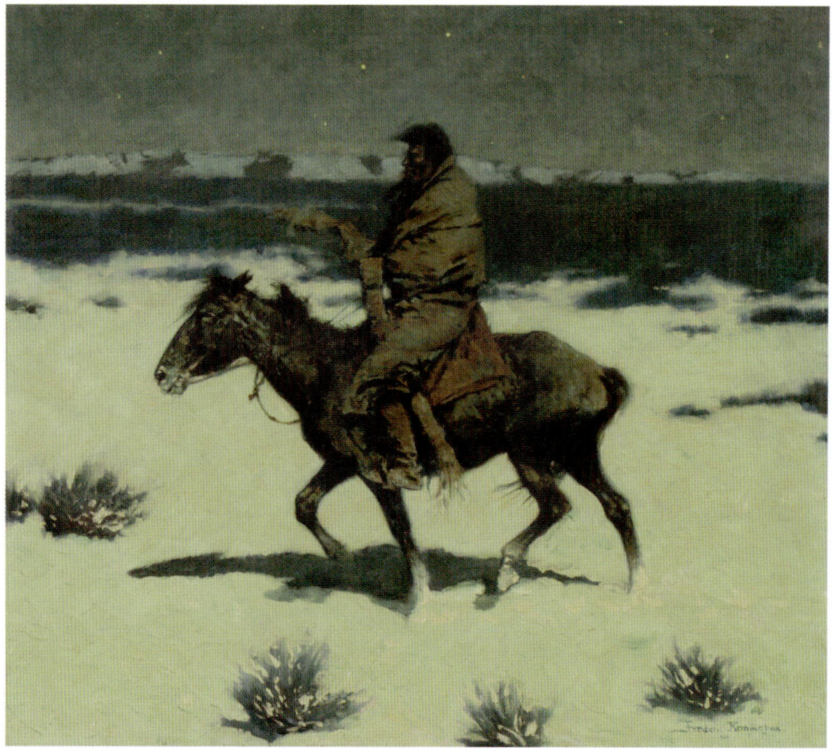

FIG. 77. Frederic Remington, *The Luckless Hunter,* 1909. Oil on canvas, 68.9 × 77.5 cm (27 × 30 ½ in.). Courtesy Sid Richardson Museum, Fort Worth, Texas.

FIG. 78. Frederic Remington, *The Hungry Moon,* 1906. Oil on canvas, 49.2 × 65.4 cm (19 ⅜ × 25 ¾ in.). Gilcrease Museum, Tulsa, Oklahoma (0127.2331).

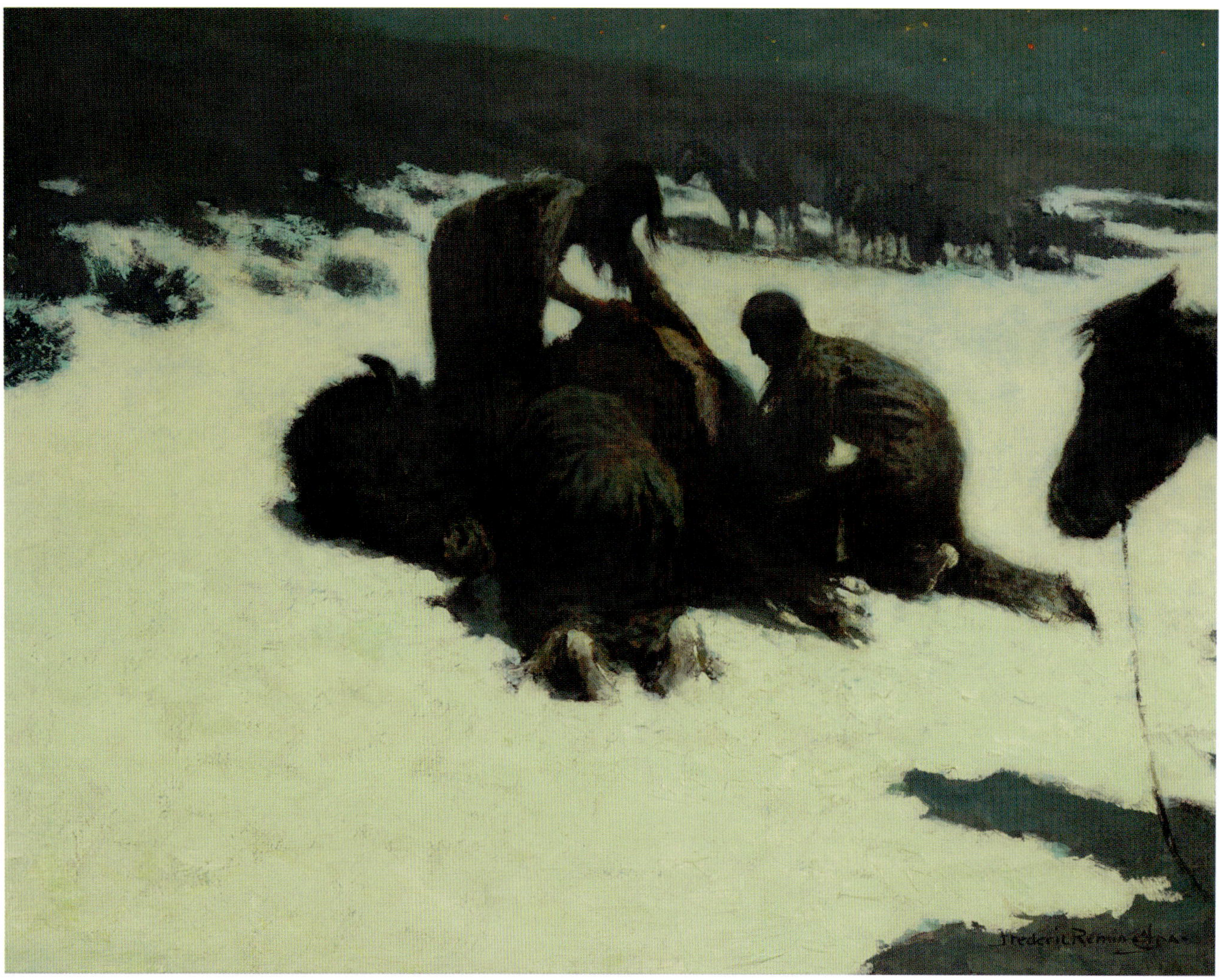

teeth."[24] But Hornaday, like almost all commentators at the time, described that annihilation as inescapable: "Before the relentless march of civilization, the wild Indian, the bison and many of the wild birds must inevitably disappear. We cannot change conditions that are as inexorable as death itself."[25] Like night following day, the vanishing of the Indian was merely a predictable phase in the natural course of things. The images of night and of the setting sun contributed toward naturalizing the Indian. The hunter was conflated with his horse in Cortissoz's remarks, and *The Hungry Moon* implicitly links the Indian women's fate to that of the bison. Once he had been driven back into the night, the figure of the Indian left the historical and political order behind. Having blended into the natural landscape, he returned to a space outside time. And yet *The Hungry Moon,* with its bodies half-buried in a snow-covered landscape, bears a disturbing resemblance to a photograph of the site of Wounded Knee taken a few weeks after the massacre there of dozens of women, children, and the elderly, worn down and starved by the U.S. Army (fig. 80). Remington might have witnessed that scene even before seeing the photograph, since he was sent there as a reporter for *Harper's Weekly.*[26] The nocturnal atmosphere of the painting, even as it covers the scene with an aestheticizing veil that makes the historical event seem more remote, also brings it closer to the monochromatic tones of the photograph. Bodies, barely discernible in the foreground of the photograph, resurface in *The Hungry Moon* as the silhouettes of the kneeling women and the dead bison. Remington, playing on formal similarities, attempted to reactivate the emotional charge of the event by means of a known image likely to bring to mind the tragic echoes of the massacre. Yet though he shifted the responsibility for the vanishing of the Indians onto an environmental phenomenon, the pathos of the visual vocabulary he used reveals the very thing he intended to conceal. *The Hungry Moon,* showing what it seeks to hide, takes the form of a veiled confession.

The paradox, as I began to suggest above, lies in the uneasy relationship between vanishing and representation: that contradiction creates a permanent back-and-forth motion, an inconsistency between the various moments of the process. The imagery of the vanishing Indian opens a breach between the bygone past and its commemorative representation, between what is declared to have vanished and what persists in front of one's eyes. The nocturne, by its ambiguity, furnishes a vocabulary able to fill that gap: in the gray zone of night, the Indian is not altogether there, but he also has not yet entirely vanished. In that sense, rather than speak of the "last" images of the Indian (as in "the last of the Mohicans"), one ought perhaps to evoke the notion of a more complex aesthetics of the "next-to-last." In the nocturne, the image may be at once projective and retrospective, embodying an anticipatory nostalgia—what Brantlinger calls the "future perfect"—of the mythic saga of the West.[27] The type of contemplation the nocturne imposes on its beholder, who is forced to peer into the darkness to gradually make out the outlines, is a particularly effective

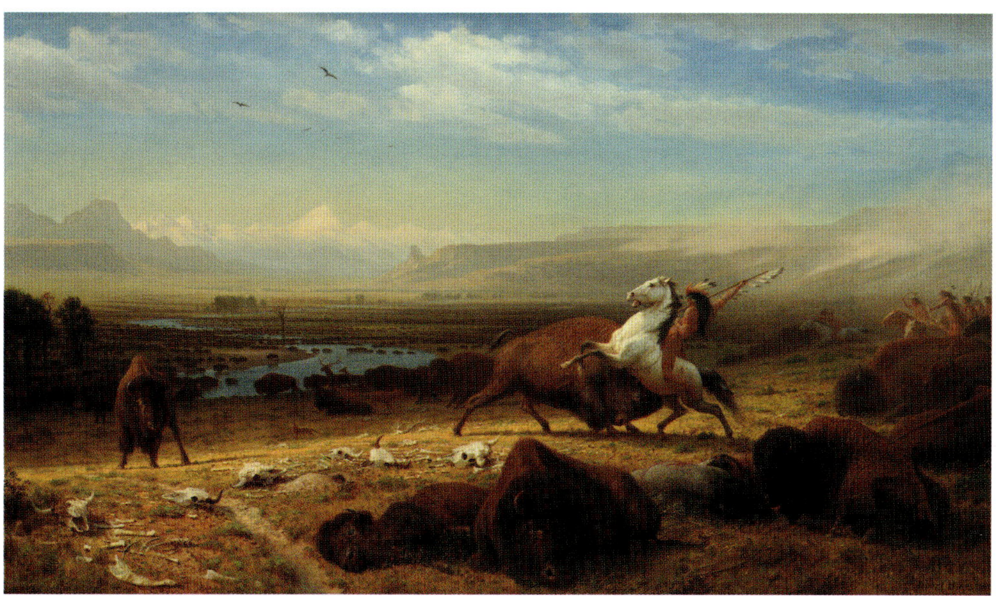

FIG. 79. Albert Bierstadt, *The Last of the Buffalo,* 1888. Oil on canvas, 180.3 × 301.6 cm (71 × 118 ¾ in.). National Gallery of Art, Washington, D.C., Corcoran Collection (Gift of Mary Stewart Bierstadt [Mrs. Albert Bierstadt]), 2014.79.5.

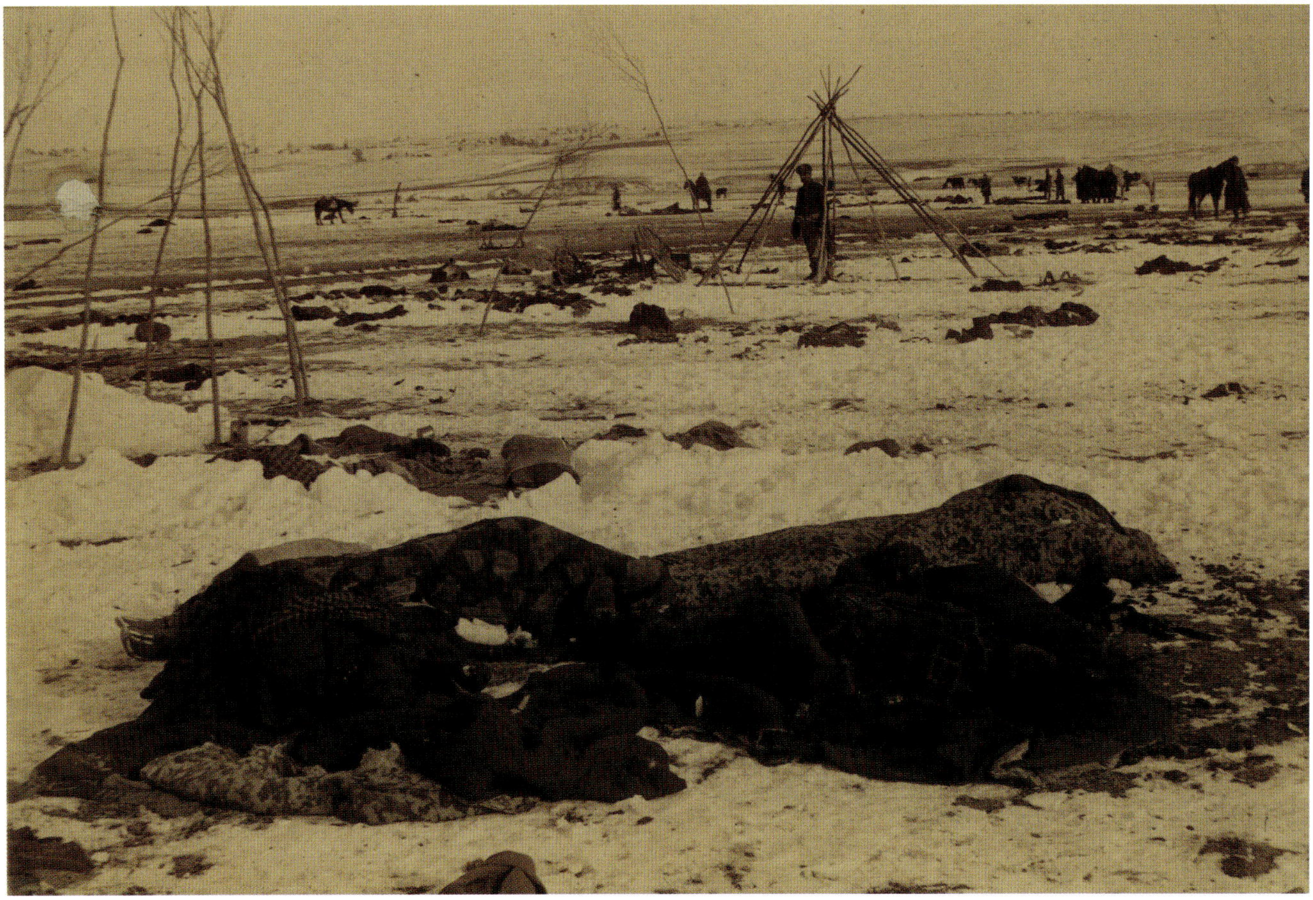

FIG. 80. "Big Foot's Camp Three Weeks after the Wounded Knee Massacre (Dec. 29, 1890)," 1891. Albumen photograph, 22.9 × 27.9 cm (9 × 11 in.). Library of Congress, Prints and Photographs Division, Washington, D.C.

medium for conveying disappearance, which is ambiguous by definition. The Indian vanishes *in and before the eyes of* the white beholder, which is to say, both in that beholder's interpretation and in her line of sight. The vanishing occurs in the span of time that contemplation requires, and the beholder is its necessary witness. Without her, the vanishing would not take place, since it would have no purpose. That spectacular vanishing—a contradiction in terms—accommodates itself perfectly to the paradoxical visual functioning of the nocturne. Just as the nocturne, in turning away from direct and precise representation, set out to deploy a vision that reflected the beholder's inner life, here the nocturnal landscape of the West, which shows Indians while hiding them at the same time, turns the beholder's gaze back toward the past. Like that of Manifest Destiny, the discourse of the supposedly vanishing Indian was created by and directed toward the white settler: the dark veil of vanishing actually concealed a mirror.

White Dawn, White Twilight

Nocturnes, even as they gave a particular visibility to the vanishing of the Indian, bore witness as well to a parallel and equally ineluctable vanishing: that of the white frontiersman. In that respect, the nocturnes by Charles Rollo Peters that were inspired by the landscapes of the Monterey Peninsula, where a colony of tonalist artists had settled,[28] speak volumes. The vanishing they depict is more akin to desertion; it leaves the landscape in an ambiguous state of semi-occupation. Peters used the same formula again and again, organizing his composition around a building, sometimes in ruins, placed in the middle ground of the image, along a road that guides the eye through the canvas (fig. 81). Unlike Remington, who persisted in incorporating human figures, Peters emptied the landscape of any human presence. This more circumspect treatment may derive from an especially violent regional history: as historian Benjamin Madley has shown, Californian Indians were the victims of an organized,

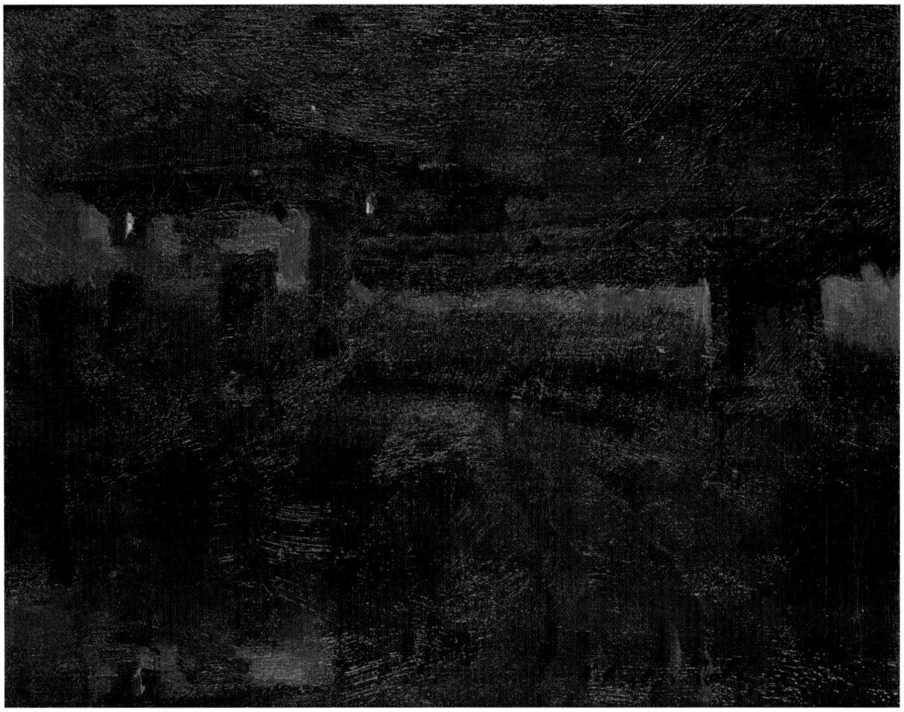

FIG. 81. Charles Rollo Peters, Untitled (*Nocturnal Landscape with Adobe Building*), n.d. Oil on canvas, 33 × 40.6 cm (13 × 16 in.). Collection of the Oakland Museum of California, Gift of Concours d'Antiques, the Art Guild of the Oakland Museum of California, A65. 13.363.

state-sanctioned violence that deserves to be qualified as a genocide.[29] While the Spanish mission rule had already been very cruel, the decrease in the native population accelerated dramatically after the United States overtook the region in 1846. By the turn of the twentieth century, most commentators agreed that the artists painting the old Spanish missions and Indian villages were performing the work of "historians" as much as artists.[30] Yet the very recent history of systematic destruction of an entire population was eclipsed by a nostalgia for Hispanic culture and picturesqueness. An article in *Overland Monthly* lamented the disappearance of local traditions and peoples, apparently referring only to Spanish heritage: "But alas! the town, with its quaint old customs, its old adobes, and even its people, who spoke the soft, musical language of a nation across the seas are rapidly passing away."[31] This focus on an abandoned architecture, however, betrays a repressed memory. Indeed, the erasure is all the more significant in that the local landscape was deeply shaped by native traditions. The architecture omnipresent in Peters's paintings showcases the adobe techniques borrowed from Southwestern Indians by the Spanish colonizers. The style came back in fashion in the early twentieth century, which might also explain Peters's success.[32] An article in the *San Francisco Call,* devoted to the architecture of some of the most "artistic" dwellings of the city's elites, mentioned the vogue for the Pueblo style, discussing at length a "Hopi" house in the center of the illustrated page (fig. 82). The author specified that the earth for the house's terraces hanging over the "cliff" of Washington Street was carried up "much as the Hopis carried it in building their homes," and, seemingly unaware of the cruel irony of this appropriation, added that "over the door is the motto adapted from the Indian, 'All we ask is to be left in peace to live our own lives.'"[33] That same newspaper had already identified the tendency more than ten years earlier: "The more expensive adobe mansions that have been built in the city in the past year or two are a revival of the mission style of architecture as adapted to dwellings" (fig. 83).[34] The buildings visible in Peters's paintings symbolize the various cultures—Indian, Spanish, then American—that occupied and still occupy the Mexican border regions and that one by one adopted the adobe architecture. Contrary to most native cultures, the tribes of the Southwest, for the most part Pueblo and Navajo Indians (the tribe represented in Curtis's *Vanishing Race* photogravure), actually resisted the supposedly inexorable advance of white civilization comparatively well.[35] Displaced in the paintings of Peters and fashionable mansions of the white elite, this architectural style acts as a silent reminder of Indian presence. Peters's adobe houses thus ensure the "local color" of his

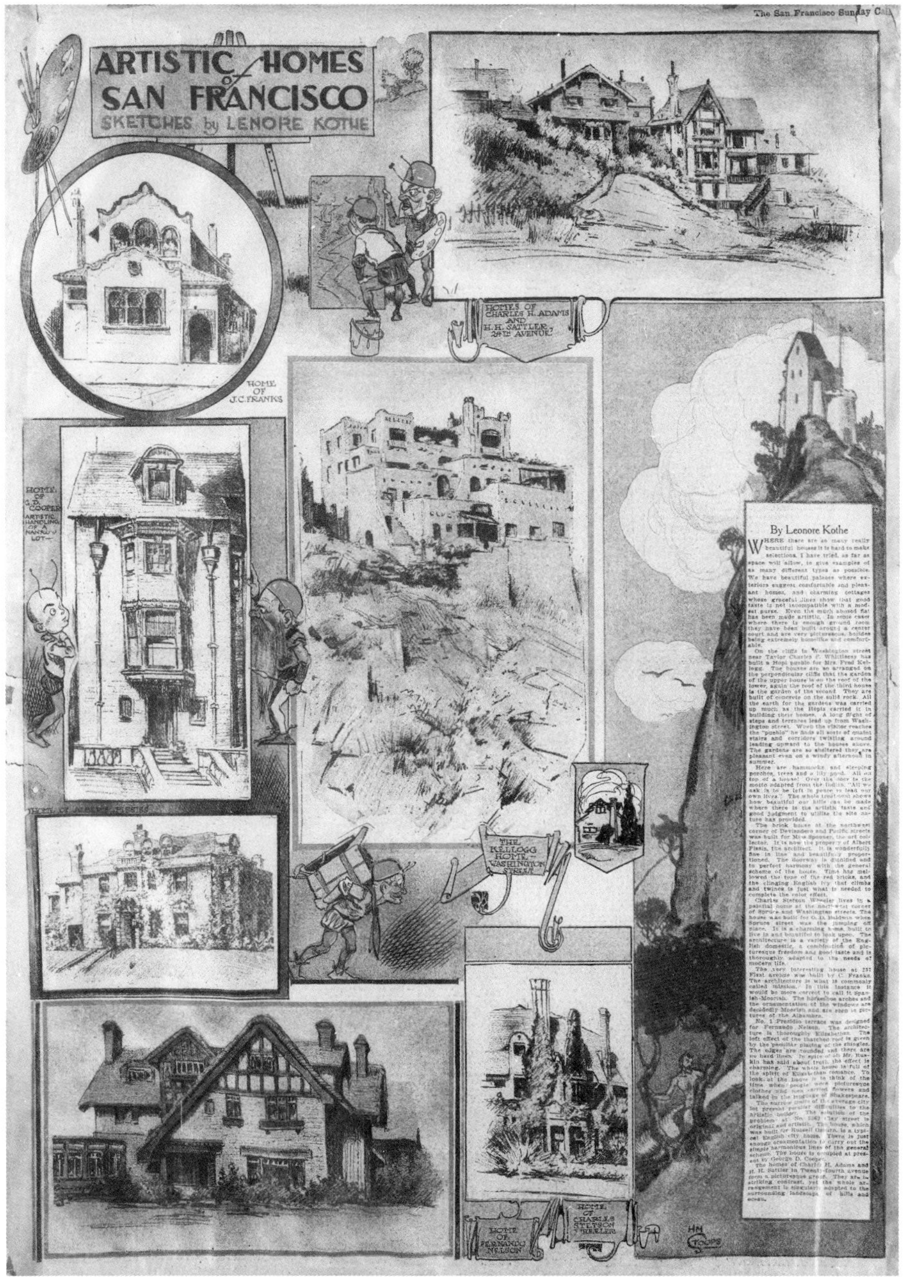

By Leonore Kothe

WHERE there are so many really beautiful houses it is hard to make selections. I have tried, as far as space will allow, to give examples of as many different types as possible. We have beautiful palaces where exteriors suggest comfortable and pleasant homes, and charming cottages whose graceful lines show that good taste is not incompatible with a modest purse. Even the much abused flat has been made artistic. In some cases where there is enough ground room they have been built around a center court and are very picturesque, besides being extremely homelike and comfortable.

On the cliffs in Washington street near Taylor Charles F. Whittlesey has built a Hopi pueblo for Mrs. Fred Kellogg. The houses are so arranged on the perpendicular cliffs that the garden of the upper house is on the roof of the lower, again the roof of the third house is the garden of the second. They are built of concrete on the solid rock. All the earth for the gardens was carried up much as the Hopis carried it in building their homes. A long flight of steps and terraces lead up from Washington street. When the visitor reaches the "pueblo" he finds all sorts of quaint stairs and corridors twisting around leading upward to the houses above. The gardens are so sheltered they are pleasant even on a windy afternoon in summer.

Here are hammocks and sleeping porches, trees and a lily pond. All on top of a house! Over the door is the motto adapted from the Indian, "All we ask is to be left in peace to lead our own lives." The whole treatment shows how beautiful our hills can be made where there is the artistic taste and good judgment to utilize the site nature has provided.

The brick house at the northeast corner of Devisadero and Pacific streets was built for Miss Spooner, the art collector. It is now the property of Albert Pissis, the architect. It is wonderfully fine in line and beautifully proportioned. The doorway is dignified and in perfect harmony with the general scheme of the house. Time has mellowed the tone of the red bricks, and the clinging English ivy that climbs and twines is just what is needed to complete the color effect.

Charles Stetson Wheeler lives in a palatial home at the northwest corner of Spruce and Washington streets. The house was built for O. D. Baldwin when Spruce street was the jumping off place. It is a charming home, built to live in and beautiful to look upon. The architecture is a variety of the English domestic, a combination of picturesque freedom and good taste and is thoroughly adapted to the needs of modern life.

The very interesting house at 237 First avenue was built by C. Franks. The architecture is what is commonly called mission. In this instance it would be more correct to call it Spanish-Moorish. The horseshoe arches and the ornamentation of the windows are decidedly Moorish and are seen in pictures of the Alhambra.

No. 1 Presidio terrace was designed for Fernando Nelson. The architecture is thoroughly Elizabethan. The soft effect of the thatched roof is given by the peculiar placing of the shingles. The edges are rounded and there are no hard lines. In spite of all Mr. Ruskin has said about truth, the effect is charming. The whole house is full of the spirit of Elizabethan romance. To look at the house is to think of the time when people wore picturesque clothes and men carried flowers and talked in the language of Shakespeare.

The narrow limits of the average city lot present peculiar difficulties to the artistic builder. The solution of the problem at No. [illegible] Clay street is original and artistic. The house, which was built for Russell [illegible], is a typical English city home. There is just enough ornamentation to carry out the simple harmonious lines of the general scheme. The house is occupied at present by George D. Cooper.

The homes of Charles H. Adams and H. H. Sattler in Twenty-fourth avenue form a picturesque group. They are in striking contrast, yet the whole arrangement is singularly adapted to the surrounding landscape of hills and ocean.

FIG. 82. Lenore Kothe, "Artistic Homes of San Francisco," *San Francisco Call*, January 1, 1911.

paintings,[36] but they also indicate superimposition of various heritages. The 1899 article in the *San Francisco Call* retraced, with the aid of photographs put to didactic ends, the various stages in the local architectural evolution, from the "adobe hut of the Mexican" to the "palace of the American," by way of the Franciscan mission. The elements borrowed from the biological evolutionist model (especially the idea of an evolution that began in the primordial mud) and the layout of the photographic montage suggest the regular and continuous unfolding of a process that culminated with white civilization. But despite the reporter's efforts to present a unified image, mud—and along with it the exotic coloration of racial difference—persists in that model adapted to American civilization: "It has aptly been termed the Americanized Moresque architecture,"[37] the writer ultimately concluded. Although he insisted on a succession over time of carefully ranked stages, the photographs reveal an implicit coexistence. Peters's deserted dwellings entail the same equivocation, hesitating between presence and absence. The nocturnal setting and the absence of human figures suggest that these houses are more or less abandoned, but the discourse remains ambiguous: by whom, exactly, were these houses occupied? As with Winslow Homer's *Searchlight,* one may wonder of what civilization these dwellings are the vestiges. Is this Indian culture, the

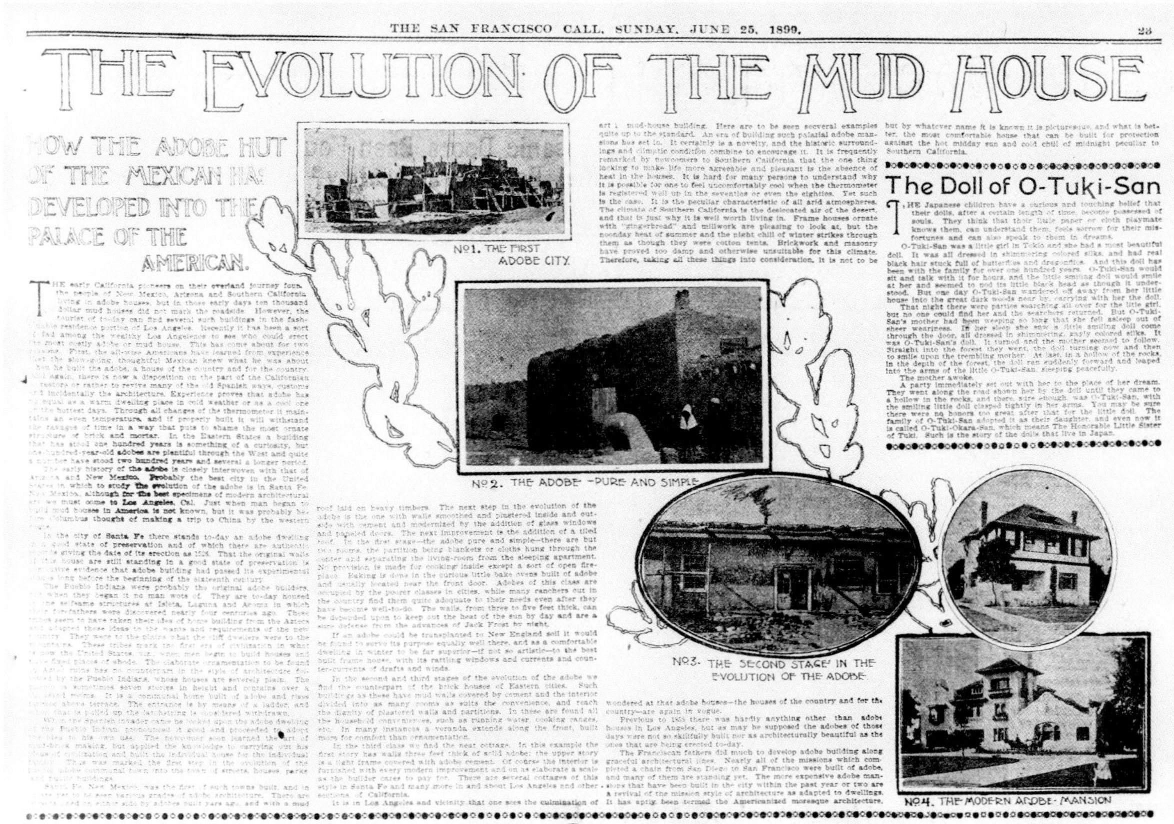
THE SAN FRANCISCO CALL, SUNDAY, JUNE 25, 1899.

THE EVOLUTION OF THE MUD HOUSE

HOW THE ADOBE HUT OF THE MEXICAN HAS DEVELOPED INTO THE PALACE OF THE AMERICAN.

The Doll of O-Tuki-San

No. 1. THE FIRST ADOBE CITY.

No. 2. THE ADOBE—PURE AND SIMPLE.

No. 3. THE SECOND STAGE IN THE EVOLUTION OF THE ADOBE.

No. 4. THE MODERN ADOBE MANSION

FIG. 83. "The Evolution of the Mud House," *San Francisco Call,* June 25, 1899.

Spanish tradition, or a certain stage of American civilization itself?

The marked interest in the picturesque architecture of the Pueblo and of the California missions is in fact symptomatic. Having arrived at continent's end, whites looked back nostalgically at what they had just destroyed. The remnants of Pueblo architecture and, in general, the Indian cultures of the Southwest seem in that respect to have been an exception to the widespread destruction of nonwhite civilizations by white American settlers. But, as Theodore Roosevelt pointed out in a passage from *The Winning of the West,* evidently inspired in large part by Frederick Jackson Turner, the vanishing of the frontier also obliterated a certain kind of white man: "As the frontiersmen conquered and transformed the wilderness, so the wilderness in its turn created and preserved the type of man who overcame it. Nowhere else on the continent has so sharply defined and distinctively American a type been produced as on the frontier, and a single generation has always been more than enough for its production. The influence of the wild country upon the man is almost as great as the effect of the man upon the country. The frontiersman destroys the wilderness, and yet its destruction means his own. He passes away before the coming of the very civilization whose advance guard he has been."[38] In the final words of the introduction he wrote for *The Winning of the West* in 1889, Roosevelt recognized this vanishing process as one that had already been under way for a long time, and that would repeat itself to affect his own generation of western adventurers: "The men who have shared in the fast vanishing frontier life of the present feel a peculiar sympathy with the already long-vanished frontier life of the past."[39] *The End of the Day,* a depiction of the everyday lives of white people on the frontier, which Remington painted in 1904 for *Collier's Weekly,* lends itself to an allegorical reading: the end of the workday coincides with the vanishing of the frontiersman's way of life, symbolized by the log cabin (fig. 84). Night and snow engulf the frontiersman and the Indian in a similar extinction.

The dawn of civilization, then, also brought with it a white death and its own share of contradictions, because, in keeping with Turner's dialectic, it abolished the very thing that made it possible. The mythology of the West developed in an ambivalent mode, always accompanied by a funereal note. Hornaday described the invasion of

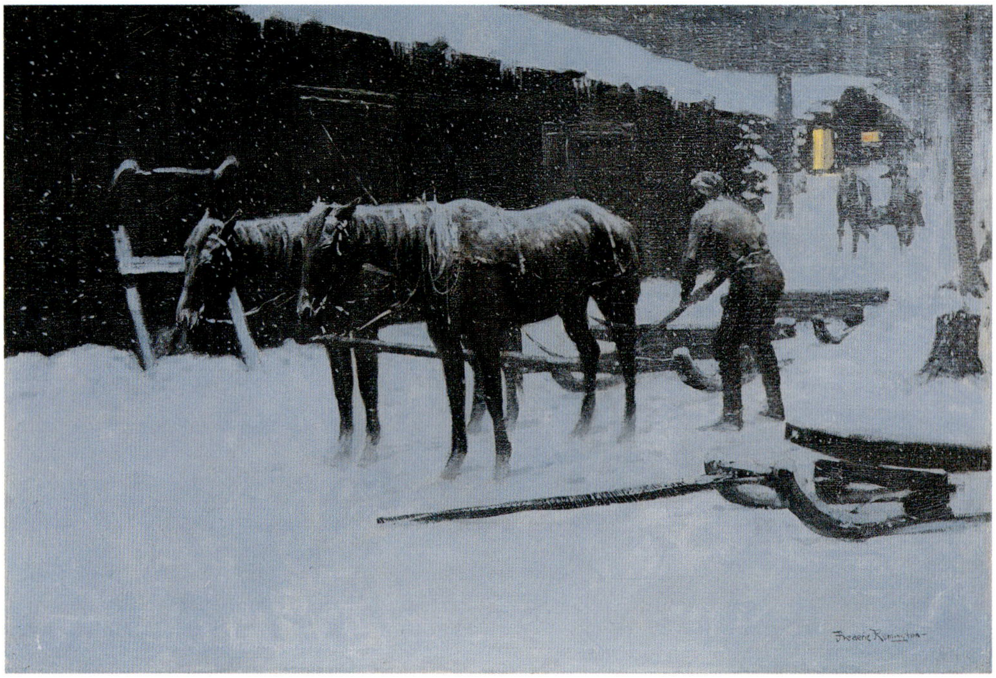

FIG. 84. Frederic Remington, *The End of the Day*, 1904. Oil on canvas, 67.3 × 101.6 cm (26 1/2 × 40 in.). Courtesy of the Frederic Remington Art Museum, Ogdensburg, New York.

civilization as extending as far as Death Valley and so irresistible that the white man had to save the continent from himself: "As civilization marches ever onward, over the prairies, into the bad lands and the forests, over the mountains and even into the farthest corner of Death Valley, the desert of deserts, the struggle of the wild birds, mammals and fishes is daily and hourly intensified. Man must help them to maintain themselves, or accept a lifeless continent."[40] And that continent, deprived of the altogether American vitality of the frontier, was transformed into an urbanized and industrialized landscape. In a revealing comparison, Hornaday commented on the inevitability of the bison's disappearance: "To-day the buffalo could not survive in Iowa, eastern Nebraska or eastern Kansas, any longer than a Shawnee Indian would last on the Bowery."[41] An article on the "old pueblo," after emphasizing the persistence of its architectural, cultural, and linguistic traditions, concluded that what ultimately made it vanish was not exactly the white settler but a different form of barbarism that came in his wake: the city and, especially, its immigrants. "In this decade the city began its migration southward. The Plaza fronts of the proud old Dons became the dens of the 'Heathen Chinee' [*sic*] and the dragon flag of the Flowery Kingdom floated over the olden time business center of the old pueblo. The passing of the old pueblo had been accomplished."[42]

The invasion of the frontiersmen was followed by the even more deadly invasion of city dwellers, whom Remington condemned in a letter, written to his wife from New Mexico, in which he threatened never to return there. Tellingly, what bothers Remington is the way newcomers have already altered the local landscape and architecture: "It is all brick buildings—derby hats and blue overhauls—it spoils my early illusions."[43] Remington, in an often-cited article in an issue of *Collier's Weekly* devoted entirely to his art, recounted a nocturnal encounter as a young man with an old frontiersman, who assured the aspiring draftsman of cowboys and Indians that the West no longer existed. The account given by Remington in the opening pages of the magazine fully participated in the aesthetic of the "next-to-last": "The old man had closed my very entrancing book almost at the first chapter. I knew the railroad was coming—I saw men already swarming into the land. I knew the derby hat, the smoking chimneys, the cord-binder, and the thirty-day note were upon us in a resistless surge. I knew the wild riders and the vacant land were about to vanish forever, and the more I considered the subject the bigger the Forever loomed."[44] The "wild riders" Remington evoked were not defined as Indians or as white frontiersmen—the term "wild" could apply to either group—and that ambiguity aptly conveyed the idea that frontiersmen and Indians were fated to vanish together. The famous illustrator, returning to his early days, lamented the defeat to come, taking the side of a "we" whose definition remained vague, but whose perspective he at least clearly shared with the old frontiersman. Both of them, now cornered, contemplated the invasion of the West by city people.

Brick buildings transformed the half-fantasized landscape of the frontier to such a degree that the choice of the nocturne can be interpreted as an avoidance strategy. Just as it reenchanted Whistler's industrial Thames, darkness temporarily suspends the disappearance of the old West by pushing the unpleasant details of urban and industrial modernity outside the frame of the painting. Scott A. Shields associates the California artists' fascination with traditional architecture with the rustic ideals of the Arts and Crafts movement.[45] He cites the remarks of a journalist vaunting the backward-looking and sentimental attitude of the artists, who in Monterey turned their backs on modern civilization: "In Monterey, where militant progress halts on the threshold, where the spirit of the past hovers over crumbling adobes, and roses, clinging lovingly, cover up the ravages of time, where romantic stories are still told as if romance had high value . . . that is where artists have loved to congregate."[46] The Monterey Peninsula, a paradise preserved in the Far West, provided a store of romantic clichés ready to be exploited by the artists who chose to live there. But that rather morbid taste for contemplating the "ravages of time" and the "spirit of the past" that inhabited the ruins like a ghostly presence also revealed the paradoxical position of the artists themselves. Although they gathered around these relics for inspiration, they were also subjected to the pressure of the advance of civilization, which transformed the landscape and reduced their art to a bubble as artificial as the ruins that attracted tourists to Monterey.

The two faces of progress and the complex relationship the image maintained with that dynamic were a commonplace in the visual culture of the time. They reappear, for instance, in the advertisement N. C. Wyeth created for Cream of Wheat. Here the cowboy, having become a postman, puts letters into a mailbox made out of an empty Cream of Wheat crate (fig. 85).[47] The title of the illustration, *Rural Delivery,* refers to a law passed by the U.S. Congress in 1898 that established mail delivery to rural areas free of charge. At a time when the United States was extending its sphere of influence to Cuba and the Philippines, progress apparently also found its way into the country's interior. In the picture, the farmlands, which may cultivate the grains that go into Cream of Wheat (a processed food manufactured more or less traditionally but in several stages in different parts of the country), are reduced to shapeless and colorless fields, which contrast with the clarity of the recycled industrial object and its logo, placed in the center of the image. The illustration announces the invasion of one America by another, as the brand's slogan underscores: "Where the mail goes, Cream of Wheat goes." Above all, the sun rising on the horizon, its circle adjacent to the crate, lends itself to a potentially contradictory reading. Its size, and its position very close to the horizon, bring to mind a harvest moon, a familiar summer-night phenomenon. Sun or moon, dawn or twilight? N. C. Wyeth gave the saga of progress an ambiguous turn in an essentially antimodern image. The advertisement, in playing on the nostalgic register of backward-looking imagery, puts forward its own visual vocabulary. The mise en abyme of the Cream of Wheat logo, which is both an element and the message of the picture, encapsulates that ambiguous and highly reflexive movement.

The melancholic simplicity of the nocturne made for a catchy pictorial vocabulary that proved easily adaptable to other settings: after the 1906 San Francisco earthquake, for instance, Charles Rollo Peters and Arnold Genthe imposed the nocturne's codes on the landscape of the devastated city. In Genthe's *Steps That Lead to Nowhere* (see fig. 54), the nocturnal setting accentuates the elegiac tone of the landscape, neutralizing the chaos produced by the catastrophe in a harmonious darkness, from which the artist (especially through the framing) brought to the fore an architectural relic invested with a symbolic value. A view of the city, published in a newspaper series of "odd photographs," shows a "ghost picture" of San Francisco, suggesting a city idealized by its very disappearance, in a process that visually inverts light and darkness (fig. 86): "The weird appearance of 'the City That Was' is accounted for by its having been printed from a positive instead of a negative. It seems to be enfolded in mystery, like a city of palaces and spires."[48] As in Whistler's *Ten O'Clock* lecture, darkness takes the beholder's imagination outside the bounds of reality, in a fantasized space and time. Three years later, Louis J. Stellman, the photographer responsible for that "odd photograph," published *The Vanished Ruin Era,* a collection of photographs accompanied by poems lamenting the "passing of the modern acropolis" of San Francisco, with recurring references to ancient Rome and Greece. In a photograph titled *A Portal of the Past,* Stellman insisted on the antique architecture of a sublime colonnade rising from the rubble, described in the adjacent text as a "phantom doorway,

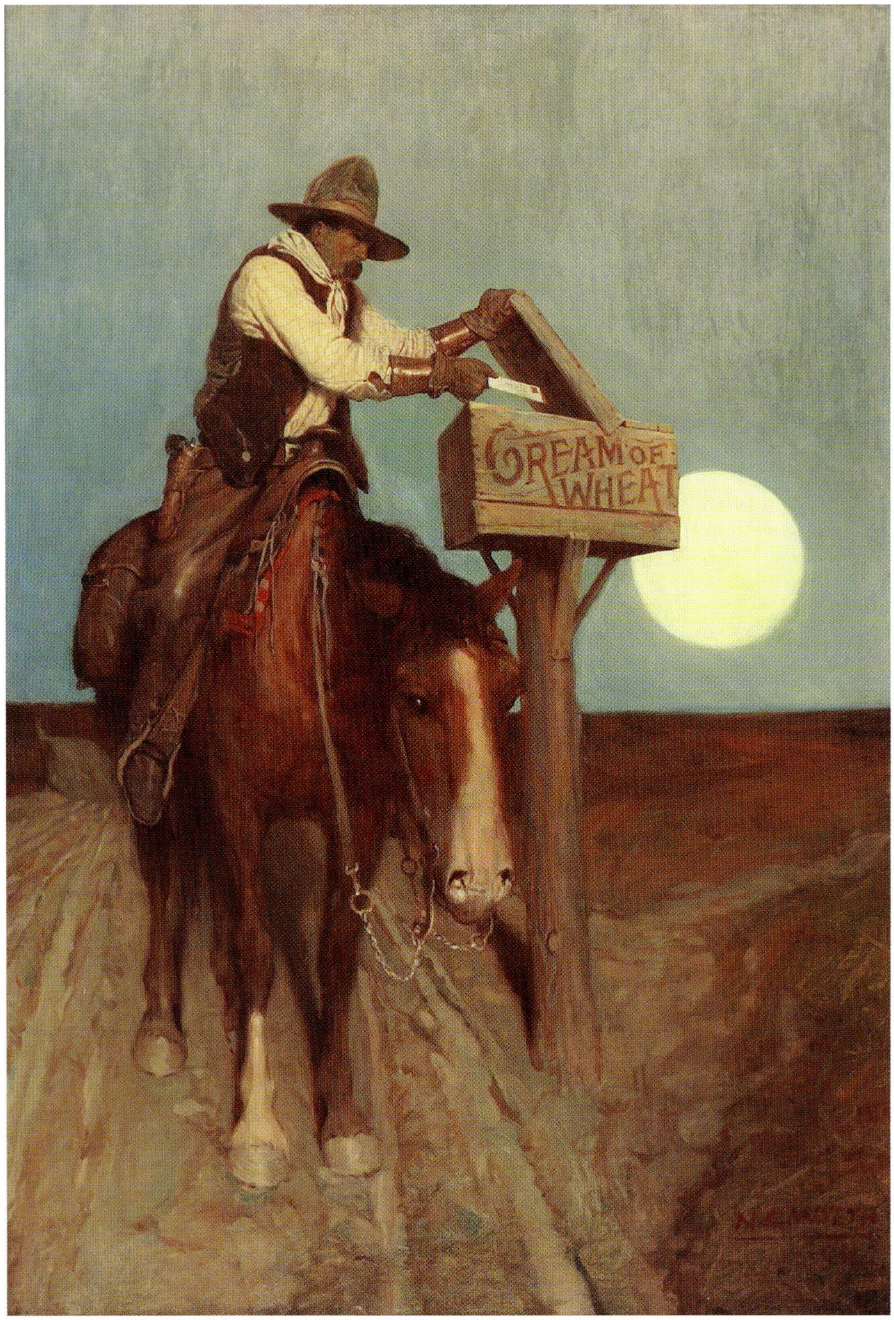

FIG. 85. N. C. Wyeth, *Rural Delivery (Where the Mail Goes, Cream of Wheat Goes)*, 1906. Oil on canvas, 112.4 × 80.96 cm (44 1/4 × 31 7/8 in.). Minneapolis Institute of Art, Gift of the National Biscuit Company (70.63).

giving on the Hall of Memory."[49] In a nocturne with an almost identical composition and title,[50] Peters depicted, between the imposing columns of the peristyle, a few skyscrapers silhouetted against a bay lit by moonlight. Here again, night allowed for anachronistic references, casting a noble aura on modernity. Yet these temporal oscillations also opened up the possibility of complete reversal. Like Cole's *Desolation*, Peters's *Portals of the Past* provides a glimpse of an ambivalent stance: seen through the prism of antiquity, the still-standing modern buildings may embody the triumphant future of American modernity, which can withstand catastrophe; but they may also be a warning, expressing the artist's anxiety about the ambitions of his own civilization, threatened, like its antique models, with decline.

THE RETURNING INDIAN

Cycle and Lineage

That imaginary return by white American civilization to its antique sources was doubly problematic. It was in the ruins, and by means of decay, that white America rediscovered a glorious past. Yet images also revealed inconsistencies in the narratives that described the evolution of civilizations. Kathleen Pyne shows that Herbert

Spencer's success in America lay in his theorization, contra Darwin, of a regular and linear progress. He assured his readers that they embodied the final stage of the evolution of species.[51] But the linearity of civilization's progress coexisted with a more uncertain model, which visualized the rise and decline of civilizations in cyclical terms.[52] Nighttime, a recurrent phase in the cycle dominated by the earth's revolutions, belongs implicitly to that model. According to the critic John Van Dyke, the cycle governs both the spheres of nature and those of culture:

> The circle is indeed nature's great working principle. Organic and inorganic matter—winds, storms, clouds, tides—all display it. . . . Yes, even the planetary system pays allegiance to it; and as the moon circles the earth, so the earth circles the sun, and the sun itself with all its planets, is following a mightier curve. . . . And is the physical or intellectual life of man any exception to the rule? Tribes travel from east to west for ten thousand years, following the track of the sun, until at last they rediscover the cradle of the race—reach the spot from which migration first started; minds build up thought for ages, advancing, as they suppose, until at last they find they are but rediscovering the truths known to the ancients. They have completed the circle, and the circumference is limited.[53]

In this context, we might compare two images that illustrated the notion of civilization (in the sense of both culture and process) in the United States during the nineteenth century. The first, a painting by John Gast that was widely disseminated as a chromolithograph, depicts a gigantic woman, an allegory for the progress of civilization and an emblem of its whiteness and power. Traversing what should be understood as the North American landscape, she moves westward, driving away darkness, Indians, and wild animals all at once, bringing with her the combined enlightenment of technology and education, symbolized, respectively, by the textbook and the telegraph wire she holds in her hand (fig. 87). A quarter of a century later, Edwin Howland Blashfield painted some of the frescoes that adorn the ceilings

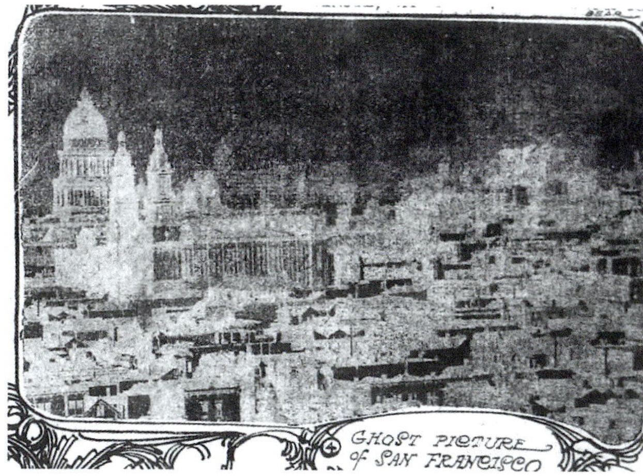

FIG. 86. Louis J. Stellman, "Ghost Picture of San Francisco," *San Francisco Sunday Call*, November 24, 1907.

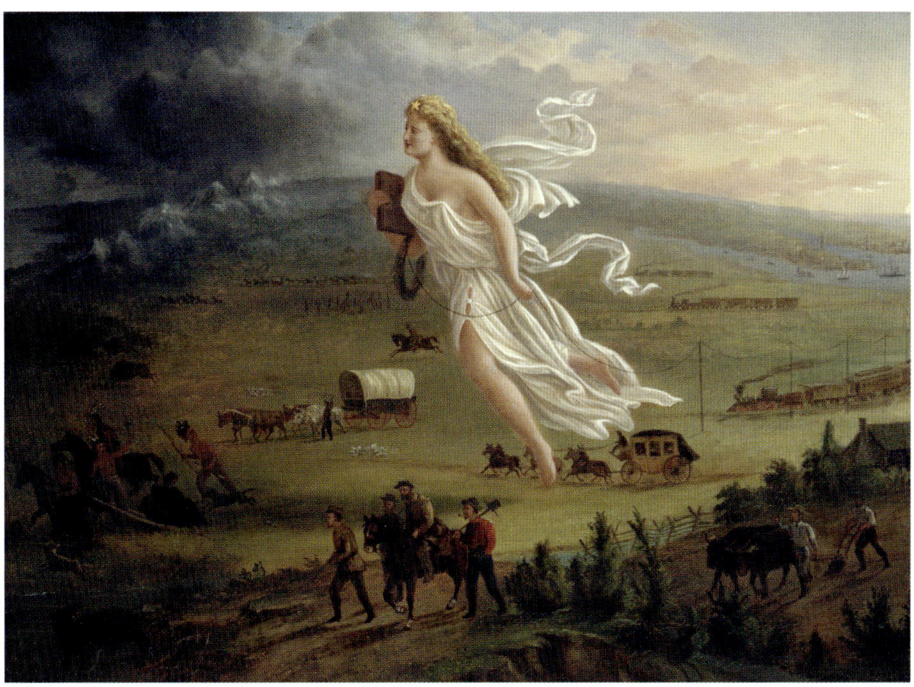

FIG. 87. John Gast, *American Progress*, 1872. Oil on canvas, 45.1 × 54.6 cm (17 3/4 × 21 1/2 in.). Autry Museum, Los Angeles; 92.126.1.

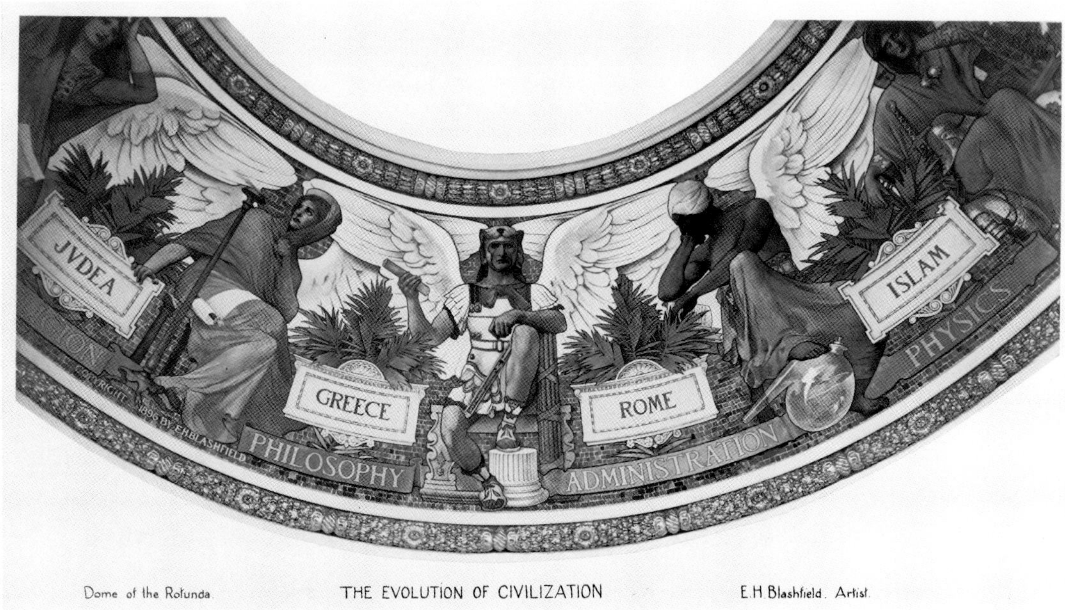

FIG. 88. Edwin Howland Blashfield, *The Evolution of Civilization, Dome of Rotunda*, c. 1896. Photograph. Library of Congress, Prints and Photographs Division, Washington, D.C.

and dome of the rotunda at the Library of Congress in Washington, D.C. Here, civilization takes on a pluralistic cast, personified by allegorical figures whose clothing, ethnic identity, and attributes are diverse (fig. 88). The civilizations thus represented, defined rather freely in terms of religion, era, and country—for example, "Islam" stands beside the "Middle Ages," which is itself next to "Italy"—seem to be arranged in chronological order, beginning with Egypt and Judea and ending with France and America. Blashfield's work represents a progression toward rule by the whitest people, but the very circularity of the fresco suggests that this progress might be a closed circle and that the course of humanity might return to its nonwhite beginnings. The words Henry A. Smith attributed to Chief Seattle in 1887 establish an explicit parallel between the Indian's decline and a decay that might befall white American civilization, a prophecy made all the more poignant by the fact that, at the time it appeared, its purported author—symbol of the vanished Indian—had been dead for several decades: "Tribe follows tribe, and nation follows nation, like the waves of the sea. It is the order of nature, and regret is useless. Your time of decay may be distant, but it will surely come, for even the White Man whose God walked and talked with him as friend to friend, cannot be exempt from the common destiny. We may be brothers after all. We will see."[54]

Significantly, the paradoxical model of the progress of civilization coincided with the temporal ambiguities that shaped the vision of the Indian. Alan Trachtenberg demonstrates that the figure of the Indian was invested with a radically different meaning beginning at the turn of the twentieth century. At a time when Turner was portraying the frontier as a crucible of Americanness, the Indian, formerly the radical "other" of white civilization, became one of the ingredients of a properly American identity: "The policy of forced assimilation that the federal government adopted in the 1880s gave rise to efforts to rehabilitate the alien native as a newly acknowledged precursor, a figure from whom authenticity might be derived for the nation itself."[55] That "alien native" as "newly acknowledged precursor" allowed Americans to, among other things, distinguish themselves from other white civilizations, even as the United States' claims internationally were becoming increasingly insistent.[56] For Theodore Roosevelt, Turner, and most commentators, the strategic redefinition of American racial identity meant affirming an interpretation of the Indian as the first American, dating back to the imaginary "mists of time." For that interpretation to prevail, however, the image of the Indian had to be kept sufficiently visible; and that rhetoric, even as it made him a dark and vanished savage, continued to express astonishment at his survival. Nocturnal imagery thus lent itself to the inclusion of the Indian within the American mythological genealogy, but it was also congruent with the more disturbing idea of his ghostly survival.

Loss and Fusion: Appropriation through Dissolution

At the turn of the twentieth century, American elites, obsessed with their class status and racial identity, dedicated themselves to genealogy or heraldry in clubs named after Saint George or Runnymede, thereby inventing medieval roots for themselves. Such roots supposedly placed them above the rest of the American population, whose origins were becoming increasingly diverse.[57] Popular illustrations, drawing largely on that imaginary conception, also pointed to the need of the white American middle class to return to the mythic sources of white Western culture. But these sources were multiple, and it was also important to find on American soil itself an ancestral lineage that would bestow on the American "race" its letters of nobility. That no doubt explains the success of illustrations that referenced the colonial period and the Revolutionary War, and of Augustus Saint-Gaudens's famous *Puritan* (fig. 89). Standing alongside the heroes of Arthurian legends and of the Revolutionary War was the Indian, transformed into a noble savage for the occasion. The character's new popularity was visible in the enthusiasm with which mainstream culture seized on the figure. Trachtenberg analyzes the example of the monument proposal put forward by Rodman Wanamaker in 1909 to commemorate the "historical" research expeditions conducted by Dixon.[58] A bronze statue, equipped with a beacon and surpassing in size the Statue of Liberty, was to stand opposite it on the shores of Staten Island, thus providing a locally produced pendant to the personification of American democracy inherited from France, motherland of the Enlightenment. As such, the new statue would commemorate the Native Americans, but it would also speak to the rest of the world, Europe in particular. It would indicate by its presence the entrance to the New World, but above all, it would affirm its cultural independence from the Old Continent. That visual language adopted the classic and spare forms of the Indian, a solitary noble savage in the twilight: "As a matter of composition, the architecture, standing on this height against the open sky, should be rugged and large in scale, without too much detail, as it will be seen mostly in silhouette against the sky." Although the monument never materialized, the program for the groundbreaking ceremonies speaks volumes: "Preceding the hoisting of the flag, Dr. Irvin J. Morgan's original Indian Music, 'The Indians requiem,' typifying the 'vanishing race,' specially composed for the Indian lectures resulting from the Wanamaker Historical expeditions, will be rendered. The requiem will follow the raising of the flag until the Stars and Stripes are mastheaded, when the combined military bands will merge into the exultant strains of the 'Star-Spangled Banner,' signifying the union of the first dwellers on the soil with the civilization of our day."[59] Having become the "first American," the Indian, who continued to be portrayed as vanishing, was immediately repatriated by means of symbols of white America. This is suggested by the final orchestration, which united Indians and whites in the same patriotic harmonies.

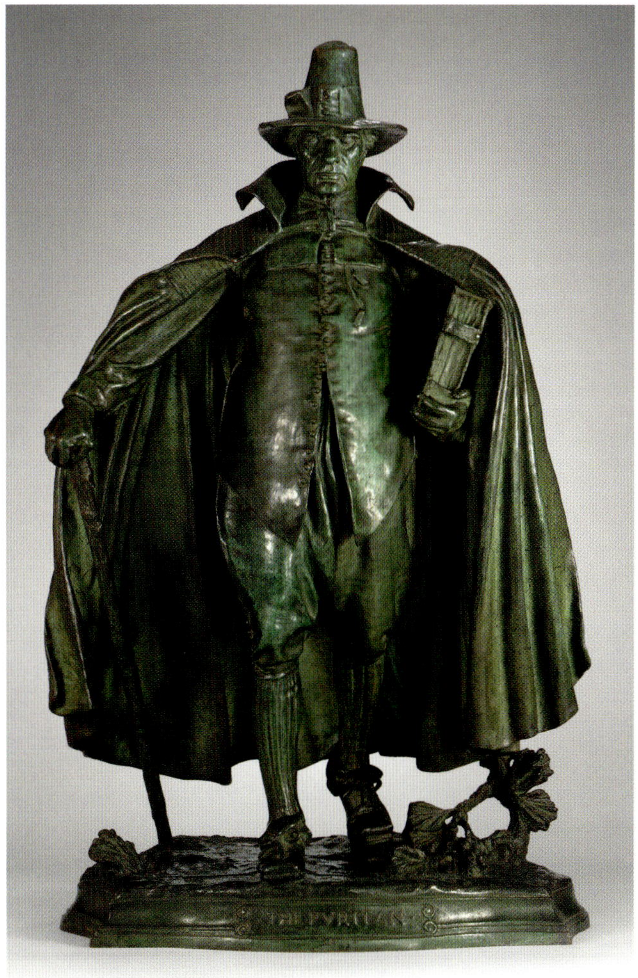

FIG. 89. Augustus Saint-Gaudens, *The Puritan*, 1883–86; this cast, 1899 or after. Bronze, 77.5 × 47 × 33 cm (30 ½ × 18 ½ × 13 in.). Metropolitan Museum of Art, Bequest of Jacob Ruppert, 1939 (39.65.53).

But that noble, light-bearing Indian contrasted with a different image of the "first"—or rather primitive—Indian.[60] Indian mythology raised the interest of white scholars: in 1898, for example, the folklorist Jeremiah Curtin published *Creation Myths of Primitive America*,[61]

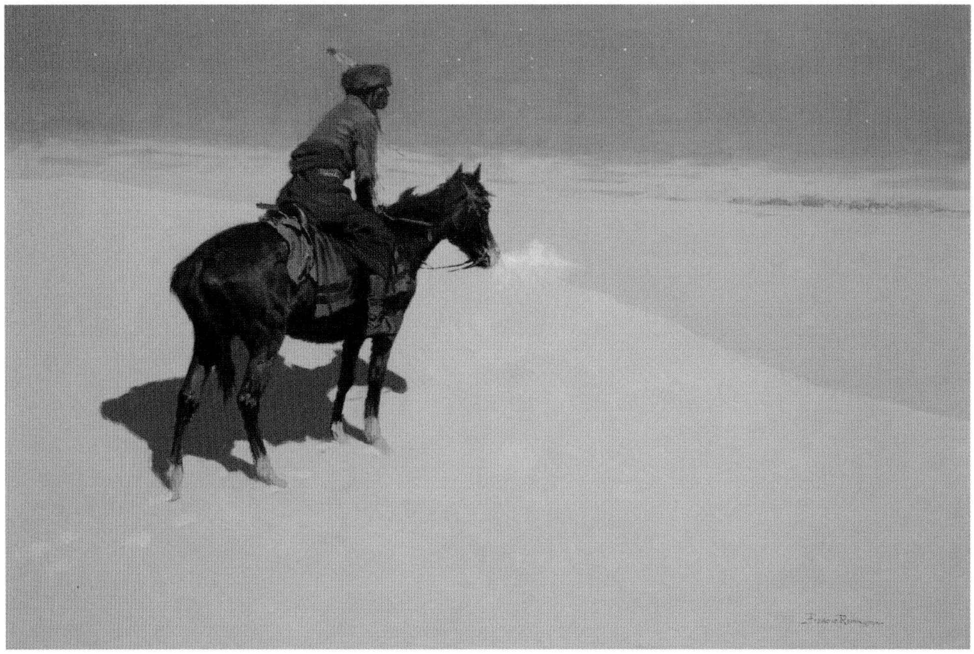

FIG. 90. Frederic Remington, *Friends or Foes? (The Scout)*, 1902–5. Oil on canvas, 68.6 × 101.6 cm (27 × 40 in.). Sterling and Francine Clark Art Institute, Williamstown, Massachusetts (1955.12).

a collection of the cosmogonies of various Indian tribes. Edward S. Curtis inserted these myths into his entries for *The North American Indian.* This entailed, first, clearing away the Indians' immediate history (Curtis announced in the introduction of his book that he would not retrace the history of the crimes that whites had committed against Indians)[62] and retaining only an apolitical image of them. But the interest white Americans showed in that folklore, even as they imagined the Indians to be symbolic ancestors, produced a sort of interweaving of origin stories and identities.

The appropriation of Indian origins translated into images in which darkness facilitated assimilation. Yet, often, the identities and positions of the characters remained equivocal. This is the case with Remington's nocturnes, which increasingly cultivated uncertainty.[63] Take, for instance, his *Friends or Foes? (The Scout):* at first glance, the painting is an inquiry into the nature of a presence that remains invisible to us (fig. 90). The rider's dark complexion, accentuated by the brightness of the snow in moonlight, leaves no doubt that he is an Indian. And the question he seems to be asking himself—is he observing an enemy or an ally?—can be transposed onto his own person: the beholder is implicitly invited to place herself in the environment depicted by Remington and to wonder whether the figure in the painting is himself friendly or hostile. Nancy Anderson, in the catalogue for the exhibition devoted to Remington's nocturnes, shows that the painting *The Stranger* repeats an earlier composition by Remington, except that the figure of the Indian stranger approaching a camp has been replaced by a white man, and day has become night.[64] Anderson attributes the substitution and the general ambiguity surrounding the identity of these figures observed in the night to a shift toward less narrative paintings on the part of Remington. But this blurring of identities is also symptomatic of the general change in attitude toward Indians at the time. Night, particularly because it erases all-too-visible ethnic markers, contributes to that imaginary fusion. The silhouettes of the white man and the Indian on the horizon seem, indeed, almost interchangeable: *The Luckless Hunter* (see fig. 77) repeats, in a slower, more crepuscular tone, the composition of *Against the Sunset,*[65] replacing the frontiersman with an Indian figure, and symbolically merging both shadows in one equivocal identity.

The Specter of the Indian

The form that the nocturne conferred on the Indian, wavering between absence and presence, was consistent with another series of clichés associated with the trope of the vanishing Indian, that of the ghost. In *The National Uncanny: Indian Ghosts and American Subjects,* Renée Bergland shows that the imagery of the ghostly Indian, which she sees as a kind of repression, served to constitute white American identity.[66] According to Bergland, that rhetoric, which transformed Indian subjects into mere specters, corresponded to a program of symbolic extermination, which grew up parallel to and in support of their actual elimination. She insists especially on the ambivalence inherent in that imagery, which she calls "unsuccessful repression."[67] Although her particular object of study is American literature from the first half of the nineteenth century, in the concluding chapter Bergland points out the particular resonance that imagery acquired after the massacre of Wounded Knee in 1890.[68] That massacre put an end to Indian resistance, which in its final years had crystallized around the Ghost Dancers religious movement. The Ghost Dance, popularized by the Paiute prophet Wovoka, combined a messianism inspired by Christianity with traditional Indian ritual practices. Wovoka called on his faithful to live in peace among themselves and announced the rebirth of Indian cultures through the return of the bison and the resurrection of dead Indians, accompanied by the imminent disappearance of whites. The strange complexity of that new religion, its intermingling of Indian and Christian themes, its virulence against whites, and the success of the movement in many Indian tribes caused uneasiness among white Americans, which no doubt contributed to the violence of the Wounded Knee massacre. The Ghost Dance continued to fascinate the white American public long after it had ended: in 1894, for example, the Edison Company devoted one of its first films to the phenomenon, using actors from the Buffalo Bill show to perform the dance.[69] Two years later, the anthropologist James Mooney published a book on the subject.[70] The prophetic conclusion of Chief Seattle's speech took on troubling and crepuscular overtones: "And when the last Red Man shall have perished, and the memory of my tribe shall have become a myth among the White Men, these shores will swarm with the invisible dead of my tribe, and when your children's children think themselves alone in the field, the store, the shop, upon the highway, or in the silence of the pathless woods, they will not be alone. In all the earth there is no place dedicated to solitude. At night when the streets of your cities and villages are silent and you think them deserted, they will throng with the returning hosts that once filled them and still love this beautiful land. The White Man will never be alone."[71] (The fact that these words are almost undoubtedly a forgery composed by a white man only shows the depth of the anxieties whites felt when reflecting on their relationships with Indians.) The white man, whose eye is less sharp than the Indian's, cannot see the magnitude of the haunting he himself has caused. Bergland points out that Wovoko's prophecy derived much of its effectiveness from the myths constructed by whites . Mooney too underscored that affinity in the last section of his book, which established a parallel between the beliefs of the Ghost Dancers and the doctrines of other religions, especially the various Christian churches.[72] In reality, the Ghost Dance embodied an exaggerated and vengeful version of the ghostly Indian invented by whites.

The accounts of Ralph Blakelock's experience in Indian territory illustrate the ambiguous, fanciful perception whites had of Indian cultures. In the case of Blakelock, commentators imagined his travels West as a return of the white man to a primitive and irrational stage, implicitly linking his imaginative gifts, his "eccentric" use of colors, or the "witchery of his genius" at the end of his career to his internment in a psychiatric hospital.[73] In 1914 Elliott Daingerfield commented with a certain uneasiness on Blakelock's picture *The Vision of Life*, better known under the title *The Ghost Dance* (fig. 91). Although he acknowledged the visual ambiguity of that scene, in which the white silhouettes, engulfed in a dark landscape, are difficult to distinguish, Daingerfield strove to reorient the work toward a white aesthetic, alluding to the tropes of the Christian religion and to the Western painting tradition derived from it. In the undifferentiated mass of the composition, he discerned the figures of a woman and a child, which he interpreted as a reference to the Virgin and Christ.[74] The artist's vision remained elusive, however, because Daingerfield interpreted the vague forms as the result of a hesitation, a withheld revelation. It was up to the beholders to complete the painting, "if our eyes are not darkened to all imagination." Here the word "darkened" took on a dual meaning, given that it was precisely through darkness that Blakelock appealed to his beholders' imagination. Above all, in encouraging his readers to see *The Ghost Dance* as a luminous vision full of life, at the center of which he detected a messianic figure in the form of a Virgin and Child, Daingerfield reactivated Wovoka's prophecy in spite of himself.

In the end, whites projected the fantasy of their own spectral fate onto the Indian ghost. In November 1890, at the height of the movement, a reporter from the *Pittsburgh Dispatch* explained that the Ghost Dancers movement was to be understood as a direct threat: "The very motive of the ghost dance is the resurrection of all the braves who have gone to the Great Spirit

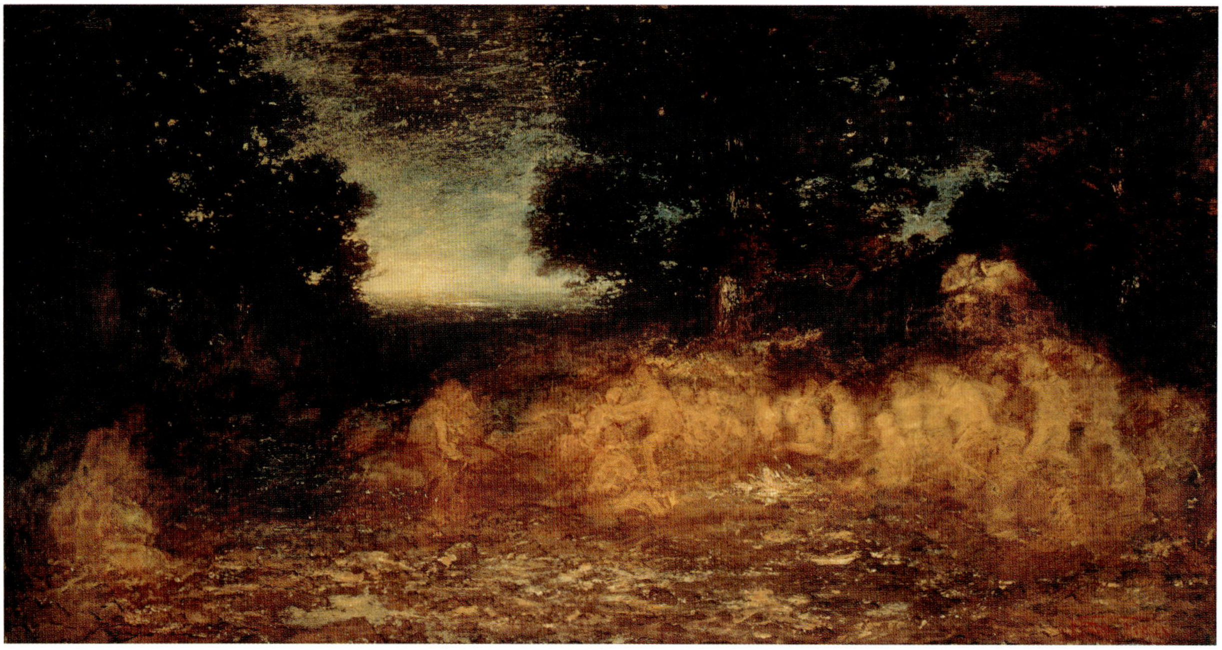

FIG. 91. Ralph Albert Blakelock, *The Vision of Life*, 1895/97. Oil on canvas, 53.7 × 100 cm (21 ⅛ × 39 ⅜ in.). Art Institute of Chicago. Charles H. and Mary F. S. Worcester Collection (1947.55).

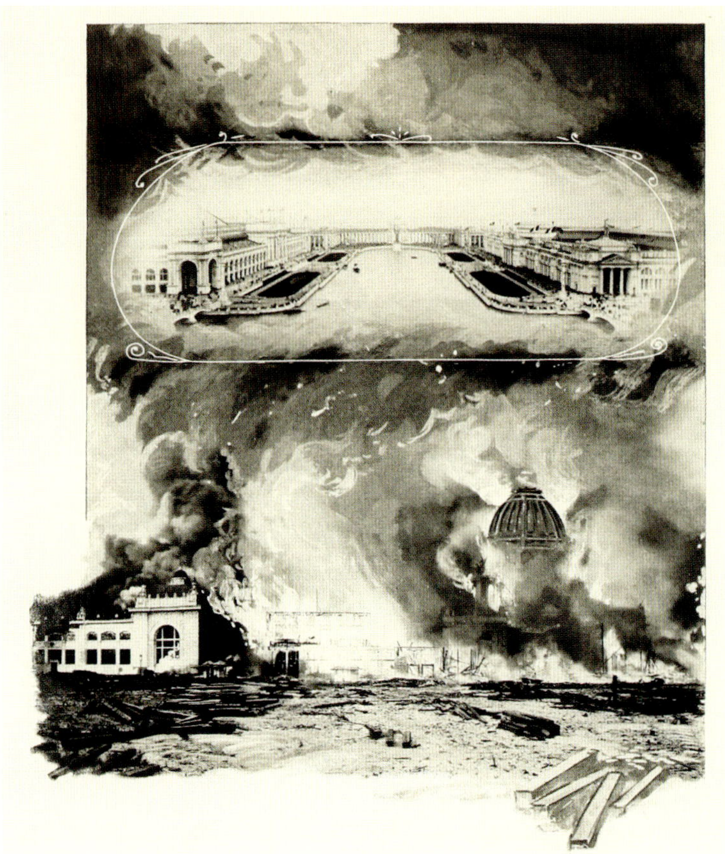

FIG. 92. William and Charles Ottman, "Burning of Administration and Mines Buildings, with Eastern View of Court of Honor and Peristyle," in H. H. Van Meter, *The Vanishing Fair* (Chicago: Literary Art Company, 1894). Library of Congress, Washington, D.C.

since the white man first set foot on American soil and the extermination of the whites."[75] Whites constantly pictured Indians as ghostly presences; in turn, the Indian religious vision threatened to transform whites themselves into ghosts. In a pamphlet published for the World's Columbian Exposition in Chicago, the artist J. A. Mitchell compared the two sorts of Americans, whites and Indians, in a text that revealed both anxiety about the difficulty of defining a white American identity and an ambiguous relationship to the Indian, considered a legitimate presence but immediately repressed with disdain. Mitchell commented on the diverse backgrounds of the Americans who streamed onto the fair's walkways and depicted the viewpoint of a fictive Indian, who, he said, "is the American." "He is the only one among us who had ancestors to be discovered. He is the aboriginal; the first occupant and owner; the only one here with an hereditary right to the country we are celebrating. Perhaps the native realizes this in his own stolid fashion. As he stalks about among the dazzling structures of the Fair, and tries, or more likely, does not try, to grasp the innumerable wonders of art and science that only annoy and confuse him, it may require a too exhausting mental effort to recall the fact that his own grandfather very likely pursued the bounding buffalo over the waste of prairie now covered by the city of Chicago."[76]

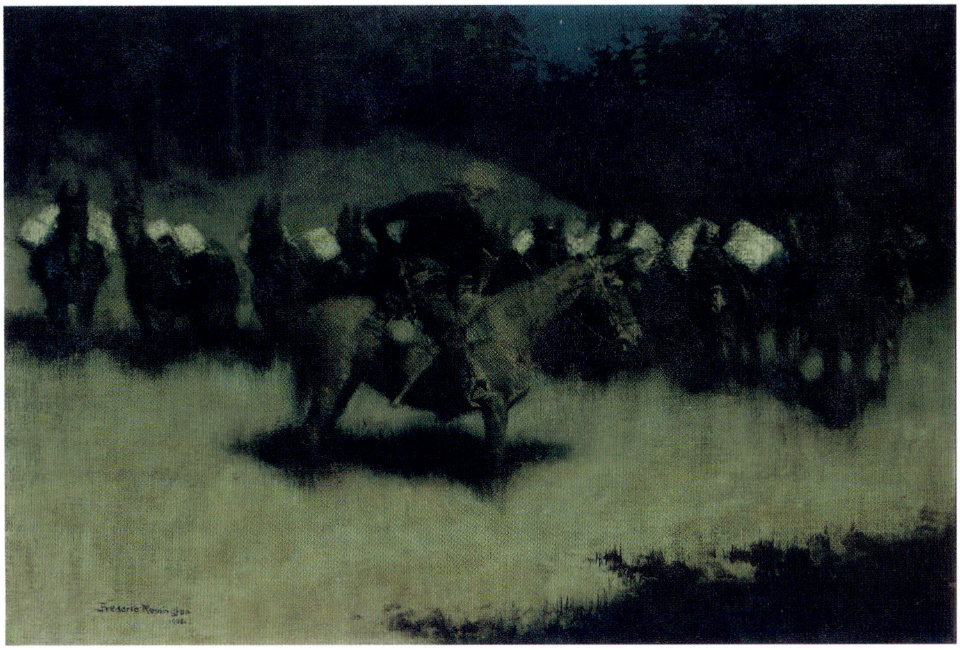

FIG. 93. Frederic Remington, *Scare in a Pack Train*, 1908. Oil on canvas, 68.6 × 101.6 cm (27 × 40 in.). Private collection.

Mitchell's illustration at the beginning of his chapter shows an Indian on horseback, astonished at the site of the White City rising up from the prairie. Although Mitchell undoubtedly wanted to express the Indian's confusion at the fair's "dazzling structures," this Indian, whom he imagined incapable of thought, suggests another possible point of view. The White City, which materialized as if by magic from the marshland of Jackson Park, could also quickly vanish, just as white Americans could be eclipsed by a reaffirmed legitimacy of the Indians. In fact, the fragility of white American civilization was an important underlying theme in publications and commentary on the Columbian Exposition. They focused in particular on the ephemeral nature of the White City. An illustrated pamphlet produced in 1894, after fire destroyed most of the fair's buildings, exploited all the poetry and pathos of that sentiment. *The Vanishing Fair*[77]—an evocative title if ever there was one—laid out almost naively the American white middle class's objects of anxiety, establishing a parallel between images of the fire of the White City's pasteboard buildings (fig. 92) and the blazes set during the Pullman Strike, which shook the city of Chicago a few months after the fair had ended. As social strife seemed to pose the threat of anarchy throughout the city, the white middle and upper classes became conscious of their own fragility. The black activist Frederick Douglass, one of the voices that rose up in 1893 against the authority and legitimacy of the white ideals represented by the Columbian Exposition, appropriated for his own ends the metaphor of the ghost, renaming the White City a "whited sepulchre."[78] The space of the nocturne lent itself particularly well to that reversal of perspective. Frederic Remington's *Scare in a Pack Train* acts, in this regard, as a pendant to Mitchell's Indian. The painter noted in his journal that one of his clients waxed enthusiastic about the work, calling it a "ghost painting" (fig. 93).[79] The rider in moonlight, a figure of white civilization on the lookout for potential assailants, maintains a defensive position guarding a team of horses, whose white packs stand out in the darkness. He watches the shadow seemingly advancing toward him from the lower right-hand corner of the painting. Anxiety persists: Are these ghosts whose presence he perceives? Or is he himself already reduced to a ghostly existence? *Scare in a Pack Train* is representative of the nocturnes of the American West, where the white man looks at himself through the prism of the vanishing Other.

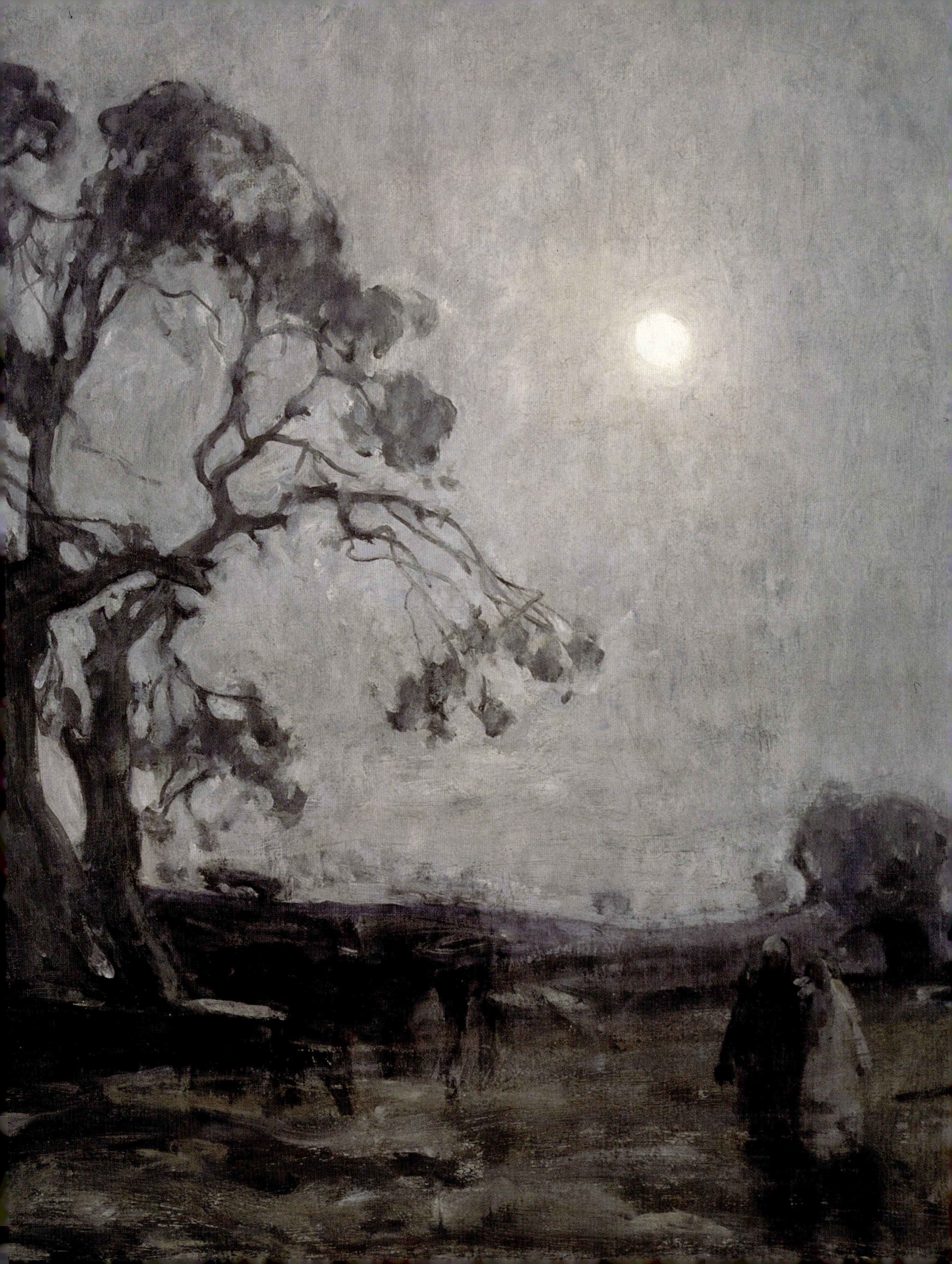

7 A Blueblood Landscape

The Nocturne as White Art in Jim Crow America

The ethnic Other preoccupying American culture during this period was not just the figure of the Indian or the inhabitant of future American colonies. There were also the African Americans, whose status deteriorated dramatically in the late nineteenth century. Amy Kaplan places African Americans at the center of the imperial question, underscoring the continuity between the various colonial conflicts: for instance, the black troops sent to the Cuban and Filipino fronts were recruited from among the Buffalo Soldiers who had participated in the Indian Wars in the late 1880s and the early 1890s.[1] Although the white racist point of view formed the thread connecting African Americans to Indians, Cubans, and Filipinos, and though the metaphor of darkness extended to all these groups, major differences persisted. Unlike the Filipinos and Cubans, African Americans were not a remote and largely imagined presence, and, unlike the Indians, they did not seem to belong to a bygone or vanishing era. That may explain the silence about them in the art of the nocturne. Thomas Eakins and Winslow Homer occasionally painted genre scenes of African American life, but these subjects constituted a relatively marginal subcategory within the canon of late nineteenth-century American art. In visual culture, African Americans appeared more often in racist caricatures.[2] The nocturne provides almost no explicit examples of blacks' presence, and though indirect allusions can be detected, the connections are obscured. For that reason, the racial connotations of nocturnes can only be considered hypothetically. The importance of the race question at the time in the United States cannot be denied, however: the memory of the Civil War was still alive, and Jim Crow laws were undoing in their entirety the political gains achieved upon emancipation. After 1901, the restrictions imposed on black suffrage ultimately ousted every African American member of Congress, and that body would remain entirely white until 1929.[3] Not only did African Americans lose their rights, but in the Southern states racial segregation was set in place. Its legality was confirmed by the Supreme Court's 1896 ruling in *Plessy v. Ferguson*. And, adding to the ordinary violence of segregation were lynchings, which killed thousands of African Americans. In 1919 the National Association for the Advancement of Colored People (NAACP) published a damning report, which listed 3,224 deaths by lynching, including those of 2,522 blacks, between 1889 and 1918.[4]

Fig. 104 detail

Although lynchings continued until the late 1960s, the turn of the twentieth century was notable for the intensity of their violence and for their number.

That context of racial tensions found expression in the visual culture of the period. In 1903 W. E. B. Du Bois announced that the "color line" was *the* problem of the twentieth century.[5] The notion of a color line was the first in a series of metaphors by which the paradoxes of visibility and invisibility, brightness and darkness, came into sharper relief. For Du Bois as for racist whites, the question of racial difference was raised first in visual terms, whether that consisted of making visible the blacks hidden by a segregated culture or, conversely, of unmasking an individual's ethnic identity and exaggerating the contrast between whites and blacks. Popular racist imagery, in repeatedly linking African Americans to night and invisibility, revealed these preoccupations: while wishing to relegate African Americans to the most profound darkness, these illustrations manifested a certain uneasiness about the stability of racial identities. The "color line" between light and dark, repeatedly thematized in visual and textual culture, was in reality not so simple: slippages, overlaps, and reversals accumulated, forming a complex network of meanings. An equivalence between skin pigment and the dark of night would seem to be too predictable and crude for nocturne artists to have made use of it. But it also appears unlikely that they could have been unaware of the symbolic charge of nighttime. As Toni Morrison argues, "invisible things are not necessarily 'not-there'"[6] and the African American presence sometimes manifested itself implicitly. Although the nocturne did not speak of black people, its silence can be interpreted as a discourse in its own right, whose avoidance strategies are themselves telling.

"ONE DROP OF NEGRO BLOOD"

Henry Ossawa Tanner, the only African American painter among the nocturne artists, exemplified, both in his career as an artist and in his art, the multiple displacements through which the nocturne both incorporated and rejected the African American presence. In the first place, the painter chose exile in Paris, where he could practice his art shielded from racial prejudice: "In Paris . . . no one regards me curiously. I am simply 'M. Tanner, an American artist.' Nobody knows nor cares what was the complexion of my forbears. I live and work there on terms of absolute social equality. Questions of race or color are not considered—a man's professional skill and social qualities are fairly and ungrudgingly recognized."[7] Tanner rightly voiced his objections to the racial prejudices that hampered his career in the United States, initially in his reply to Eunice Tietjens, when she declared his palette of blues ill-suited to his ethnic identity. The artist's reaction was directed against the entire system for defining race in force at the time in the United States: "Now am I a Negro? Does not the 3/4 of English blood in my veins, which when it flowed in 'pure' Anglo-Saxon men and which has done in the past effective and distinguished work in the U.S.—does this not count for anything? Does the 1/4 or 1/8 of 'pure' Negro blood in my veins count for all? I believe it, the Negro blood counts and counts to my advantage—though it has caused me at times a life of great humiliation and sorrow—that it is the source of all my talents (if I have any) I do not believe, any more than I believe it all comes from my English ancestors. I suppose according to the distorted way things are seen in the States my blond curly-headed little boy would also be 'Negro.'"[8] The measures to which Tanner was referring concerned the so-called "one-drop rule."[9] The theory, commonly accepted but implicit in the nineteenth century, was made official by *Plessy v. Ferguson*, which denied Homer Plessy the right to travel in whites-only railroad compartments in Louisiana, despite the fact that he had only one black great-grandparent and could pass for white. Tanner found himself in a similar situation. The newspaper articles devoted to him after his success at the Paris salons continually remarked on his light complexion: "In his personality there is little or no trace nor suggestion of African ancestry. His clear, gray eyes are of the Aryan type; his complexion is a clear white, bronzed by the sun in an active outdoor life. His features are of the classic Roman mold, his carriage, attire and manner that of the modern Parisian. His thick, dark, curly hair, brushed carelessly back from a fair, broad brow, suggests the southern Latin races rather than types of tropical origin."[10] Another reporter wrote, "This young man belongs to that race of which the great novelist, Dumas, was the glory; he is a mulatto. Beard and hair are crinkly; his regular, thin and handsome features are yellow."[11] These descriptions oscillated between the desire to pin down the individual by attributing an ethnic identity to him (putting to use a vocabulary drawn from the racist pseudosciences of the time) and the need to justify Tanner's extraordinary career by pointing to the complexity of his ethnic origins, listing his affinities with prestigious personalities and cultures.

Tanner's reaction to Tietjens's article was itself complex, a sign of the difficulties he had with the fallacious logic of racial classification. Tanner first noted the contradictions of the one-drop rule and, insisting ironically on how the proportion of black and white blood was measured, highlighted the absurdity of a principle that purported to be grounded in scientific reasoning. As Alan Braddock points out, Tanner placed the words "pure" and "Negro" in scare quotes, manifesting thereby his refusal to adhere to the simplistic categorization they were supposed to determine.[12] Above all, Tanner insisted—like the reporters who described him for their readers—on physical appearances, which contradicted the so-called biological truth determined by the one-drop rule. From that standpoint, he paradoxically conformed to the racist attitude of most of his contemporaries, displaying a certain ambivalence. Tanner's letter to Tietjens continued with an anecdote about the French government's purchase of his painting *The Raising of Lazarus:* "It was telegraphed to the States 'A Negro sells picture to the French government.' Now a paper in Baltimore wanted a photo of this 'Negro.' Of course they had none. So out they go and photograph the first dock hand they come across, and it looked like maybe some of my distant ancestors when they once came from Africa."[13] Here, Tanner distanced himself from the white reporters steeped in prejudices, but also from the African American dockhand, whom he seemed to consider with equal disdain. In Tanner's words, the dockhand, by his skin color or occupation, was symbolically assimilated to the human cargo of slave ships, freshly disembarked on American soil. Tanner reproduced whites' racist contempt by insisting on the inferiority of that laborer at Baltimore Harbor, an inferiority marked as much by his social situation and his location as by the color of his skin.

Tanner's need to distinguish himself by using exactly the same racist criteria from which he had suffered attests to the obsession at the time with the (in)visible dimension of race, which the incoherence of the *Plessy v. Ferguson* ruling only underscored. Tanner not only disputed the clear division between "whites" and "blacks"; he also condemned the contradictory attitude of whites, who, while constantly scrutinizing individuals for ethnic markers, refused to see distinctions within each of the two categories. The hit song "All Coons Look Alike to Me," though supposedly in the voice of a black woman, was in reality complicitous with a point of view shared by whites (fig. 94). That consigning of all blacks to a uniform darkness concealed the uneasiness of whites when confronted with a more dangerous confusion between "whites" and "blacks." Indeed, blackness appears to have been an elusive quality more than a stable criterion. Here again, there were multiple reversals: advertisements for Ivory soap, which organized their entire rhetoric around the theme of whiteness, praised the soap for being 99.44 percent "pure" (fig. 95). On its own terms, the slogan called into question the soap's declared purity: What about the minuscule proportion left over? Would "one drop" of impurity suffice to compromise the whole? At the other end of the spectrum, an advertisement for a hair straightener urged readers of *Colored American* to "be not deceived," reinvesting with commercial meaning a formulation that could be addressed to whites anxious about the possibility of being "deceived" by a black passing for white (fig. 96).[14] In that context, the dark of night made the distinction even more difficult. Darkness made the Other, whose appearance could no longer be studied altogether reliably, doubly invisible and indiscernible. That, for example, is indicated by the rhymes and metonymic slippage of meaning that drove popular racist songs. Many of them systematically emphasized the stereotypical association between African Americans and the night—for example, "The Man in the Moon Is a Coon"[15]—but also the awkward feelings elicited by that association. "The Moon, the Coon, and the Little Octoroon" declares in its first verse: "A yaller moon, a dusky coon, it ain't no good combination."[16] The illustration on the cover of the sheet music for "Appearances Dey Seems to Be Against Me" shows a black character caught stealing chickens by a white farmer in the middle of the night (fig. 97). The title of the song has its own irony: appearances were (and still are), by definition, always against African Americans from the start. Although the image depicts a comic scene in which the black figure is unmasked, it also betrays a malaise, further reinforced by the innocence that the thief feigns without great conviction.

Theories of evolution contributed to that uneasiness, by suggesting to whites concerned about genealogy that they might have black ancestors. "Désirée's Baby," a short story by Kate Chopin published in 1893, taps into that anxiety. The blackness of the child to which Désirée gave birth is not, as the young mother is led to believe, the

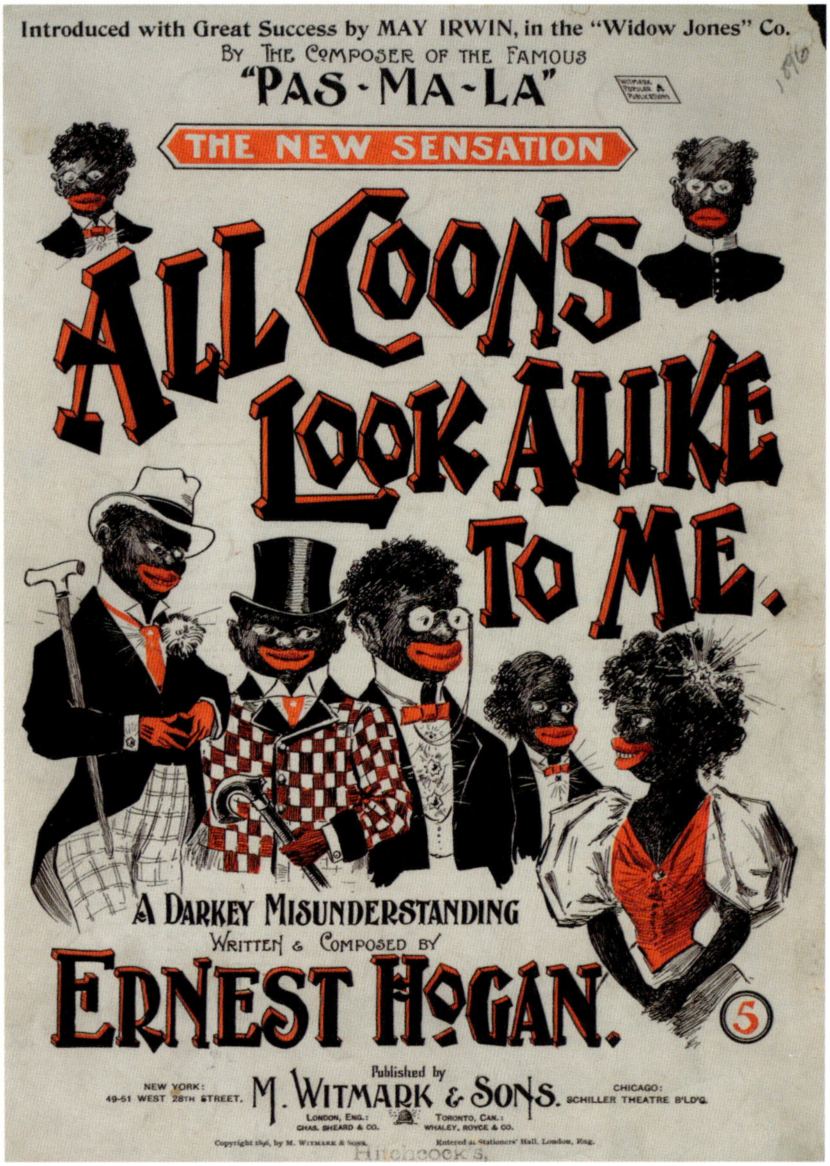

FIG. 94. *All Coons Look Alike to Me,* 1896. Musical score cover (music and lyrics by Ernest Hogan), New York, Witmark and Sons. Music Division, New York Public Library for the Performing Arts, Astor, Lenox and Tilden Foundations.

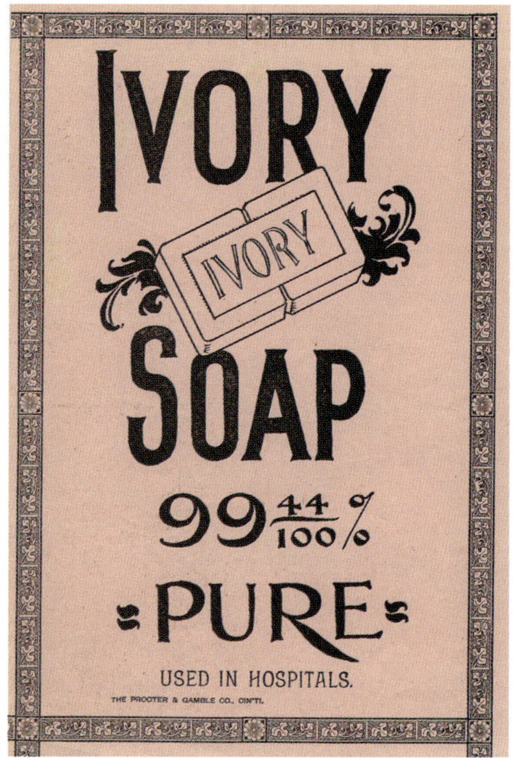

FIG. 95. "Ivory Soap, 99 44/100% Pure," c. 1890–1910. Advertisement, 19 × 12.5 cm (7½ × 4 15/16 in.). Ivory Soap Collection, Archives Center, National Museum of American History, Smithsonian Institution, Warshaw Collection of Business Americana, Washington, D.C.

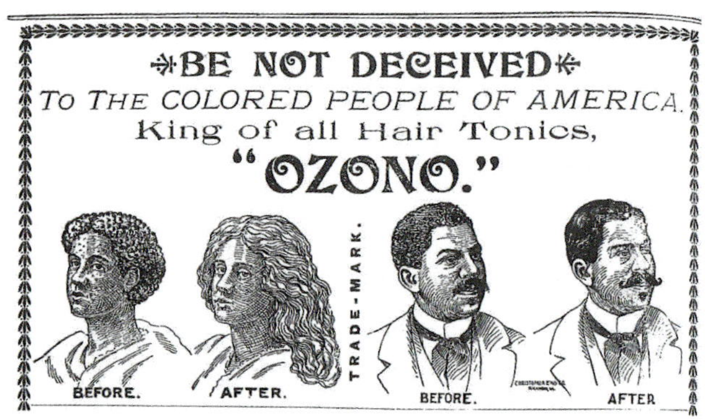

FIG. 96. Ozono, "Be Not Deceived," 1900, *Colored American,* November 10, 1900.

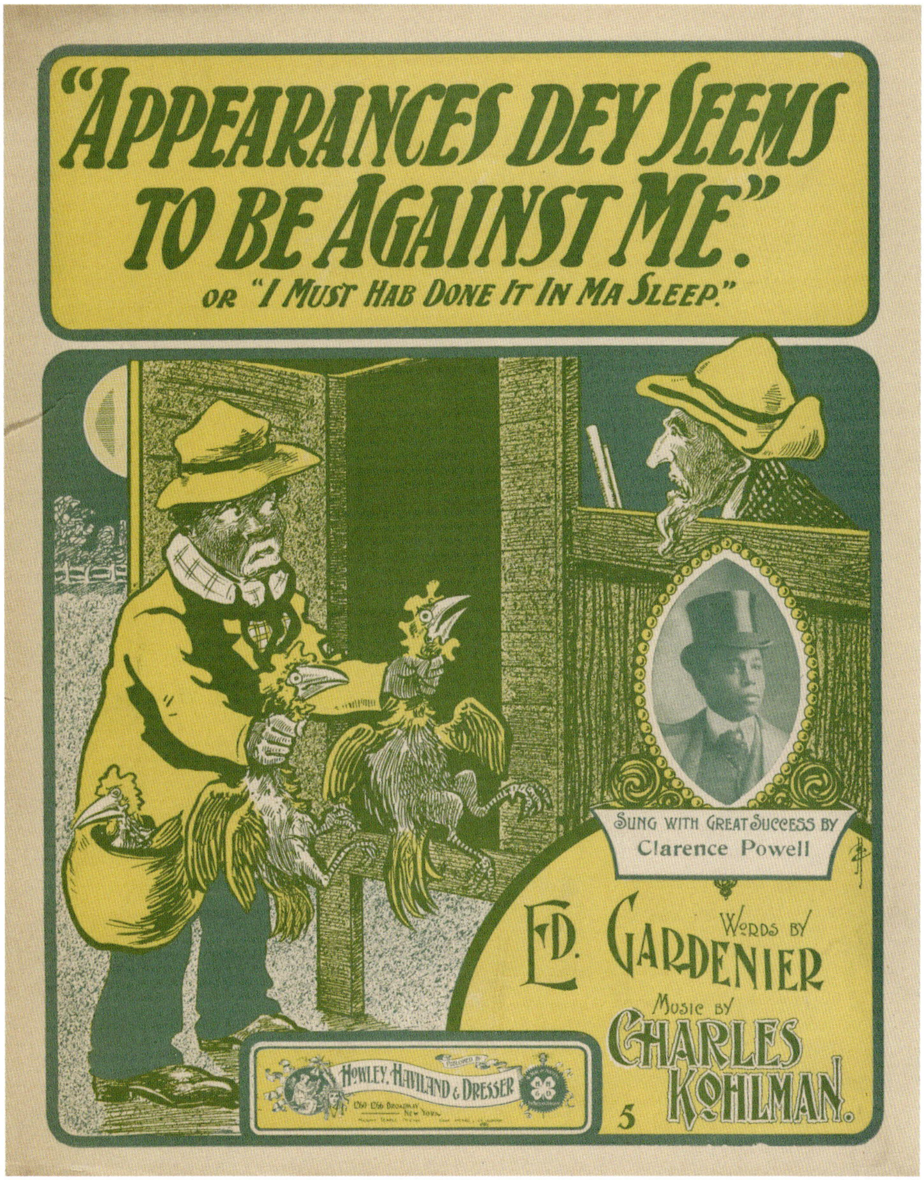

FIG. 97. *Appearances Dey Seems to Be Against Me or I Must Hab Done It in Ma Sleep,* 1901. Musical score cover (words by Ed. Gardiner, music by Charles Kohlman), Chicago, Howley, Haviland & Dresser/Maurice Richmond Music Co. Music Division, New York Public Library for the Performing Arts, Astor, Lenox and Tilden Foundations.

result of her own ancestry, which remains unknown. The end of the short story reveals the African genealogy of an elderly, remote, and concealed figure, the mother of her husband, Armand Aubigny.[17] When Kate Chopin's short story appeared, the idea was spreading that whites' ancestors could have been dark-skinned and that they might represent a primitive state of humanity, might even be the "missing link" between apes and human beings. For example, the racist theorist Madison Grant, ten years before publishing *The Passing of the Great Race,* in which he worried about the future of the "Nordic" race, put the Congolese pygmy Ota Benga on display in a section of the Bronx Zoo. Caged alongside chimpanzees and orangutans, Ota Benga was labeled "Missing Link."[18] The *Literary Digest* warily debated the genealogy question: "While some would have us believe that primitive man was fair-complexioned, there seem no less cogent reasons for maintaining that his skin was of a darker tint. It is not necessary for us to accept the extreme position, and thereby assume that he was black. A middle course is open, as suggested by Dr. A. R. Wallace, who advances the view that primitive man was probably of mongoloid stock, and that his subsequent modification into the white, and brown, and black varieties was due to his migrations into geographical areas where he was subjected to the influence of varied conditions and climates."[19] Although the reporter held out the possibility that we need not accept the "extreme position" of certain scientists but may rather choose a "middle course," he was forced to acknowledge the biological continuity between whites and blacks. Their skin color resulted from a single pigment, whose quantity increased or decreased depending on the environment. In addition to that troubling revelation, there was the even more disturbing possibility that the appearance of individuals could be altered, especially by means of electric technology, itself obscure and invisible. Another article from an 1899 issue of the *Literary Digest,* for example, examined the capacity of electricity to erase marks on the skin and pigmentation: "These facts are perhaps not easily explained, but they are undeniable, and although the laws that govern them remain hidden in obscurity they none the less manifest themselves by visible and tangible effects, one of the most common of which is decoloration." The reporter averred that "it is neither impossible nor even improbable that electricity acts on the pigment." He nevertheless reminded his readers that these theoretical speculations were far from being put into practice and concluded, reassuringly, that blacks might in reality prefer to remain as they were.[20] These debates about racial identity and its possible evolution, about the definition of ethnic categories and their permeability, show how the efforts by whites to maintain strict segregation between ethnic groups were undermined by contradictions. The clarity of the boundary between whites and blacks was called into question on a daily basis, making way for a series of ambiguous cases. For Tanner, night served as a space of negotiation, offering a visual form supple enough to accommodate an entire set of identities.

OVERLAPPING IDENTITIES

Although Tanner's genre scenes of African American life had already assured the artist a certain success at the start of his career, in the 1890s he displaced the center of gravity of his art, devoting himself to religious painting. But if he conspicuously avoided subjects focused on the question of ethnic identity, he did so only to return to them by roundabout means, which may have offered him more freedom. Several art historians have put forward racial readings of Tanner's religious paintings. Dewey Mosby suggests we understand his works as parables in the manner of gospel songs, whose religious themes actually conceal subversive reflections on the African American condition. For example, Mosby interprets *Nicodemus* (fig. 98) as a reference to the clandestine nocturnal religious practices of slaves before emancipation, and *The Raising of Lazarus* as a parable of emancipation itself, arguing that Lazarus's features are reminiscent of Abraham Lincoln's.[21] Alan Braddock links that formal ambiguity to Tanner's complex position as a light-skinned black in exile in France.[22] That reading takes the interpretation beyond parable and allegory, to reveal on the canvas itself Tanner's project for a utopia of "perfect race democracy."[23] Braddock focuses his analysis on the figure of Christ, explaining that it reflects an effort at a racially mixed representation, its aim being a sort of ethnic universality. He links several paintings, in which Jesus' ethnic identity is visually undefinable, to theories of the time that Christ may have belonged to a black race.

Braddock's analysis can be extended to Tanner's oeuvre as a whole. Characters whose faces are immersed in shadow appear repeatedly in his paintings: in addition to *Nicodemus Visiting Jesus,* there is *Daniel in the Lions' Den* (fig. 99), whose motif is replicated in almost identical form in two different paintings, and *Salomé* (see fig. 62), whose racial ambiguity I have already pointed out. In each of these paintings, the character stands in a space of contrasting light, which sets up an opposition between brightly illuminated clothing and a face concealed in darkness. *Daniel in the Lions' Den* provides the most striking example of Tanner's formal play with light and shadow. The prophet is depicted standing in a dark room, sunlight streaming through square openings in the ceiling. Here, as in his *Annunciation,* Tanner gave a luminous but stylized form to the divine presence: just as the archangel Gabriel is incarnated as a vertical beam of light in the *Annunciation,* the projected light is an incarnation of the divine presence that protects Daniel from the lions. The chiaroscuro effect presents narrative elements that can be interpreted in two different ways. The dazzling light carves out very regular geometrical shapes in the darkness, drawing a square on the ground and extending out into a triangle, whose far corner covers Daniel's bound wrists. This detail emphasizes his imprisonment but at the same time indicates the miraculous reversal of his imminent freedom. As Mosby shows, the prophet exiled to Babylon, then unjustly imprisoned, symbolizes as well the fate of African Americans held in bondage and oppressed by Jim Crow laws. Daniel was in fact one of the biblical figures most often cited in Negro spirituals, which almost systematically reinterpreted the gospels in contemporary terms. One of the most famous established an explicit analogy, asking, "Didn't my Lord deliver Daniel? An' why not-a every man?"[24] In choosing that highly symbolic figure, Tanner situated himself within the African American religious tradition. And, in covering Daniel's face with a veil of shadow, he maintained uncertainty over the figure's ethnic identity: immersed in that equivocal darkness, Daniel personifies both the biblical prophet and the African American.

That overlapping of identities is also reminiscent of a cultural practice common in Tanner's time, that of blackface in minstrel shows, when white actors played stereotypical black characters such as Jim Crow, who gave his name to the era. Although the practice is now denounced for its racism, the legacy of blackface is two-sided: the minstrel shows also represented and disseminated to the rest of society certain elements of African American culture, especially dance and music. W. T. Lhamon Jr. points out the complexity and internal contradictions that drove the phenomenon, which he considers a field contested by several sociocultural groups with conflicting agendas: "Blackface performance became a social rite that elites wanted to harness and gradually did. What had begun as a way of registering cross-racial charisma and union then became *also* a way of registering racial separation and disdain. As a maturing cultural form, blackface places into compact tension, at once, both charisma and disdain, in a continually adjusting but never completely erasing process. The meanings pile up."[25] In the three paintings considered here, the spectacular effects of light projected onto the human figures, like footlights onto a darkened stage, bring to mind the theatrical context of minstrel shows, here oddly incorporated into the

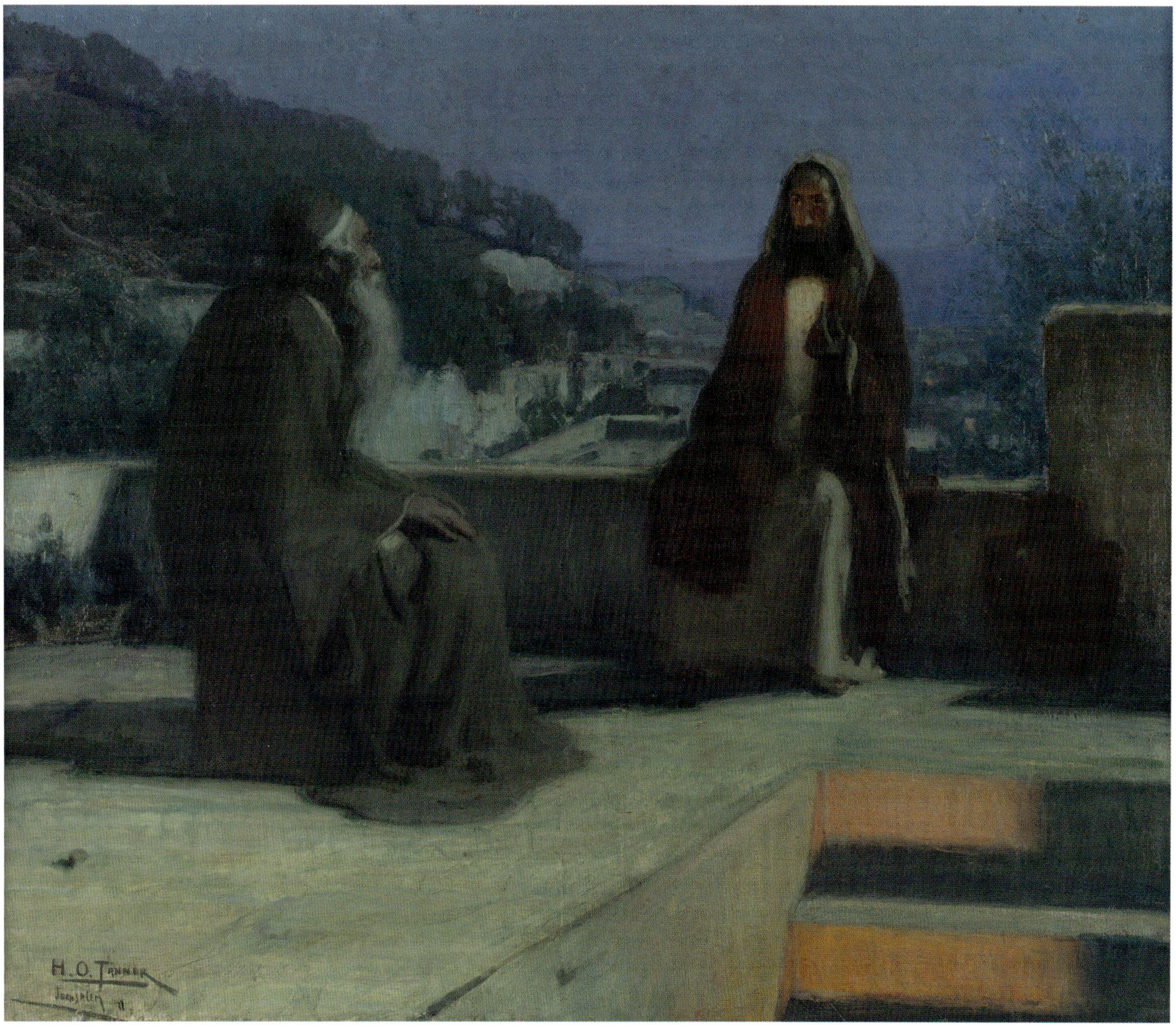

FIG. 98. Henry Ossawa Tanner, *Nicodemus*, 1899. Oil on canvas, 85.6 × 100.3 cm (33 11/16 × 39 1/2 in.). Courtesy of the Pennsylvania Academy of the Fine Arts, Philadelphia. Joseph E. Temple Fund (1900.1).

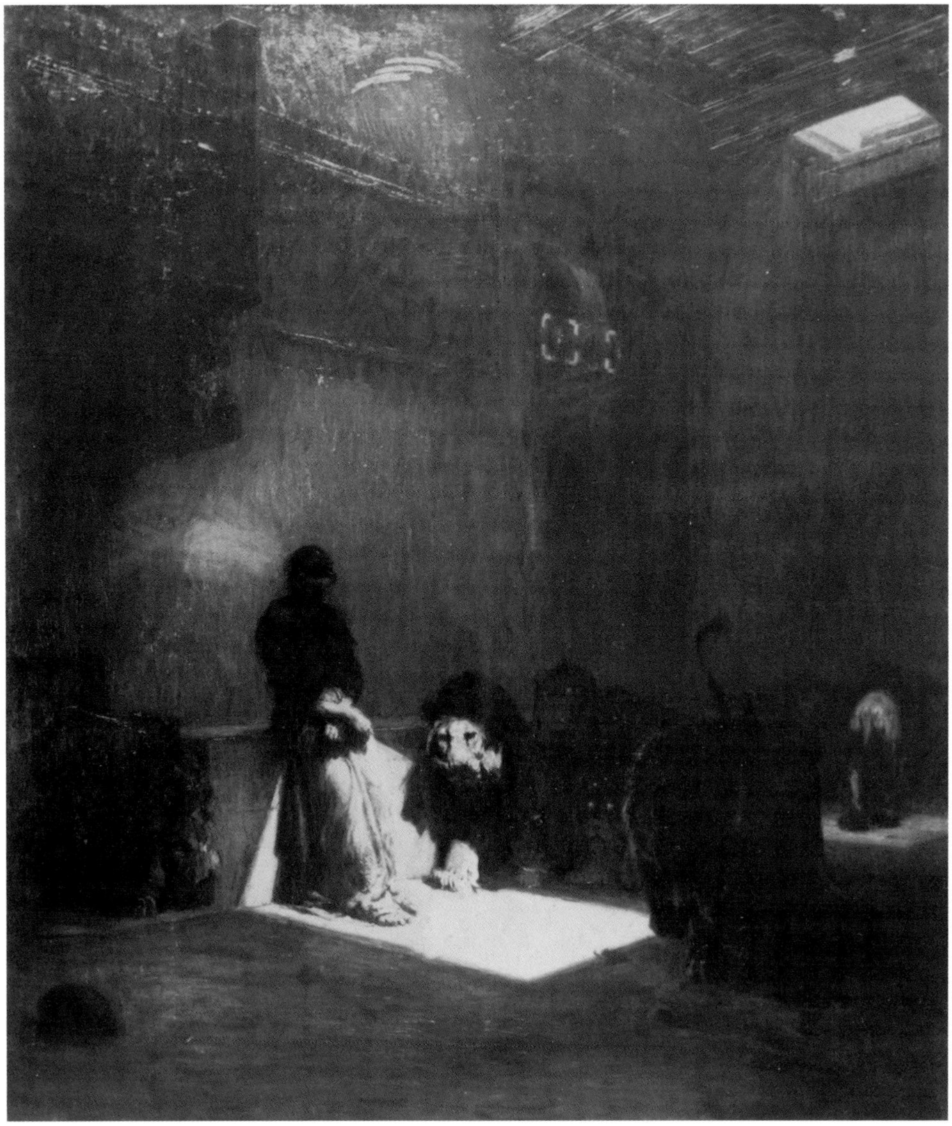

FIG. 99. Unknown photographer, *Daniel in the Lions' Den,* by Henry Ossawa Tanner. Courtesy of the Pennsylvania Academy of the Fine Arts, Philadelphia. Dorothy and Kenneth Woodcock Archives.

religious paintings of the gospels. Further complicating that juxtaposition is the fact that Tanner used the night to reappropriate a genre invented by whites: Jesus, Daniel, and Salomé would thus all appear to possess a dual identity, each side seemingly unable to overshadow the other completely. Although the contrasts are stark in appearance, the definition of identities proves to be as changeable as the variations between shadow and light.

"SPECTACULAR SECRETS": THE NOCTURNE AND NIGHTS OF LYNCHING

The twists and possible interpretations accumulate, however, beyond blackface itself. Tanner, in painting *Salomé* (see fig. 62), projected the shadow of lynching onto the biblical figure. At Salomé's feet, the artist painted, by way of contrast, the head of John the Baptist. The formless mass enveloped in a yellowed piece of cloth is indicated with just a few brushstrokes, but its color is evocative. Dark brown tones mingling with the bloody red can be made out, which suggest that the skin of the beheaded prophet was dark. The story of Salomé resonated with news events of the day. It was the desire aroused by that overexposed female body that, in a triangular relationship, motivated King Herod's murderous act. Likewise, a large proportion of the victims of lynching were black men accused of having raped or merely desired a white woman. Tanner, in juxtaposing that phantasmal (female and white) body with the image, blurry but with a solid presence, of a mutilated (male and black) body, rendered silently present a bloody reality that affected him personally as an African American. But here, as in blackface, contemporary history was told only through masks and indirections.

Lynching, a spectacular outburst of racial violence, was one of the most prominent elements of visual culture that addressed relations between whites and blacks in the United States. That practice, which often took place at night, was, like nocturnal landscape painting, dominated by strong tensions between visibility and invisibility. It turned the unwatchable into a spectacle, which was then disseminated through images circulating in secret. Lynching was widely documented by amateur photographers,[26] especially on photo cards—photographs printed on postcards, which were then mailed by their creators. The 1912 ban on circulating images of lynching in the photo card format only confirms their power of fascination and the scope of their diffusion; and the presence of photo cards created after that date in photographic archives demonstrates the strength and persistence of the phenomenon. These violent images, in which gangs of white onlookers gathered together around the mutilated bodies of their victims, smiling and winking at the camera, seem very remote from the refined and detached aesthetic of the nocturnes. Nevertheless, they combined this aggressive hypervisibility with a form of invisibility. The historian Jacqueline Goldsby links lynching to a sensationalist visual culture, while pointing out how its representations paradoxically omitted the violence. In the first place, because these images, created by and for the use of individuals who are now unknown to us, circulated in great volume but somewhat discreetly, they created a kind of secret society.[27] Photographs of lynching, a spectacle both impossible to ignore and impossible to watch, cultivated a conundrum somewhat similar to the absence-presence of the Indian in Curtis's and Dixon's photographs, elusive but still visible.

The culture of lynching corresponded to a visual regime halfway between the explicit and the implicit. For example, in "The Monster," a novella published in *Harper's Magazine* in 1898, Stephen Crane tells the story of a black man caught between invisibility and monstrous hypervisibility.[28] The text recounts what appears to be a symbolic lynching in reverse, in which the black character, Henry Johnson, is punished by the community in the small town of Whilomville for having performed a good deed, the rescue of the white son of his employer, Dr. Trescott, from a house fire. Henry emerges from the accident disfigured and insane, which leads all the residents of Whilomville, blacks and whites together, to reject him. The rescue scene, which places Henry in the middle of the conflagration, clearly evokes a lynching. Consider the description of the flames engulfing the house: "After a moment the window brightened as if the four panes of it had been stained with blood, and a quick ear might have been led to imagine the fire-imps calling and calling, clan joining clan, gathering to the colors. From the street, however, the house maintained its dark quiet, insisting to a passer-by that it was the safe dwelling of people who chose to retire early to tranquil dreams. No one could have heard this low droning of the gathering clans."[29] That gathering of "clans," luminous in the darkness but invisible to the passersby outside, is somewhat suggestive of the acts of arson committed at night by the Ku Klux Klan, called the "invisible empire" by its members.[30] Henry, who survives the fire disfigured, becomes a "monster," a visual contradiction, as he is by definition seen by all but unbearable to look at. The novella can be read as a parable: Henry, a man whose features have turned into indistinguishable ugliness to most, and whom most consider unable to think rationally, is unjustly punished; but he is also a monster in the sense that he personifies the violence of the African American condition.

Lynching was discussed directly by a number of commentators, who tried to use the scandal to bring about reform. But there were also many cultural products that, like Crane's novella, dealt with lynching indirectly, through a series of displacements. Hence lynching seems to have occupied the same place in American culture at the turn of the twentieth century as its monstrous victim: it was visible and repugnant, and so had to be concealed. But there was also a risk it would resurface unexpectedly. The rhetorical figures adopted by opponents of lynching, whether euphemism or ironic antiphrasis, exacerbated the contradictions of white racist ideology, which promoted itself as an enlightened civilization even while tolerating the barbarism of lynching. These rhetorical strategies also reveal the dynamic of repression surrounding the question of lynching, which remained difficult to address directly, even by those who denounced it. An illustration from the *Crisis,* the newspaper of the NAACP, shows the implicit inversion of American democratic values: the last traces of human remains are being consumed in a bonfire, while, in the background, a group of agitated men retreat in the moonlight (fig. 100). The title of the image is taken from the first lines of the "Star-Spangled Banner": "O say, can you see by the Dawn's early light, / What so proudly we hailed at the Twilight's last gleaming!" The image eloquently

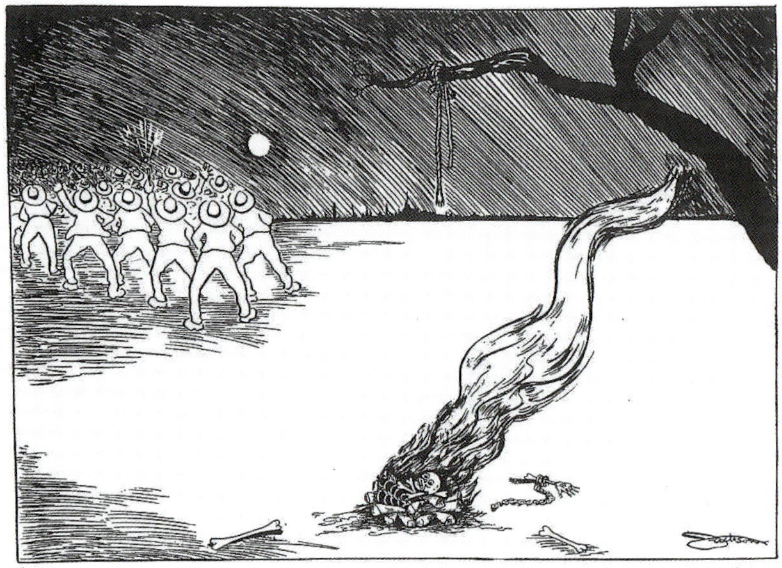

"O say, can you see by the Dawn's early light,
What so proudly we hailed at the Twilight's last gleaming!"

FIG. 100. "O Say, Can You See by the Dawn's Early Light,/What So Proudly We Hailed at the Twilight's Last Gleaming!" *Crisis* 9, no. 4, February 1915.

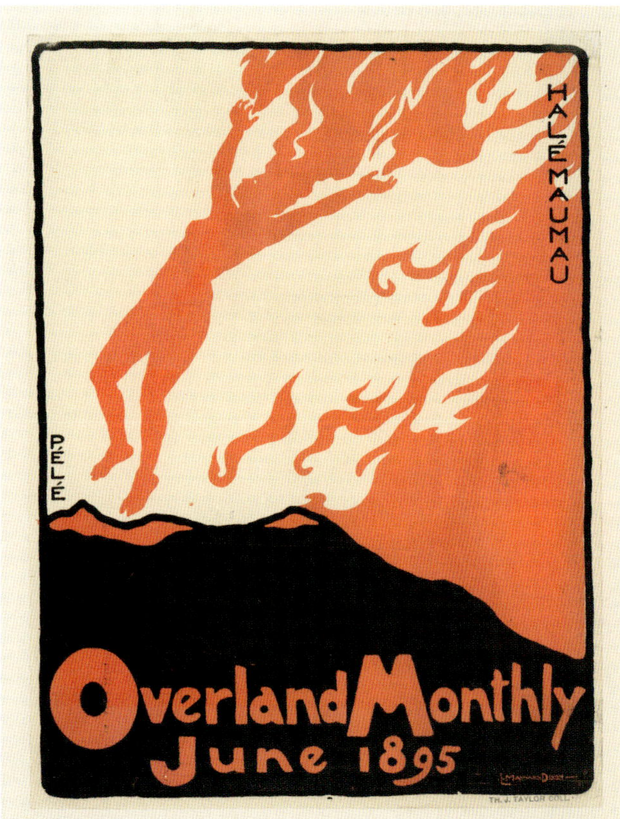

FIG. 101. Maynard Dixon, *Overland Monthly*, June 1895. Art and Architecture Collection, Miriam and Ira D. Wallach Division of Art, Prints and Photographs, New York Public Library, Astor, Lenox and Tilden Foundations.

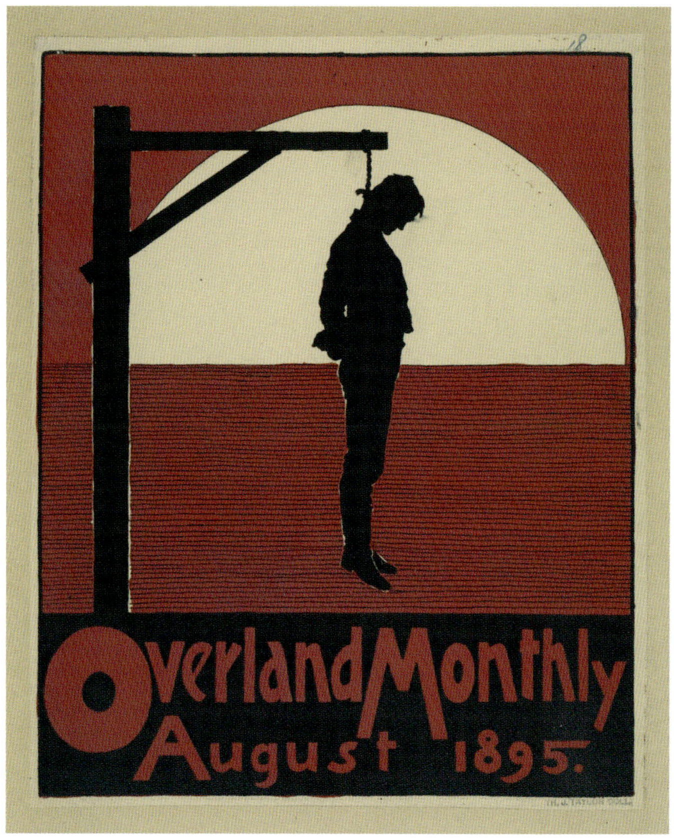

FIG. 102. Maynard Dixon, *Overland Monthly*, August 1895. Art and Architecture Collection, Miriam and Ira D. Wallach Division of Art, Prints and Photographs, New York Public Library, Astor, Lenox and Tilden Foundations.

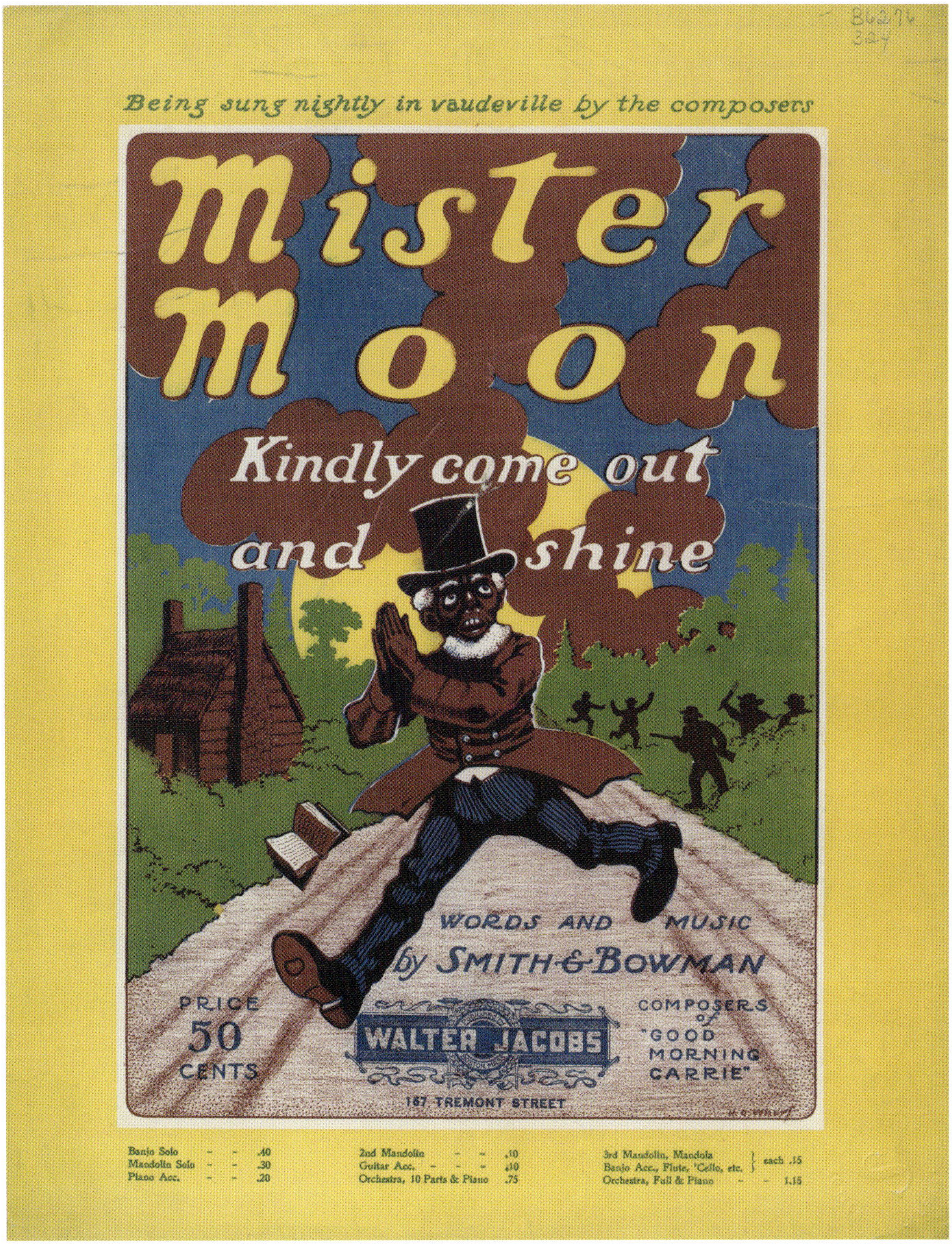

FIG. 103. *Mister Moon: Kindly Come Out and Shine,* 1903. Musical score cover, Walter Jacobs, Boston. Frances G. Spencer Collection of American Popular Sheet Music. Crouch Fine Arts Library and Baylor University Digital Collections, Baylor University, Waco, Texas.

suggests the elision, between twilight and the glorious dawn, of a barbaric night, which American citizens would have had trouble "proudly" hailing.

Other images, similar to Crane's text in that regard, more or less consciously reactivated the imagery of lynching, while transferring it to a different context. This can be discerned, for example, in two covers of the *Overland Monthly* (figs. 101, 102). Both illustrations are very stylized: the first shows a woman's body, drawn in silhouette, in the flames of a volcano; the second, a hanged man against the setting sun. They refer, respectively, to an article on the possible annexation of Hawaii and one on the gold rush of 1849. Nonetheless, they use a visual vocabulary that, in 1895, when the United States had just experienced the four deadliest years for lynching,[31] was a reminder of another dimension of white supremacy. None of the articles in these issues directly addresses the question of lynching or the situation of African Americans; yet it is difficult to imagine that readers of the magazine, upon seeing images that supposedly refer to bygone days or distant territories, would not have thought of lynching as well. Another illustration, for the cover of the sheet music for the popular song "Mister Moon," depicts in a humorous vein something similar to

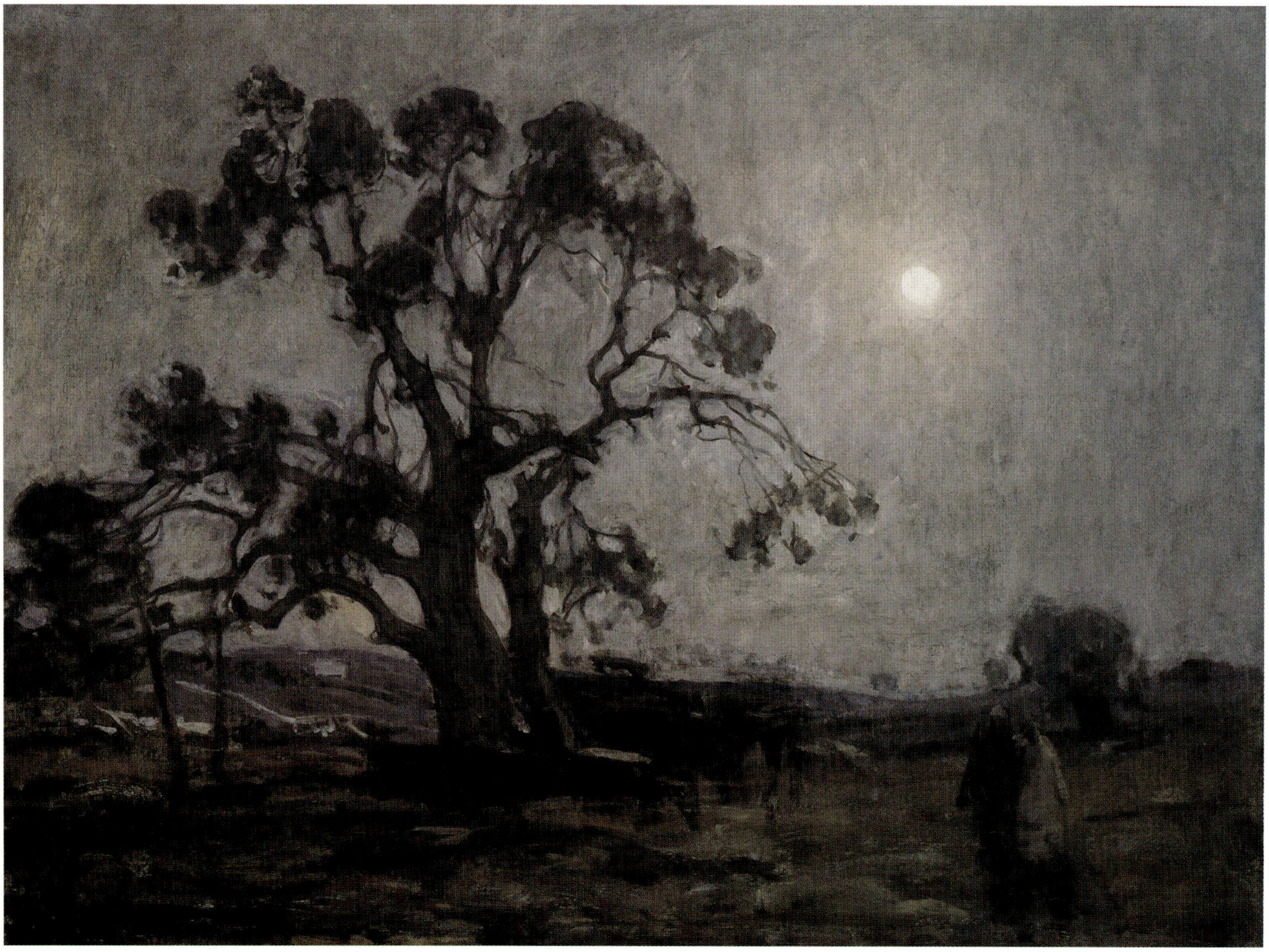

FIG. 104. Henry Ossawa Tanner, *Abraham's Oak*, 1905. Oil on canvas, 54.4 × 72.8 cm (21 ⅜ × 28 ⅝ in.). Smithsonian American Art Museum, Gift of Mr. and Mrs. Norman Robbins (1983.95.185).

a scene of lynching (fig. 103). If we are to believe the lyrics, the main character, a black pastor frightened by the village children who play tricks on him, begs the moon to come out and light his way home. But the silhouettes appearing on the horizon hardly bring to mind the innocent amusements of local young rascals. The figure closest to the victim is clearly armed with a rifle, which is more suggestive of the nocturnal stalking by lynchers than of schoolchildren's pranks. Hence lynching reappears in different forms, displaced in time and space or poorly concealed behind sick jokes. In that sense, it can be said that visual culture, to borrow an expression favored by Toni Morrison, was haunted by "a dark and abiding presence" to which it was blind but of which it was unable to rid itself.[32]

From that standpoint, some nocturnes can be considered potentially haunted by the memory of lynching. The figure of a lone tree, which recurs in nocturnal landscapes, though it may seem at first glance to suggest an atmosphere of silence and serenity, could thus refer to the reality of the violent acts perpetrated against African Americans. The night would act both as a veil concealing the bodies of the victims hanged from the tree and as an evocation of the morbid atmosphere of nocturnal lynching. In a certain way, these works might constitute a logical sequel to the caricature in the *Crisis.* Once the agents of violence have left the scene, and the bodies of their victims have completely vanished in the darkness, a heavy silence falls over the scene. Night would thus seem to introduce an elision of the violence comparable to the dissimulations and displacements of popular imagery or of Crane's novella. The only trace of the monstrosity of lynching would be the solitary silhouettes of trees, discreet markers of memory that both blend into the nocturnal landscape and are singled out for the beholder's eye.[33] This motif was taken up by Henry Ossawa Tanner.

According to Joseph Pennell, one of his classmates at the Pennsylvania Academy of the Fine Arts (and later a close friend of Whistler's), Tanner himself was the victim of a hazing that took the form of lynching, carried out by the white students at the academy.[34] One evening after class, they are said to have "crucified" him on his easel, abandoning him in that position in the middle of the street. The act contains its share of symbolic displacements, and it is very probable that the artist who painted *Abraham's Oak* years after that episode put something of that memory into the painting—or at least, something of the awareness of the violence inflicted on African Americans generally (fig. 104). On the left side of the image, two vertical marks, probably braces to prop up the tree's drooping branches, suggest ropes used for hanging. That tree, afflicted by the weight of centuries of anguish, brings to mind the punishment of the oak, as rendered in Paul Laurence Dunbar's poem "The Haunted Oak," written two years before Tanner's painting was created. The poet questions a bare oak tree, bringing it out of its silence. The oak says: "I saw in the moonlight dim and weird / A guiltless victim's pains," and "I feel the rope against my bark, / And the weight of him in my grain."[35] Although Tanner moved the tree to the Holy Land, the haunting that marks Dunbar's poem persists. In linking Abraham's name to the tree, Tanner referred as much to recent American history, particularly that of African Americans, as to the biblical figure of Abraham and Palestine. Just as at Gettysburg Abraham Lincoln had transformed a place and a moment of meditation and mourning into political discourse, investing his acts with the invisible power of the dead,[36] here too, contemplation may quietly suggest a discourse turned toward an urgent contemporary affair. As it happens, the "unfinished work" of which Lincoln spoke, the emancipation of blacks that was supposed to lead to a more perfect union, had not yet come to fruition forty years later. Read against this background of indirect references, Tanner's nocturne stands as a silent testimony, mourning innumerable, invisible, and anonymous deaths in subdued yet insistent tones.

PART III

Landscape Reconfigured

Urban Nocturnes

At a time when the United States was embarking on imperial conquest overseas, another frontier opened in urban territory. The city already constituted a new, difficult-to-navigate space, but at night it assumed the wild and threatening aspect of a "jungle," to borrow the title Upton Sinclair chose for his fictional chronicle of the daily lives of immigrants employed in Chicago slaughterhouses in 1906.[1] Americans were facing the altogether new reality of a rapidly spreading urbanization. "We are now a nation of cities,"[2] noted the general secretary of the City Vigilance League of New York in 1895. The statement raised its share of questions. "What shall we do with our great cities? What will our great cities do with us? These are the two problems which confront every thoughtful American." So declared Reverend Lyman Abbott in his introduction to *Darkness and Daylight* (1896), a collection of narratives by three explorers of the New York slums.[3] For a good number of Americans, cities generally became a major concern, from the exemplary cities built for the world's fairs, to the futurist utopia of Edward Bellamy (who, in *Looking Backward,*[4] imagined urbanization on the model of department stores), to ideal cities such as the one constructed by George Pullman for his employees on the outskirts of Chicago.[5] Their reflections, whether on discovering, constructing, or reforming the urban space, were accompanied by work in the visual field that attempted to define through the image that unprecedented phenomenon.[6]

The novelty of the urban spectacle was not confined to the United States,[7] but Americans cities were distinguished from other Western metropolises in several crucial ways. In the first place, electrification reached new levels there. In addition, American architecture made a radical break from Old Continent models. Then too, there was the speed of change in the American urban landscape, a direct consequence of the mass immigration during that period and the relative youth of American cities. As the sociologist John M. Gillette explained in 1913, "We have had other city ages in the history of mankind, but none on such a universal scale, nor any in which in any state the cities were so numerous, so large, or so essentially a vital part of the social mechanism as is now the case." Gillette calculated the increase in the American urban population between 1900 and 1910 at nearly 12 million.[8]

Within a few years, Americans witnessed the emergence and definition of a modern urban landscape, a testing ground to which major symbolic values were attributed. The late nineteenth and the early twentieth centuries were thus marked by the renunciation of the

Jeffersonian ideal of a nation of small farmer landowners. The American nocturne, though it at first avoided urban views and simply imitated Cazin's or Corot's rural landscapes, eventually returned to the urban views that had inspired Whistler's London nocturnes. The urban night provided a sort of middle course between the obsolescence of the pastoral ideal and the visual shock of the city in broad daylight. The vision Whistler developed in *Ten O'Clock* already makes explicit the function of reenchantment that the nocturne attributed to the night: the "poor buildings" disappear, while the chimneys and warehouses take on the aspect of "campanili" and "palaces." Night covers and transcends the ugliness of the urban landscape, making it a "fairyland."[9] Yet this section will demonstrate that while Whistler saw the nocturne as a way to detach himself from the city's prosaic reality, the enchanting spectacle he described was in reality intimately connected to the technological and commercial development of American capitalism.

◆ ◆ ◆

The urban night, a transitional space, was populated by ambiguities and uncertainties, which for the most part were rendered visually. Spectacular and sensational, it was also the site of every sort of dissimulation. The city thus constituted a multifarious world, and its observers admitted they had trouble making sense of it. Nathalie Cochoy, in a study on the figure of the urban *passante* (female passerby) in nineteenth- and twentieth-century American literature, shows how the urban environment forced the writers she studies to redefine their writing strategies. The attitude of Theodore Dreiser and Stephen Crane, as Cochoy describes it, is close to the ambivalent renunciation apparent in nocturnal antivision. "The American writers prefer not to copy New York," she explains, but that very refusal to represent opens the way for an adaptation:

> Again and again, they devote themselves to an anamorphic distortion of description, leading to a reiterated renunciation of the task of naming the city. The city, under cover of snow or of night, is often invisible in their narratives. But the occultation of description gives rise to a reflection on the limits of language. Poets and novelists therefore constantly remind the reader that New York City evades the rigidity of words and grammars. For Whitman and Hart Crane, it is "untranslatable"; for Henry James, "unspeakable"; for Henry Adams, "senseless." And it is precisely in confessing their powerlessness to name or their resistance to naming the urban movement that they manage to demonstrate its mysterious attractions.[10]

The night privileged by artists who depicted the metropolis can be interpreted as a pictorial version of that "anamorphic distortion": it is both elusive and revealing. A number of artists dwelt on the idea that night shows the hidden face of the city, a backstage that remains to be discovered and deciphered and which provides the key to the city in daylight. Darkness, which intensifies urban anonymity, is the privileged site for a blurring of identities and of interpersonal relationships. That reformulation of identities and social relations coincided with a major reworking of the urban space and the appearance of radically new forms, symbolized by the skyscraper. Representations of the urban night responded to these unprecedented developments and acted as spaces of reflection, in which a simultaneous reconfiguration of social relations and of vision occurred. Although it is not possible to retrace here the history of American urbanization at the turn of the twentieth century, or even to give an exhaustive account of contemporary representations of the city,[11] I will consider how the visual vocabulary of the nocturne reflected and altered the perception of these transformations.

Night inspired groups of artists who considered the urban landscape from diverse, even opposing, aesthetic and ideological positions. The question arose of what constituted the urban "landscape," whether it was best characterized by its population or its architecture. Two general tendencies took shape: on one hand, tonalist painting and pictorialist photography privileged atmospheric effects and formal explorations in often-deserted views of the nocturnal city; on the other, painters from Robert Henri's realist school were intent on representing the city in all its turbulent activity and made its residents a main focus of their attention.[12] That approach, often politically engaged, and the marked interest artists in that group manifested for the daily lives of the popular masses earned them the name "the Ashcan School."[13] Their works, often genre scenes depicting an overcrowded urban night, led to a reevaluation of the notion of landscape as profound as the formalist explorations of tonalism and pictorialism. To better understand how artists, by means of nighttime, visualized the changes in urbanized and industrialized space, I shall confine myself, in most of the examples considered, to a definition of the urban landscape as an outdoor view, giving interior scenes only a complementary, illustrative role. Other types of images, such as Jacob Riis's photographs documenting urban poverty, postcards, and popular illustrations, will provide points of comparison by which to reconstruct the visual context of these works, in order to highlight their potential ideological importance in particular. I will pursue the analysis of nocturnes in dialogue with one last type of artifact drawn from the visual culture of the time: the world's fairs and amusement parks such as Luna Park in Coney Island. These idealized forms of the American city will be used to bring to light some of the political content that the nocturne passes over in silence.

One of the major differences between the artists of the Ashcan School and the tonalists and pictorialists has to do with their relative distance from or proximity to their subject matter. At first sight, the Ashcan School artists adopted a position marked by sympathy, producing images that thematized the proximity between individuals, while the tonalists and pictorialists refrained from evoking too insistently the human presence. I will seek to understand these two types of representation of the nocturnal city in conjunction with each other, endeavoring to demonstrate that the main lines separating them conceal more complex attitudes and that the space between them constantly fluctuates. The imagery of the nocturnal city was in fact shaped by the perpetual distancing and foreshortening effects produced by darkness. The novelty of the urban experience was conveyed in terms of contrasts and unusual connections among heterogeneous elements, which produced both indignation and wonder. The overcrowding and anonymity that governed relations between individuals in the urban environment also gave rise to spectacular fluctuations between the near and the far, and required an adjustment of vision, a problem that was compounded by nighttime. The urban night, a simultaneously expanded and contracted space, was aptly represented in the ambiguous dynamics of the nocturne and its characteristic oscillations between rejection and assimilation.

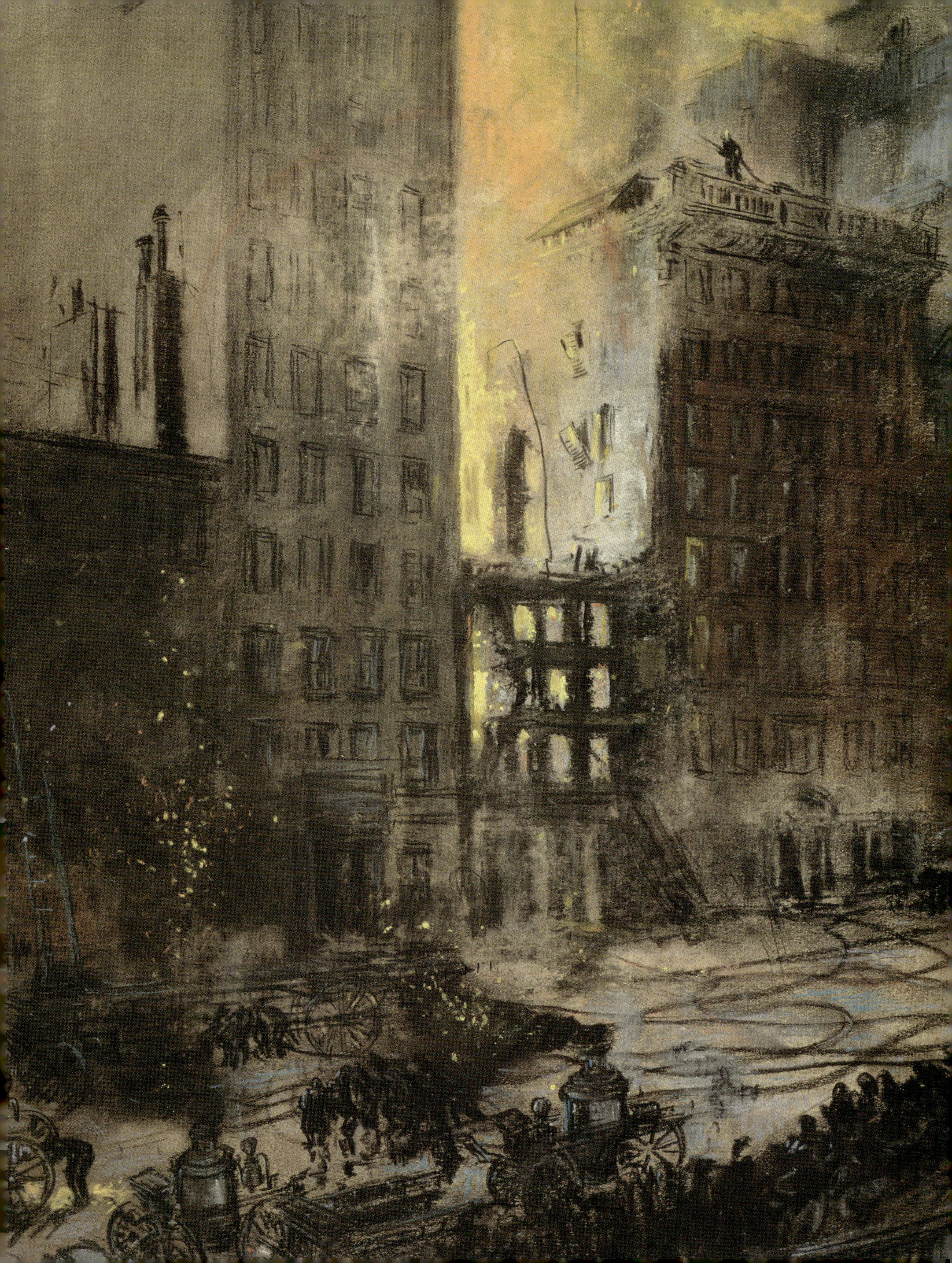

8 Contrast, Confrontation, and Spectacle

The Alterity of Urban Nights

At night in the metropolises, Americans discovered not only a new environment but also a new social experience. The urban night revealed or intensified, even exaggerated, social transformations, whether the spectacular growth of immigration, women's emancipation, or the development of what was beginning to be defined as a society of leisure. The first pages of Theodore Dreiser's *Sister Carrie,* which depicts his heroine in a state of reverie as she approaches the metropolis, make obvious the dual aspirations of an entire class of migrants. They had come to look for work in the city, but they were also attracted by the recreation the night promised them there: "To the child, the genius with imagination, or the wholly untravelled, the approach to a great city for the first time is a wonderful thing. Particularly if it be evening—that mystic period between the glare and gloom of the world when life is changing from one sphere or condition to another. Ah, the promise of the night. What does it not hold for the weary! . . . Says the soul of the toiler to itself, 'I shall soon be free. I shall be in the ways and the hosts of the merry. The streets, the lamps, the lighted chamber set for dining, are for me. The theatre, the halls, the parties, the ways of rest and the paths of song—these are mine in the night.'"[1]

For contemporary observers, the urban space offered a concentrated vision of the transformations driving American society in general. Lyman Abbott wrote, for example, "Thus the city presents in microcosm all the contrasts of our modern life. . . . The city is not all bad nor all good. It is humanity compressed, the best and the worst combined, in a strangely composite humanity."[2] Indeed, contrast and condensation dominated the perception of the city and its visual representations: the city was regularly portrayed as a dual entity, the night being its hidden and mysterious face, or as a kaleidoscopic environment, filled with colorful and jumbled elements. The various descriptions of the urban night wavered between an insistence on the distance separating the observer from the observed and an enthusiastic descent into a universe where he was accosted from all sides. The two types of perception were not contradictory but complementary: if the city was by definition a "land of contrasts," these contrasts were multiplied ad infinitum, which forced the beholder constantly to rethink her own position.

Fig. 113 detail

THE EXTREMES OF DARKNESS AND LIGHT: THE CITY AS A SPACE OF CONTRASTS

Although American cities were equipped with unrivaled public lighting systems, which promised to change night to day,[3] darkness and landscape still had to be rethought together. Joachim Schlör, in his history of the urban night in Paris, London, and Berlin in the late nineteenth and early twentieth centuries, includes a chapter in the form of a "digression," in which he addresses the question of urban lighting.[4] Was it light or darkness that defined the urban night? Although light created an enchanting and novel landscape, it also plunged the city's least lighted neighborhoods into what seemed an even more profound darkness. In reality, the nocturnal city seems to have been characterized by that dialectic between bright and dark; it even emerged from that very contrast. For example, in the guidebook he composed for the World's Columbian Exposition in Chicago of 1893, the British journalist James Muirhead portrayed the city of Chicago as a space with a geography of profound contrasts, in which darkness and light reflected disparate economic and social realities: "In some respects Chicago deserves the name City of Contrasts, just as the United States is the Land of Contrasts; and in no way is this more marked than in the difference between its business and its residential quarters. In the one—height, narrowness, noise, monotony, dirt, sordid squalor, pretentiousness; in the other—light, space, moderation, homelikeness."[5] The image of the nocturnal city as a dark double of the daytime city—in both the moral and physical sense—was well established in the nineteenth century and gained currency in several metropolises (think, for example, of Eugène Sue's *Mystères de Paris*).[6] But in the United States of the late nineteenth century, it acquired a new intensity, notably with the pressure that immigration exerted on urban growth. The genre of the sensationalist investigation had thrived in American publishing houses since the mid-nineteenth century: it set out to reveal in broad daylight, under the cover of investigative reporting or advice for tourists, the hidden, more or less clandestine, and illicit face of the nocturnal city.[7] As of the 1890s, such texts were accompanied by many photo illustrations, reproduced as halftones.[8] The best-selling book *Darkness and Daylight*, by Helen Campbell, Thomas Wallace Knox, and Thomas Byrnes, which presents in succession the points of view of a missionary, a journalist, and a former police officer, eloquently illustrates the increasingly visual dimension of these investigations, where the gaze is thematized and organized in a series of contrasts between day and night (fig. 105). Its approximately 250 illustrations drawn from photographs, some of them taken by Jacob Riis, play on the sensationalist appeal of the images, and especially on their contrasts. They propose to show to one half of American society its dark Other. But the night city was also, conversely, the spectacular and enchanting city of light. Whereas the night of toil and of the slums required surveillance, the night of leisure activities was dominated by spectacle: the gaze intent on controlling was replaced by a contemplation filled with wonder.[9] There again, representations of the night unfolded as discovery and contrast, systematically setting the electric wonderland in opposition to the prosaic reality of everyday life. The night enhanced by electric lighting opened up a world of leisure, a time of sociability detached from daytime activities, where hierarchical relations, economic issues, and cultural practices were entirely reconfigured.[10] From Gotham's depths to the bright lights of Broadway, from the slums of the Lower East Side to the never-ending festivities at Coney Island, Americans of the time witnessed the formation of a multifaceted city. Several different populations, engaged in diverse activities, moved about in the same space at various times, which made for contrasting visual environments. The nocturnal city gave rise to new social practices concomitant with new modalities of vision, which required constant readjustments. Although the visual products to be discussed here do not always belong to the artistic realm proper, they are part of a discourse that formed the context of the works produced by nocturne artists. I will consider them as a point of entry of sorts into the analysis of representations of the urban night in the fine arts, by showing how these images collectively reflected and shaped the perception of the new urban experience.

The urban night provided artists with a new space for formal experimentation and breathed new life into the objects of their art, but their gaze was still marked by a certain distance, on which the aesthetic context of the nocturne allowed them to capitalize. Both the city of illuminated pastimes and the poor neighborhoods scrutinized by the reporter were worlds in their own right, detached from the urban middle class's daily life. They existed in the first place as images and were apprehended primarily through the media. The duality of the city accentuated a visual regime divided between two

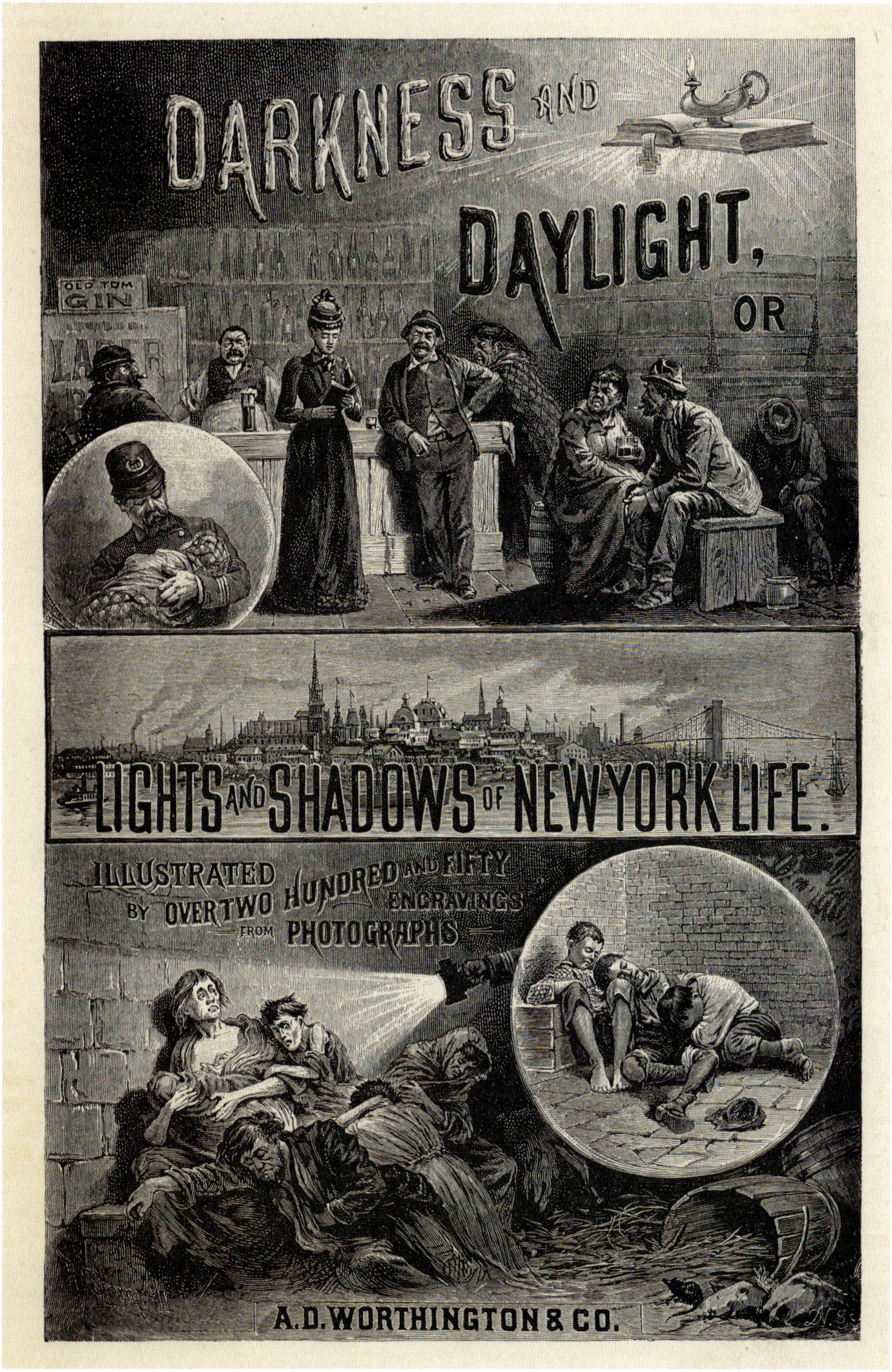

FIG. 105. Title page from *Darkness and Daylight, or, Lights and Shadows of New York Life* by Helen Campbell, Thomas Wallace Knox, and Thomas Byrnes (Hartford, CT: A. D. Worthington, 1900). Rare Book and Manuscript Library, Columbia University, New York.

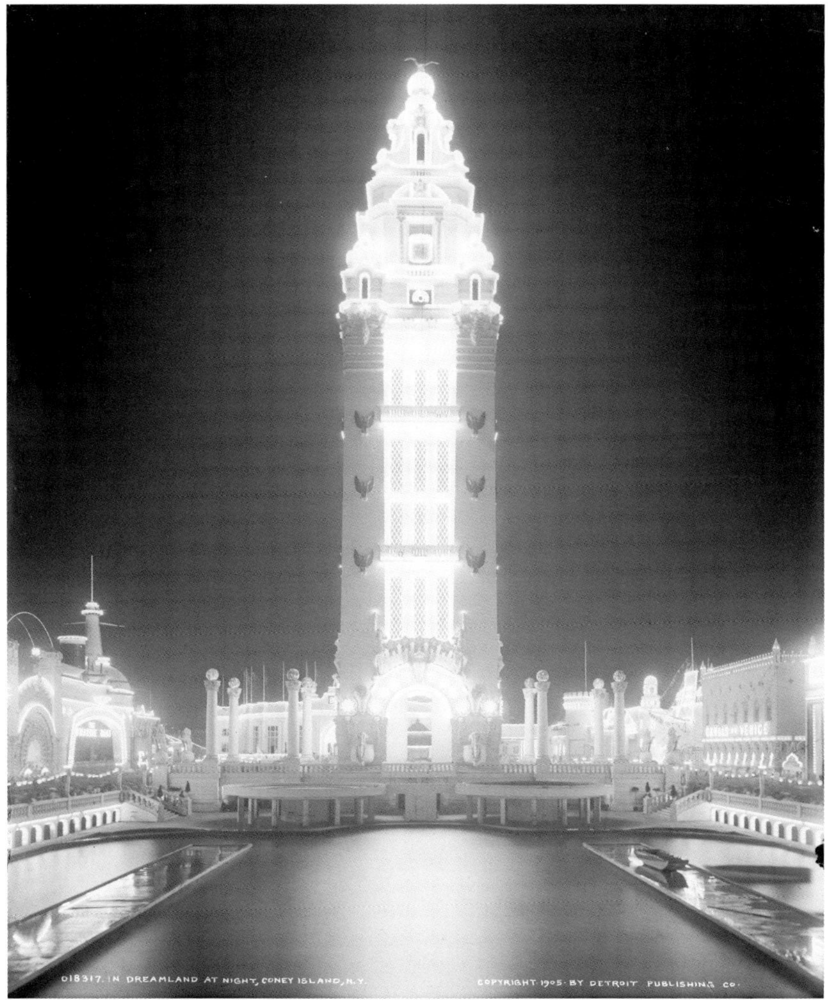

FIG. 106. *In Dreamland at Night, Coney Island, N.Y.,* Detroit Publishing Company, c. 1905. Glass negative, 20.3 × 25.4 cm (8 × 10 in.). Library of Congress, Prints and Photographs Division, Washington, D.C.

extremes: the invisible, which had to be uncovered, and the hypervisible, to be consumed on a large scale. In both cases, images thematized the distance, whether that separating the outside observer from poor immigrants or that contrasting the dream life of the city of leisure and the daily life of its visitors. Nighttime was congruent with that distancing effect and reinforced it, adding a supplementary symbolic and visual screen and redirecting the gaze toward the extraordinary.

Cities of Light: Night and the Urban Spectacle

In 1907 the Russian writer Maxim Gorky gave an account of his visit to Coney Island (fig. 106). In a text that has become famous, he showed his readers the apparition at night of what he called a "city all of fire," which electric lighting brought forth from the darkness as if by magic: "With the advent of night a fantastic city all of fire suddenly rises from the ocean into the sky. Thousands of ruddy sparks glimmer in the darkness, limning in fine, sensitive outline on the black background of the sky, shapely towers of miraculous castles, palaces and temples. Golden gossamer threads tremble in the air. They intertwine in transparent, flaming patterns, which flutter and melt away in love with their own beauty mirrored in the waters. Fabulous and beyond conceiving, ineffably beautiful, is this fiery scintillation. It burns but does not consume. Its palpitations are scarce visible. In the wilderness of sky and ocean rises the magic picture of a flaming city."[11] The nocturnal city appeared first as a luminous, "miraculous" fantasy, so essentially visual it could not even escape a narcissistic contemplation of itself. Along with it, an environment characteristic of the rapidly growing society of leisure developed, in opposition to the city of daily toil. Indeed, though a part of society continued its work after sunset, a majority of city dwellers discovered that the time available for recreation could now extend into the wee hours of the night. The industrial, technological, and social growth that governed urban expansion also gave rise to a real visual explosion as a result of artificial lighting, whose development accompanied the opening of new spaces of sociability. In 1899 Thorstein Veblen published his *Theory of the Leisure Class*, in which he showed the reworking of social relations, now organized around frivolous and conspicuous consumption rather than necessary economic exchanges.[12] The nocturnal city, a world of lavish illumination, spectacle, and entertainment, was the exemplary environment for that new set of sociocultural attitudes. At the dawn of the twentieth century, Americans discovered the pleasures of outdoor nighttime amusements, whether the world's fairs, regularly open at night beginning with the 1893 World's Columbian Exposition in Chicago, or amusement parks such as Luna Park, or simply neighborhoods and entertainment spots (public parks or rooftop beer gardens) scattered throughout the city, all intimately linked to the use of artificial lighting.

Leisure activities and nocturnal lighting converged, first, at the world's fairs, which in several respects served as urban testing grounds.[13] These artificial cities, built within a span of a few weeks and designed to last for only a season, were regularly compared to the "real cities" read as their dark counterparts. They were the embodiment of an ideal vision that was supposed to compensate symbolically for the urban problems affecting the era and to inspire remedies. For example, the editor of the *New England Magazine* contrasted the "White City" of the 1893 Columbian Exposition to the "Black City" of Chicago and to the working-class neighborhoods of other American metropolises: "Here, for the first time, was a veritable city, springing suddenly into existence, like the baseless fabric of a dream, in a night for but a day, conceived and constructed and controlled upon the principles of beauty and of reason, a city where throughout was regard for the fitness of things. This was indeed unlike what the man from Boston or Philadelphia or New York had left behind, in Broadway or the Bowery, and he had a right to be overpowered. It was indeed a contrast to the Chicago into which he plunged when the street car or the steamboat bore him away."[14]

In 1893 the organizers of the World's Columbian Exposition in Chicago decided to illuminate the exposition solely with electric lights. Every evening, they deployed a dazzling spectacle, accentuated by the uniformity of the white façades on the fairground. The historian David E. Nye points out the scale and cultural importance of the event: "The Columbian exposition in Chicago had more lighting than any city in the country. Some visitors saw more electric light in a single night at the fair than they had previously seen in their entire lives."[15] The journalist Murat Halstead described the spectacle of the White City in the magical terms that Gorky and many others also used, but he took his flights of fancy to such an extreme as to make electricity the very substance of the fair: "When the whole casket is illuminated, the cornices of the palaces of the *White City* are defined with celestial fire. The waters that are at play leap and flash with it. There are borders of lamps around the Lagoon. The spectacle is more resplendent than the capitals of Europe ever saw when ablaze with festivals to celebrate triumphant peace or victorious war. It is all an electrical exhibit."[16] In comparing that illuminated city to the European capitals, Halstead showed how, for observers at the time, the White City was equivalent to a blueprint for a future American city. More than a spectacle, it provided visitors to the fair with the brand-new experience of a grandiose urban landscape, through which they could move freely at night. The White City was vaunted as the paragon of the modern and rational city, where order and cleanliness reigned. Subsequent world's fairs went even further than the Chicago exposition, using increasingly elaborate lighting systems, and commentators constantly regarded them as idealized "cities" associated with variegated light effects: the Pan-American Exposition in Buffalo, for instance, was renamed the "Rainbow City" and the "City of Lights," and the 1915 Panama-Pacific International Exposition of San Francisco was dubbed the "Jewel City."[17]

Although the Chicago fair staged carefully orchestrated light displays to promote the intellectual and moral elevation of its visitors, it coexisted with a series of artificial cities oriented toward more suspect pleasures. For many visitors the Midway Plaisance, where the private concessions of entertainers, from belly dancers to Buffalo Bill, were assembled (this section of the fair was carefully cordoned off from the main fairground), turned out to be more attractive than the majestic solemnity of the White City. Whereas the grand and orderly architecture of the White City sought to impose refined cultural values on visitors, the Midway Plaisance catered to the public's taste for the sensational, the sensual, and the odd. Because entertainment prevailed over culture there, the Midway Plaisance probably provided a faithful representation of the interests of Americans at the time and also proved effective at influencing them. The amusement parks that grew up around the large urban centers were the direct heirs of the Midway Plaisance: they perpetuated and transformed the experience introduced by the artificial cities at the World's Fairs. In the early twentieth century, many "White Cities" conspicuously reproduced the electric illumination and spectacular aspects of the Chicago fair, but, in a movement that seemingly subverted the intentions of its creators, they declared no other ambition than to amuse the crowds. In his book on Coney Island, John F. Kasson explains that Frederick Thompson, the creator of the famous Luna Park, was inspired by the White City, yet his reinvention of it led to a complete reversal: "The spectacle intensified visitors' sense of Coney Island as a magical realm that violated conventional rules. Luna turned night into day, a feat which symbolized its topsy-turvy order."[18] The same year that Kasson published his book, Rem Koolhaas proposed a second interpretation of Coney Island: according to him, it was a "fetal Manhattan." More than the White City, he declares in his "retroactive manifesto," it was the disorderly and excessive world of the city of pleasures that served as a prototype for the (post)modern metropolis.[19]

In these urban recreational areas, every aspect of the real city was turned into a spectacle, including the most harrowing elements of urban dwellers' daily lives. In Coney Island, the crowds thronged every day to witness the "Fighting the Flames" show, a staging of a fake fire in a building modeled on the tenements in the city's working-class neighborhoods. Beginning in the late nineteenth century, these squalid, overcrowded, and overpriced apartments in the slums of the metropolises, such as New York's Lower East Side, became a veritable institution in the exploitation of the working classes. Rundown buildings regularly caught fire, an event that often made headlines. The most infamous no doubt was the fire at the Triangle Shirtwaist Factory in 1911.[20] In that sense, the artificial city allowed spectators to live or relive vicariously a daily life that was quite close at hand, to transcend tragic but ordinary reality through an extraordinary but harmless event (ironically, the amusement park itself went up in flames in 1911). The nightlife experienced in these places of *re-creation* became visible through the spectacle and the image, as attested, for example, by the countless postcards that depict Luna Park by night—images of images, reality to the second or even third degree. Electric lighting underscored the artificiality of these nighttime experiences, which were appreciated precisely for their artificiality. Nevertheless, the lights never fully obliterated the dark reality, against which they stood out in contrast. By a strange detour, "Fighting the Flames," a popular entertainment that took place in bright light, and the darkness of the urban slums were united in the eyes of spectators. Readers of Jacob Riis's accounts of slum life or visitors to Luna Park from the white urban middle class consumed both the spectacle of a city of light that revealed their aspirations and the images of a dark city that uncovered their anxieties.

The implicit contrast that distinguished these cities of pleasure from the urban darkness was more clearly visible within the cities themselves, in the neighborhoods specifically devoted to nighttime entertainments. For example, New Yorkers discovered the wonders of electricity on Broadway, which, on the model of the White City, was quickly renamed "the Great White Way."[21] Young writer Rupert Hughes thus marveled at the illuminations at the heart of Manhattan in 1904: "Broadway was one long cañon of light. Even the shops that were closed displayed brilliantly illuminated windows. In some of them all the trickeries of electricity were employed and rhapsodies of color glittered in every device or revolved in kaleidoscopes of fire. From most of the buildings hung great living letters. Some of these winked out and flashed up again at regular intervals. Others of them spelled bulletins in sentences that flared automatically. . . . The hunt was always for something new, something different, something that caught the eye by its super-ingenuity, its hyper-phosphorescence, among all the other radiances. Broadway, the most brilliant street in all the world, was aglow, agleam, ablaze."[22] Here again, artifice dominated, especially in the theater districts. Carrie, the title character of Theodore Dreiser's novel, ultimately achieves success under the bright lights of Broadway. The last scene of the novel shows her at the height of her career as an actress, "amid the tinsel and shine."[23] At the same time, however, she has become a spectator, a stranger to her own life. The pivotal chapter in the novel, which announces a reversal of fortunes of Carrie and her lover Hurstwood, who is condemned to a life of poverty, is eloquently titled "Of Light and Shadows: The Parting of Worlds." The penultimate section of Stephen Crane's novella *Maggie, a Girl of the Streets* shows the decline and suicide of a woman whom the reader suspects is the heroine. The author, who in this chapter keeps the character at an anonymous distance, also plays on the register of contrast, juxtaposing the lights of the theater and its wealthy audience with the more ambiguous glistening of the poverty nearby: "Electric lights, whirring softly, shed a blurred radiance. A flower dealer, his feet tapping impatiently, his nose and his wares glistening with rain-drops, stood behind an array of roses and chrysanthemums. Two or three theatres emptied a crowd upon the storm-swept pavements. . . . People having been comparatively silent for two hours burst into a roar of conversation, their hearts still kindling from the glowings of the stage. . . . An atmosphere of pleasure and prosperity seemed to hang over the throng, born, perhaps, of good clothes and of having just emerged from a place of forgetfulness. In the mingled light and gloom of an adjacent park, a handful of wet wanderers, in attitudes of chronic dejection, was scattered among the benches." The following pages trace a descent into the city's darkness, following the path of the young prostitute, whose potential clients embody one after another every rung of American society, down to the lowest. The last stage of that journey plunges the heroine into a bleak environment, where the landscape itself is weirdly more human than the individuals she meets: "Further on in the darkness she met a ragged being with shifting, bloodshot eyes and grimy hands. She went into the blackness of the final block. The shutters of the tall buildings were closed like grim lips. The structures seemed to have eyes that looked over them, beyond them, at other things." Crane takes care to evoke one last time the contrast and distance that separates the young woman from the space in which she had been moving a few moments earlier—"Afar off the lights of the avenues glittered as if from an impossible distance"—while at the same time emphasizing the proximity of the two worlds (in reality, the distance is far from "impossible").[24] These examples show a city of light that incessantly invokes its own shadow, without which it could not exist, but they also underscore the fluidity of the contrasts and the proximity of the Other.

Cities of Shadow: The "Other Half" of American Society

For a portion of the city's population, the urban night sparked fear and mistrust of what Jacob Riis called its "other half," which, in the American metropolises, consisted primarily of immigrants newly arrived from eastern Europe and the Mediterranean and living in overcrowded tenements. City dwellers from the middle and upper social classes, the descendants of earlier generations of immigrants from western and northern Europe, looked askance at this increasingly foreign population, growing at an unprecedented rate only a short way from their homes. Rampant urbanization brought the reality of the toiling classes within their sight, and they discovered simultaneously the existence of these classes and their living conditions. In 1908, in an article in the *Atlantic Monthly,* the racial theorist William Z. Ripley explained the unusual nature of that immigration, which he contrasted to the settlement of Europe: "In America the people, one may almost say, have dropped from the sky. They are in the land, but not yet an integral part of it. The population product is artificial and exotic. It is as yet unrelated to its physical environment. A human phenomenon unique in the history of the world is the result. . . . It is not alone the rapid increase in our immigration which merits attention. It is also the radical change in its character, in the source from whence it comes. Whereas, until about twenty years ago, our immigrants were drawn from the Anglo-Saxon or Teutonic populations of northwestern Europe, they have swarmed over here in rapidly growing proportions since that time from Mediterranean, Slavic, and Oriental sources."[25] Ripley considered this "horde" of immigrants "eruptive," evoking the imagery of an invasion, which Thomas Bender has shown was characteristic of the time,[26] and which was also found, for example, in Louis Dalrymple's illustration for the magazine *Judge* a few years earlier (fig. 107). Dalrymple's caricature, in representing the flood of immigration reaching the coasts of the United States by night, shows how common the symbolic association was between atmospheric darkness and the supposed benightedness of immigrants, whose sinister faces are labeled with comments such as "anarchism," "pauper," "illiterate," or "Mafia."

Photojournalism, such as Riis's *How the Other Half Lives*[27] and *The Pittsburgh Survey,* with documentation by Lewis Hine,[28] though they did not share Dalrymple's hysterical alarmism, also reflected somewhat the point of view toward the new arrivals held by white middle- and upper-class Americans (figs. 108, 109). The photographers set out to establish a panorama of the proletariat,[29] showing that, with the recent technological developments, the capitalist regime was extending labor's reach to populations, spaces, and times that had previously been little affected by economic activity. Hine and Riis added a compassionate and moralizing discourse to the discovery of the Other, which had usually been marked by fear

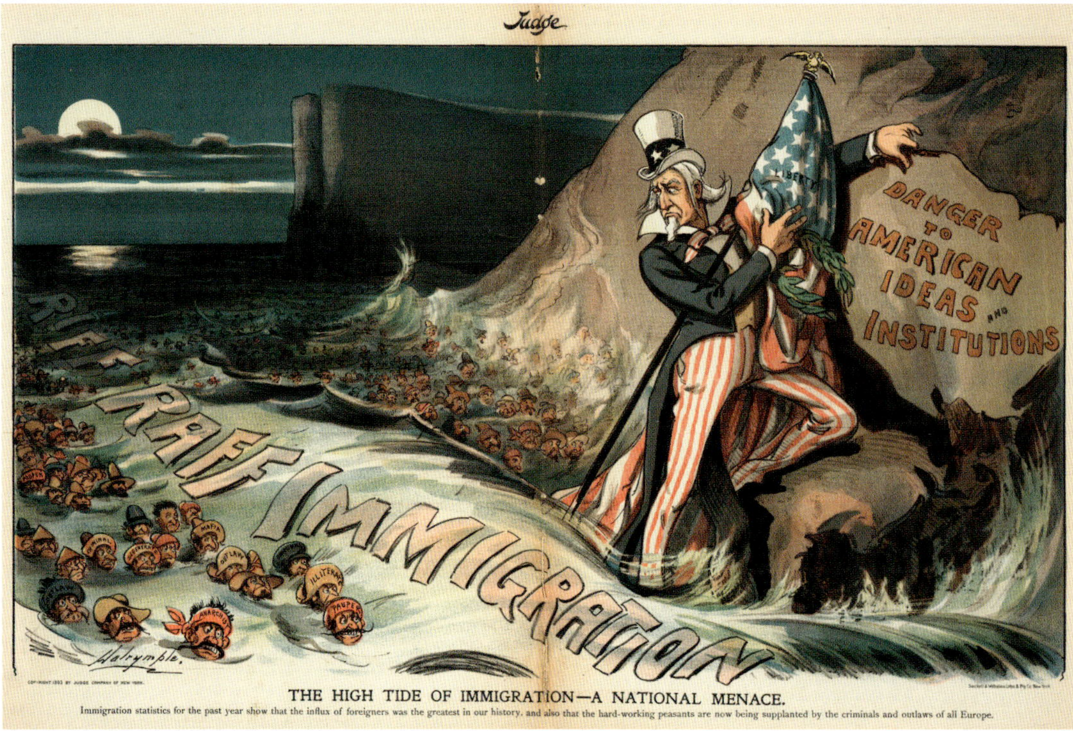
Judge
DANGER TO AMERICAN IDEAS AND INSTITUTIONS
RIFF RAFF IMMIGRATION
ILLITERATE
PAUPER
ANARCHIST
Dalrymple.
THE HIGH TIDE OF IMMIGRATION—A NATIONAL MENACE.
Immigration statistics for the past year show that the influx of foreigners was the greatest in our history, and also that the hard-working peasants are now being supplanted by the criminals and outlaws of all Europe.

FIG. 107. Louis Dalrymple, "The High Tide of Immigration," *Judge Magazine* 45 (August 22, 1903). Chromolithograph, 31 × 46 cm (12 1/8 × 18 in.). Ohio State University, Billy Ireland Cartoon Library & Museum.

and disgust, and they encouraged their readers to support the social reform movement. The few photographs that Hine made for *The Pittsburgh Survey,* for example, show women and children doing night work, performing tasks created by the new economic developments. In *Why Night Shifts Are "Necessary": Wrapping and Mailing after Midnight,* Hine forces his audiences—magazine readers no doubt—to face the unpleasant underside of the illustrated press industry and, above all, by calling into question the necessity of that work for society as a whole. As Upton Sinclair had done explicitly in *The Jungle,* Hine suggested a direct link between the development of capitalism and the urban poverty that engulfed laborers. In extending modern visual culture's power of representation to these nocturnal social spaces, Hine and Riis exhibited the desire to reestablish an overarching vision of American society, a complete cycle that would comprehend (in both senses: understand and include) the nighttime as well as the daytime of contemporary economic and social realities.

The imagery of the urban night conveyed in books such as Riis's was marked by ambivalence, notable in the first place in the use made of light and darkness. At a time when racist and evolutionist theories were focusing on the environment's influence on individual development, the exploration of the city's dark slums also revealed how the upper classes of American society perceived their new fellow citizens. The ambient darkness of the tenements seemingly tainted the morality of the individuals who inhabited them, while the reformists who descended into the working-class neighborhoods to bring virtue and hygiene were associated with light. In that respect, the progressivist conquest of the big cities adopted the familiar vocabulary of imperialist invasion and, like it, was sometimes armed with light produced by new technology. Such was the case for the cover illustration (see fig. 105) and the frontispiece to the chapter on criminality (fig. 110) in *Darkness and Daylight.* Here, light is seen as a religious and moral symbol that exposes the poverty of the disreputable neighborhoods and as an instrument of the law, a corrective incursion into a potentially dangerous darkness. The illustration shows the police confronting a row of individuals pushed up against a wall, caught in the beam of a flashlight. It brings to mind the familiar images of mug shots, thus leading the reader to understand that these men and women are already considered guilty. The progressive reformers who set out to transform the urban environment, whether

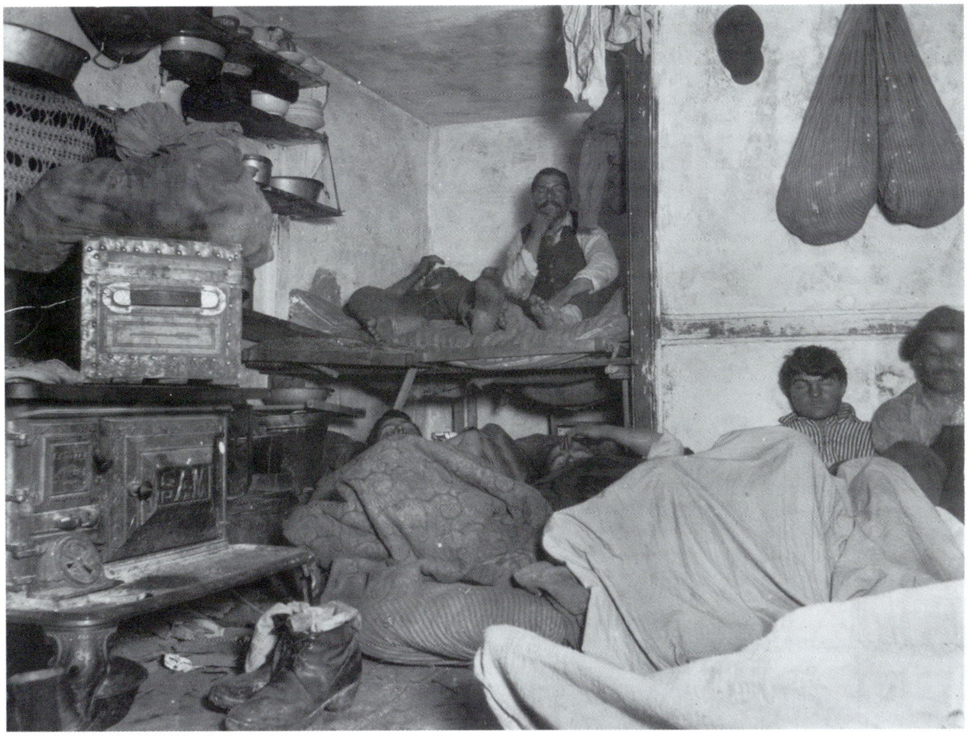

FIG. 108. Jacob August Riis, *Lodgers in Bayard Street Tenement, Five Cents a Spot*, 1889. Gelatin silver print, printed 1957, 15.7 × 12 cm (6 3/16 × 4 3/4 in.). Museum of Modern Art, New York. Gift of the Museum of the City of New York.

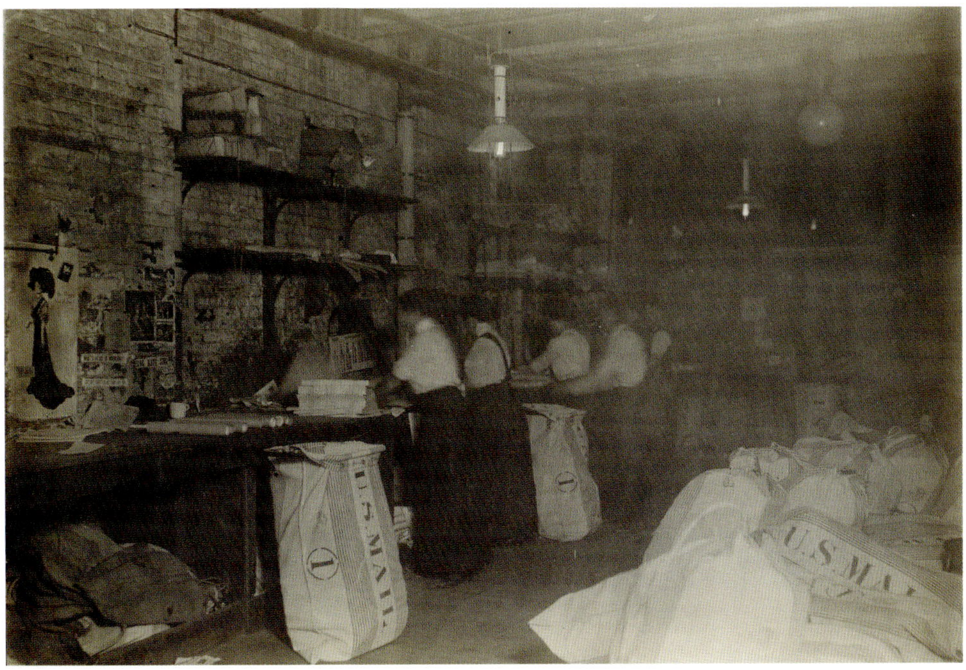

FIG. 109. Lewis Wickes Hine, *Why Night Shifts Are "Necessary": Wrapping and Mailing After Midnight*, 1907–33. Photography Collection, Miriam and Ira D. Wallach Division of Art, Prints and Photographs, New York Public Library, Astor, Lenox and Tilden Foundations.

Jane Addams with her Hull House "colony" in Chicago,[30] Helen Campbell with her Bible, or Riis with his photojournalism, considered the urban working-class neighborhoods "problems" that the volunteerism of society's upper classes had to solve.[31] The distribution of light and shadow replicates the assignment of active and passive roles. These are particularly visible in the photographs by Riis, who seized on photography to make his writings more vivid. Above all, he equipped himself early on with a flash, still a very recent technology when he published *How the Other Half Lives*. The account he gave fifteen years later of that turning point in his career gives a glimpse of the invasive dynamic driven by light: "A way had been discovered . . . to take pictures by flashlight. The darkest corner might be photographed that way. Within a fortnight a raiding party composed of Dr. Henry G. Piffard and Richard Hoe Lawrence, two distinguished amateurs, Dr. Nagle and myself, and sometimes a policeman or two,

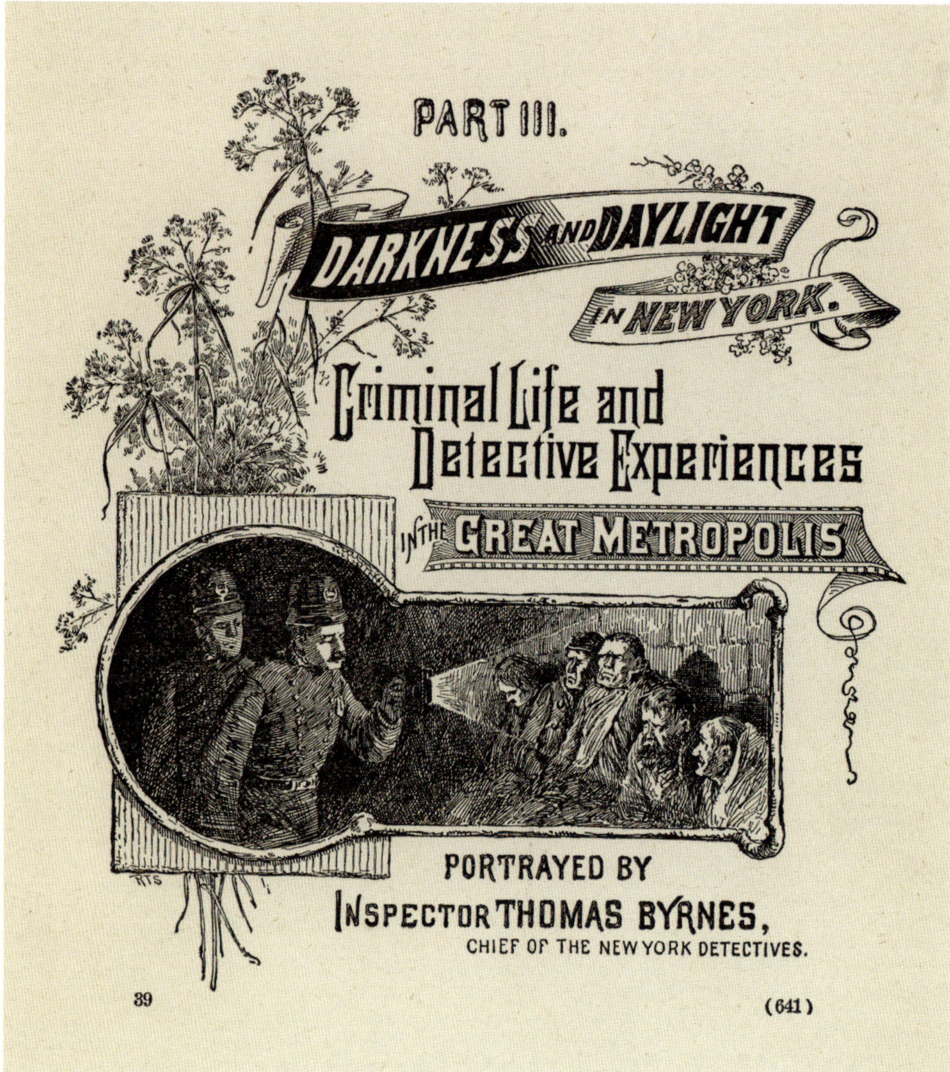

FIG. 110. Illustration from the Third Part of *Darkness and Daylight, or, Lights and Shadows of New York Life* by Helen Campbell, Thomas Wallace Knox, and Thomas Byrnes (Hartford, CT: A. D. Worthington, 1900). Rare Book and Manuscript Library, Columbia University, New York.

invaded the East Side by night, bent on letting in the light where it was so much needed."[32] The camera, wielded as a weapon, contributed to a visual distortion of relationships. The explosion of light caused by the magnesium flash accentuated contrasts, casting the exposed subjects into an even more profound darkness: "[Riis's] photographs effectively made everything seem, if possible, dirtier, more crowded, more chaotic than the reality," comments the historian Peter B. Hales.[33] In addition to the darkness, the confined space increased the impression that one was encroaching on strangers' privacy. As historians of the urban night have shown, darkness fueled fear, among the middle- and lower middle-class populations, of aggression from slum dwellers.[34] In these images, by contrast, positions seem to have been reversed: invasion and aggression are the acts of the privileged. Riis speaks of the "terror" occasioned by his photographic equipment, noting, for example, that his magnesium cartridges resembled those of firearms. Elsewhere he relates how, in clumsily handling the flash, he caused several fires in the tenements he was photographing.[35] According to Riis, the force of the camera supplanted that of the police, who were reduced to the role of spectators: "To the photographers it was a voyage of discovery of the greatest interest; but the interest centred in the camera and the flashlight. The police went along from curiosity; sometimes for protection. For that they were hardly needed. It is not too much to say that our party carried terror wherever it went. The flashlight of those days was contained in cartridges fired from a revolver. The spectacle of half a dozen strange men invading a house in the midnight hour armed with big pistols which they shot off recklessly was hardly reassuring, however sugary our speech, and it was not to be wondered at if the tenants bolted through windows and down fire-escapes wherever we went."[36]

Several historians have pointed out the surveillance

function of Riis's and Hine's documentary practice[37]: The images considered here convey, if not actual control, then at least the desire to ensure one's own domination through the gaze. In that sense, nocturnal darkness was the environment in which the tensions between different groups were exacerbated, as well as the extraordinary atmosphere that allowed for an entirely new rapprochement and, within the image itself, the medium for maintaining distance. An ambiguous game was thus set in place, based on an intense and unexpected nearness to the Other. The surprise was first and foremost felt by the individuals represented. But it also affected Riis's readers, who were confronted with these shocking images by the proxy of the photographer's gaze. Riis's photographs, in fact, underscore the dominant position of the photographer, who took over the space of the poor and captured hunched, helpless subjects dazed by the violence of the flash.[38] The same point of view is also found among artists of the Ashcan School in depictions of the Lower East Side: in Sloan's *Roofs, Summer Night,* the residents of the tenements are seen in passive poses, like Riis's subjects, captured unaware in their sleep (fig. 111). The social positions of Riis and Sloan were somewhat similar (both belonged, however marginally, to the white middle class), and both men displayed real sympathy for the men and women they portrayed. (Sloan was very active politically; for example, he was one of the main contributors to the socialist magazine *The Masses.*)[39] But these images of nocturnal encounters are also marked by an awareness of a persistent alterity. Amid the tangle of Sloan's sleepers, one man alone is awake, and he looks at his companions in that conscious state, thereby tempering the impression of an inert mass. Although the beholder of the image is invited to imagine herself, like the photographer, master of the gaze, the figures represented are deprived of the ability to see, reduced by their prostration and the overcrowded conditions to an almost animal tactility. Riis and Sloan, though they set out to represent the "other half" of American society, seemingly needed to attenuate their proximity to their subjects through a distancing effect that relied partly on darkness. In these images, residents of the Lower East Side are both forcibly exposed and concealed behind the very violence of that exposure: nighttime, even while emphasizing the abjection of their living conditions, transforms their presence into a formless and harmless vision.

Two nocturnes by Everett Shinn, *Fire Scene in the Bowery,* an etching the artist did in 1904, and *Fire on 24th Street,* a pastel with the same theme produced three years later, illustrate that remote approach to urban poverty

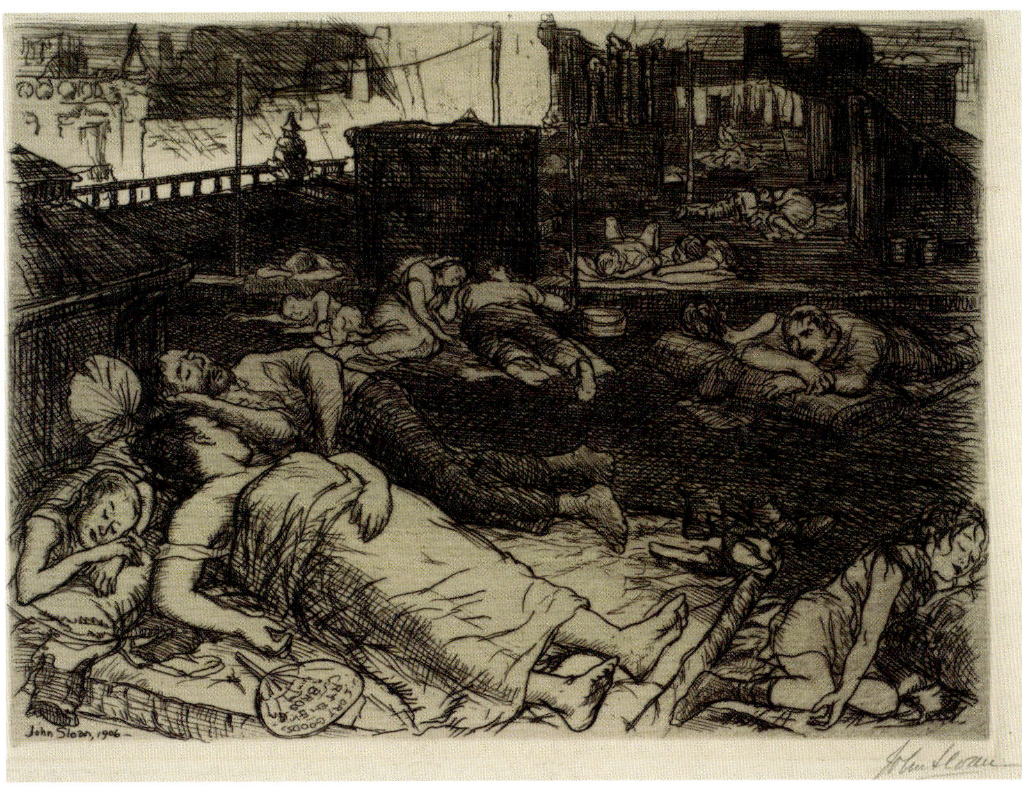

FIG. 111. John Sloan, *Roofs, Summer Night,* 1906. Etching, plate: 23.3 × 27.5 cm (5¼ × 7 in.). Metropolitan Museum of Art, Gift of Mrs. Harry Payne Whitney, 1926 (36.30.23).

(figs. 112, 113). Shinn, who during his career combined newspaper illustration with an independent artistic practice, produced two works in which the line between newspaper image and work of art appears porous. The first is a view in which darkness engulfs the drama, which is difficult to make out from the few contrasting lines of the image. It takes some time for the beholder to distinguish, in the foreground, the silhouettes of two onlookers, who thus act as visual and emotional go-betweens vis-à-vis the scene. The beholder's gaze is at street level, immersed in the darkness of the etching, which imitates the thickness of the smoke obscuring the fire. In the center of the image, a street lamp disseminates light, which is inscribed on the paper as negative space: the paper is left white at that spot. This minimal light, a bright point in the center of the scene whose gleam guides the eye through the image, accentuates the surrounding darkness more than it dispels it, and further reinforces its opacity. *Fire on 24th Street,* though it shows bright colors and the outlines of the neighboring buildings, is even more remote from its subject. The onlookers, more clearly visible but paradoxically less distinct, are dwarfed by the buildings and by the high-angle view the artist has chosen. He lingers with manifest pleasure on the decorative interlacing of the fire hoses, the glow of the flames reflected in the clouds of smoke, and the sprays of sparks emitted by the fire and the fire engines. The verticality of the image, its point of view, and its formal sobriety, are reminiscent of Whistler's famous *Nocturne in Black and Gold: The Falling Rocket* (see fig. 10). The aesthetic reference to Whistler effaces the blackness of the urban slums: just as *Nocturne in Black and Gold* depicts,

FIG. 112. Everett Shinn, *Fire Scene in the Bowery,* 1904. Etching and engraving on paper, 25.1 × 17.5 cm (9 7/8 × 6 7/8 in.). Private collection.

FIG. 113. Everett Shinn, *Fire on 24th Street,* 1907. Pastel on paper, 59 × 45.7 cm (23 1/4 × 18 in.). Private collection.

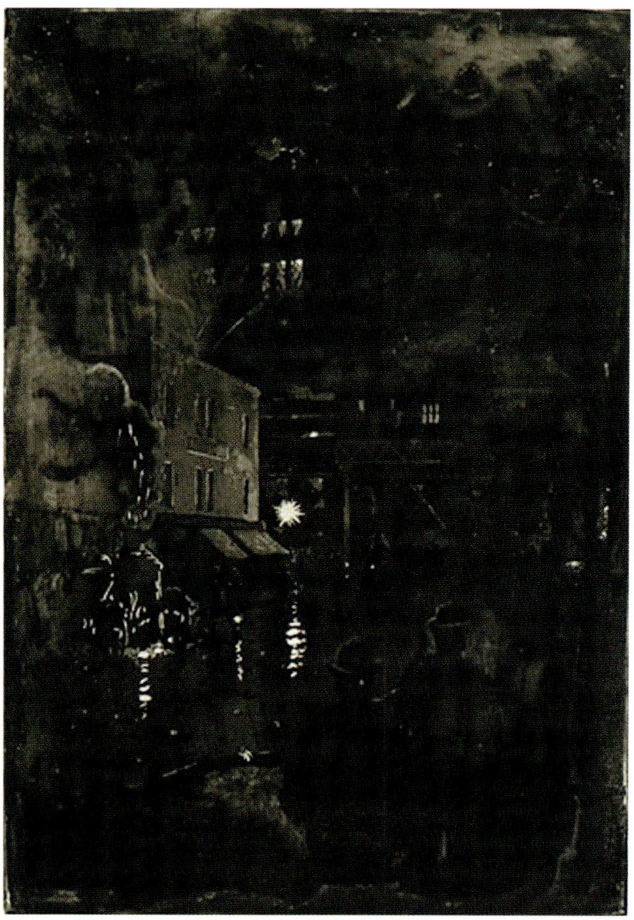

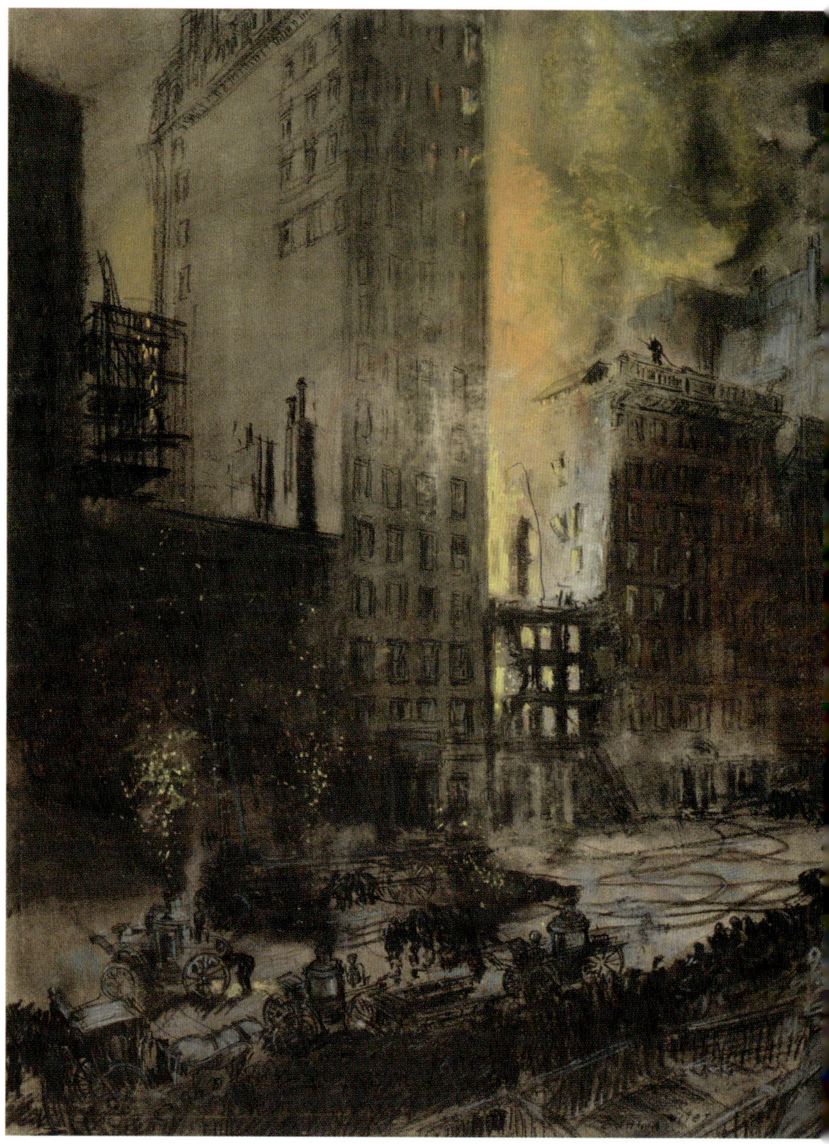

from afar, the Cremorne Gardens in London, a place of illicit pleasures, so Shinn in some sense relegates social commentary to the background. The painting seems to be a distant echo of the "Fighting the Flames" attraction, with the working-class spectacle reworked as a formal, refined pleasure.

FROM THE COSMOPOLITAN TO THE PICTURESQUE: THE WHOLE WORLD IN A CITY

Nighttime was not simply a place of contrasts, however: it also provided a visual field conducive to a much more complex series of variations between near and far. Between the radical alterity of urban poverty and the fantastic spectacle of lights at Luna Park, American city dwellers had a more mixed experience of the nocturnal city: it was both foreign and entertaining, but its different aspects were fluctuating and varied. A good number of images focused on that cosmopolitan variety, expressing another aspect of the fascination exerted by the city. Here again, the world's fairs can serve as a revealing prototype. Their visitors were invited to discover a veritable patchwork of cities, where the pavilions of every nation stood side by side with special attractions such as "Street in Cairo" at the 1893 fair, and "Streets of Mexico" and "Venice in America" at the Buffalo fair.[40] One illustration published in *Harper's,* of a crowd of nocturnal visitors on the Midway Plaisance, depicts the many incongruous connections between individuals from very different countries. The beholder makes out, interspersed among the tide of boater and bowler hats, men in Turkish, Bedouin, Germanic, Indian, or Chinese costumes (fig. 114). The composition of the image, which imitates the off-center framing of a photograph taken from only slightly above the crowd, makes the most of spatial effects: whereas the high-angle view creates an impression of detachment, the figure of the Turkish warrior advancing in the very center of the image, directly facing the beholder, establishes a striking—and somewhat destabilizing—visual connection. The folk costumes and festive atmosphere keep the scene in the realm of the extraordinary, but the suggested confrontation with the Other is disconcerting. The gender distribution in particular suggests a certain tension: the women in the crowd are all white and obviously from a relatively wealthy social milieu. The fact that all the exotic figures depicted are male (even though belly dancing and other displays of exotic beauties were among the most popular attractions at the fair)[41] suggests that the illustrator, perhaps out of prudery, preferred to eclipse the figure of the exotic woman. In so doing, however, he inadvertently made white women the only females in the potential sexual exchanges suggested by the commingling in the scene.[42]

The exotic patchwork, artificially re-created, of the world's fair concessions was, like the fairs themselves,

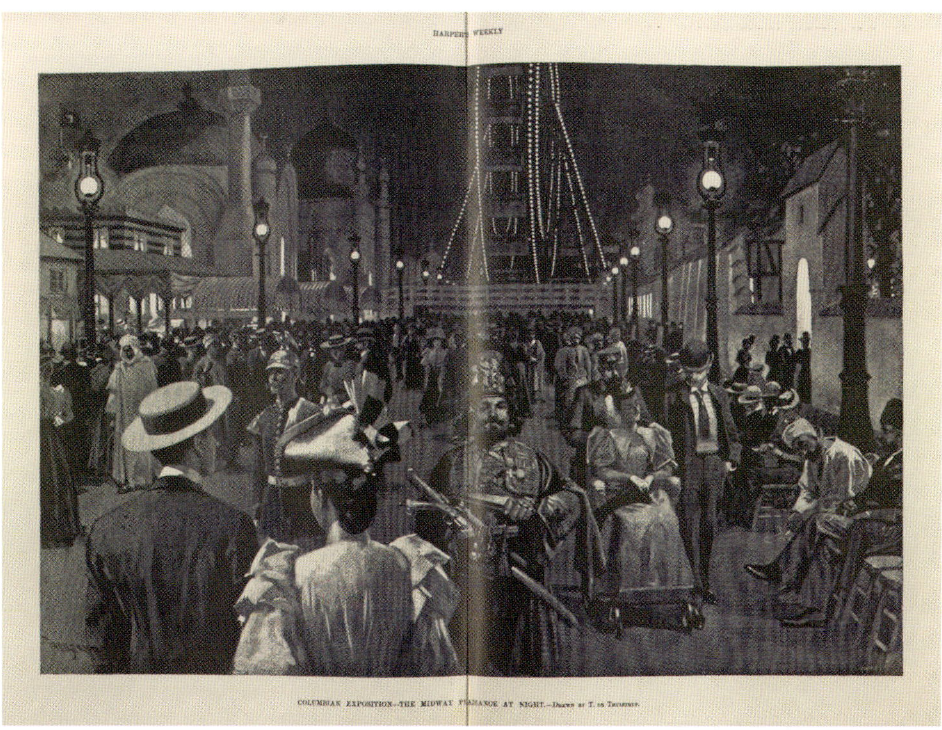

FIG. 114. T. De Thulstrup, "Midway Plaisance at Night," *Harper's Weekly* 37, no. 1920 (October 7, 1893). Beinecke Rare Book and Manuscript Library, Yale University.

one of the spectacular results of the growth of exchanges on a global scale, which resulted from imperialist expansion and the rise of international capitalism. The same factors governed the development of American industrial and urban centers and the surge in immigration to the United States, which transformed the urban in the early twentieth century. American cities took on an increasingly fragmented appearance because of immigration, with the proliferation of colorful and diverse ethnic neighborhoods: in every metropolis, the urban territory was divided up into a Chinatown, a Little Italy, an eastern European Jewish neighborhood.[43] A guide to Chicago depicts in vivid terms one of the most animated neighborhoods in the city, a true global village before its time: "[South Water Street] can hardly be called a thoroughfare, street and sidewalk being obstructed during business hours by barricades of barrels, boxes, crates, chickens coops, trucks, wagons and teams, leaving only a bare passage in the middle of the road. The traffic is heaviest during the early morning hours, and at that time the street offers an interesting spectacle of confusion, made picturesque by the characteristics of the traders, nearly all the nationalities and tongues of this world being represented among them, as is the produce of all countries and climes."[44] Riis described the visual variety of the urban landscape, seen through the prism of a variegated map: "A map of the city, colored to designate nationalities, would show more stripes than on the skin of a zebra, and more colors than any rainbow." For Riis, the overall effect was "an extraordinary crazy-quilt."[45]

That landscape of many colors was itself shifting: in the course of the various waves of immigration, communities were displaced, dispersed, or replaced by new groups. Henry James, returning to New York after many years in Europe, found himself speechless before the irreducible strangeness of the city and its newest residents: "The claim of the alien, however immeasurably alien, to share in one's supreme relation was everywhere the fixed element, the reminder not to be dodged."[46] In New York, James, who considered himself a European more than an American, felt doubly foreign. After visiting Ellis Island, where the magnitude of immigration came as a shock to him, he imagined the city as a fundamentally unstable field, where what remained of his identity as a white and wealthy American—which he expressed by a "we" that included his reader—was shaken by the presence of an "inconceivable" Other. The city looked like a polymorphous entity so complex that words failed the writer: "The ambiguity is the element in which the whole thing swims for me—so nocturnal, so bacchanal, so hugely hatted and feathered and flounced, yet apparently so innocent, almost so patriarchal again, and matching, in its mixture, with nothing one had elsewhere known. It breathed its simple 'New York! New York!' at every impulse of inquiry; so that I can only echo contentedly, with analysis for once quite agreeably baffled, 'Remarkable, unspeakable New York!'"[47] Images came to the aid of speech and offered James's contemporaries, similarly disoriented by that spectacle, domesticated visions, superimposing on the urban scenery a familiar vocabulary that allowed them to assimilate more easily these new realities. The photographs that the California pictorialist Arnold Genthe took in San Francisco's Chinatown focus on its picturesque and familiar aspects: Chinese lanterns outside the grocery store, the costumes and queues typically worn by the men in the neighborhood (fig. 115). Genthe used the easily recognizable imagery of exoticism, which, not surprisingly, reappears on a postcard from the period, supposedly representing a street in Chinatown by moonlight (fig. 116). Here, the shadows on the ground give away the fact that the photograph was taken in daylight; the developer covered the print with a bluish wash and cut openings in the images of the lanterns along the street.[48] When the postcard is placed in front of a light source, the characteristic and even caricatural elements of that exotic and urban landscape stand out. The veil of night is materialized in that object, which literally emphasizes its mediation role.

The nocturnal atmosphere poeticized and distanced the Other, which James had trouble characterizing in his familiar vocabulary. The two extremes, dark city and bright city, thus came together in a deliberately reenchanted image, activated by clichéd cultural associations, which often put to use a nocturnal aesthetic. Such was the case especially for a set of images that borrowed more or less explicitly from the theme of the *Thousand and One Nights* to consider the novelty of the urban landscape. Unexpurgated and unabridged English translations of the book were produced by John Payne and Richard Francis Burton in 1882 and 1885, respectively. Countless editions appeared between 1890 and 1917, and they also served as a reservoir of images from which modern authors drew, beginning with Robert Louis Stevenson in his collection of short stories *The*

New Arabian Nights.[49] In the United States, the theme and format revived by Stevenson were adopted by the popular author O. Henry in "A Madison Square Arabian Night," in which he humorously transposes that exotic imagery to the context of the modern metropolis.[50] In that story, the rich Carson Chalmers invites a homeless man to share his dinner in exchange for telling his life story. The man willingly plays the story-telling game and, with a hint of irony, proclaims himself the Scheherazade of that new caliph of Baghdad.[51] The same exotic interpretation of the modern city, and particularly of its marginal populations, can be found in the photographs of young children sleeping in the middle of the street, which Jacob Riis inserted into his chapter "Street Arabs":[52] the *Thousand and One Nights* served as a model to rework urban squalor into a more acceptable form. The euphemism "street Arabs," combined with the sleeping pose Riis chose to depict these poor children, distances and softens the reality of a sometimes sordid and cruel urban spectacle. Riis's homeless children are an almost tender image, and while their misery should elicit pity or outrage, the abnormality of their situation is transcended in a ready-made vision tapping into popular picturesque codes.

In George Luks's *Allen Street,* the reference to the exotic Orientalist imaginary is wholly implicit, merely suggested by the veiled silhouettes of the women and the display of food, furniture, carpets, and various other

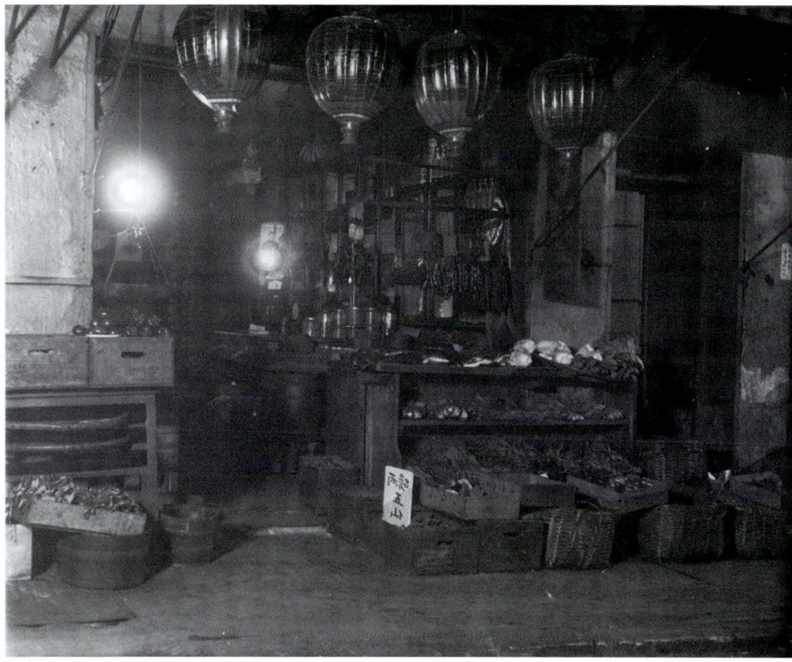

FIG. 115. Arnold Genthe, *A Grocery Shop, Chinatown, San Francisco,* c. 1896–1906. Transparency, 12.7 × 17.8 cm (5 × 7 in.). Library of Congress, Prints and Photographs Division, Washington, D.C.

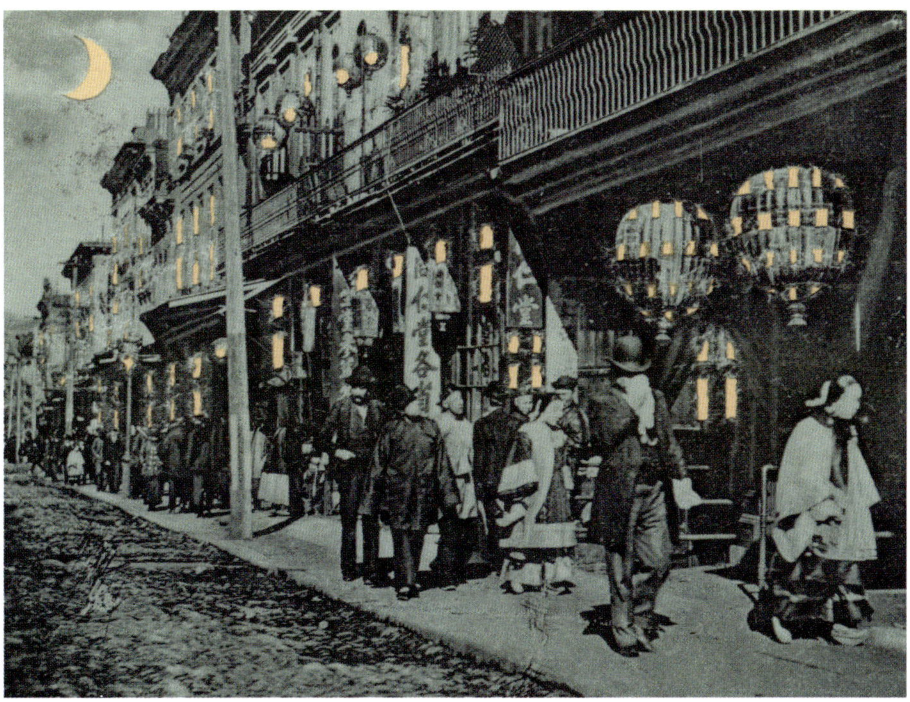

FIG. 116. Street scene, Chinatown, c. 1900. Photomechanical print, 14.30 × 8.77 cm (5 5/8 × 3 1/2 in.). Art and Picture Collection, New York Public Library, Astor, Lenox and Tilden Foundations.

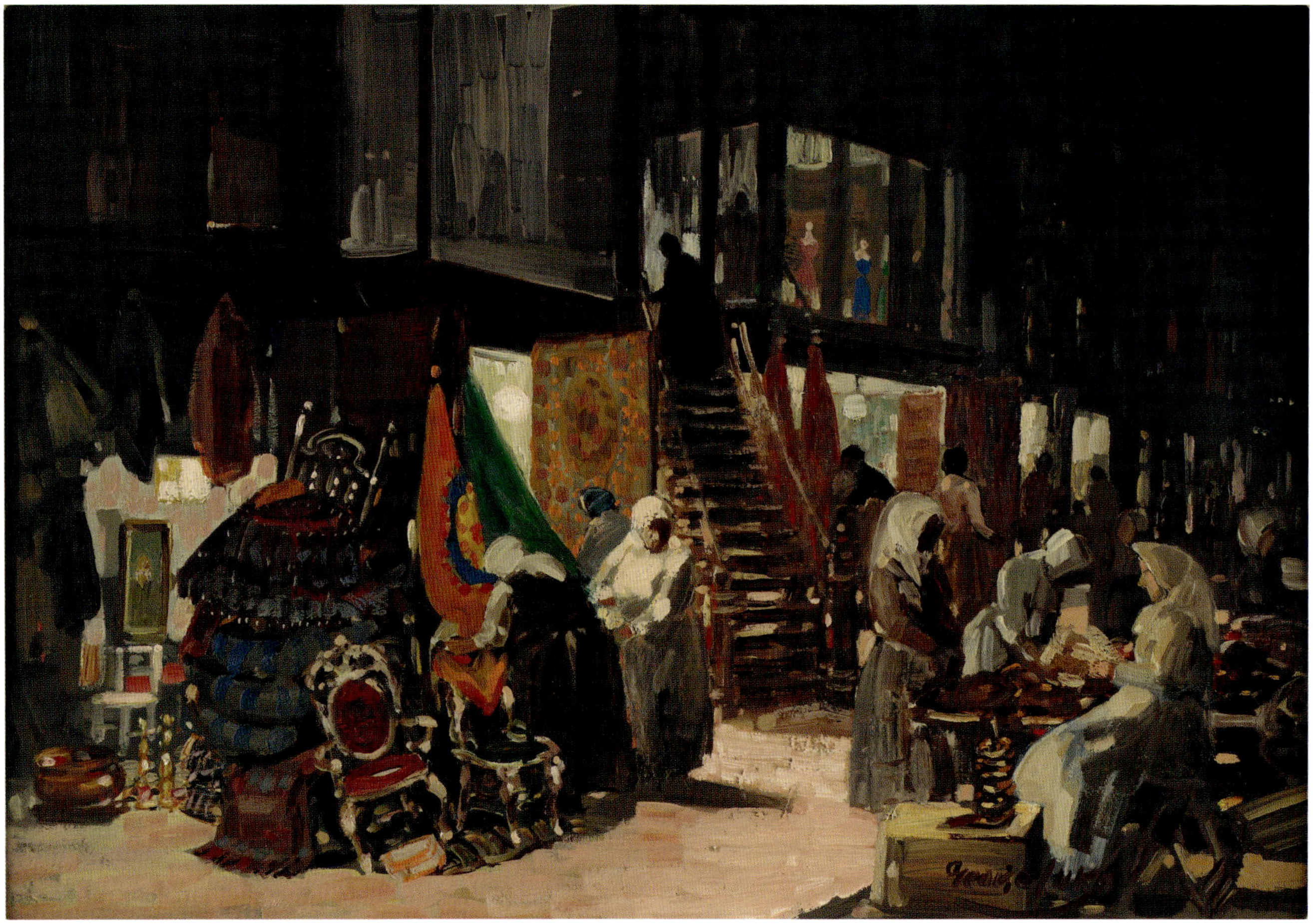

FIG. 117. George Benjamin Luks, *Allen Street,* c. 1905. Oil on canvas, 81.3 × 114.3 cm (32 × 45 in.). Hunter Museum of American Art, Chattanooga, Tennessee. Gift of Miss Inez Hyder (1956.1).

objects on the sidewalk, which bring to mind a bazaar (fig. 117). In the early twentieth century, Allen Street, on the Lower East Side, was occupied for the most part by Romanian Jewish immigrants and Sephardic Jews from Greece, Turkey, Egypt, and Syria.[53] A guidebook of the time recommended that its readers stop by the neighborhood, called "Judea," during their "ramble at night."[54] Luks, sharing that taste and quest for exoticism, deliberately painted his subjects in a setting that resembles their country of origin more than the white middle-class United States. But the visual codes he used moderate the strangeness of the scene. Seen from afar, between darkness and the artificial light of the display windows, Luks's indistinct figures take on a picturesque and acceptable appearance.[55] The nocturnal context is part of that economy of the picturesque: even while preserving difference and surprise, it provides a relatively neutral ground that mitigates the alterity.

Nonetheless, that filter imposed on the scene is incorporated into a painting that brings multiple distances into play. That urban landscape, perceived as a familiar remoteness, is itself the result of a complex spatial dynamic, revealed in the details of the image. *Allen Street* gives a glimpse of an urban territory appropriated by a distant culture and of a surprising proximity between two spaces: this improvised bazaar is illuminated by the shop windows of the metropolis, where the low-cut gowns of the mannequins contrast with the traditional costumes of the women on the street. Two ways of life, indicated by the women's clothing, along with two types of economic exchanges coexist in that environment: the nighttime market of heterogeneous goods set out on the sidewalk, and the shop windows with modern lighting and faceless mannequins. The night scene shows a different time, a different activity, outside working hours and the usual modes of social exchange of the capitalist system. But the process of appropriation and dispossession that disturbed James during his visit to Ellis Island works in both directions: if the immigrants occupy the streets and mark the urban landscape with a remote culture, that appropriation is itself reappropriated. Luks's gaze "Orientalizes" the scene in the sense Edward Said uses that term: "The Orient was Orientalized not only because it was discovered to be 'Oriental' in all those ways considered commonplace by an average nineteenth-century European, but also because it could be—that is, submitted to being—made Oriental."[56] In depicting Allen Street like an oriental bazaar out of the *Thousand and One Nights*, Luks makes it, paradoxically, a white, Anglo-American vision. And if the painting illustrates in some measure the exchanges between various groups and cultures, in itself it participates in these transactions, converting the everyday into a consumable image. Behind that vision of an exotic New York, a whole system of relations of dominance can be made out. The very presence of these immigrants in this place marks a convergence produced by the combined influences of imperialism and capitalism.[57] Thomas Bender shows the intimate connection between immigration and colonization: the immigrants arriving en masse from poor countries created the impression, among native-born Americans, that they were being colonized by these new arrivals,[58] even as the economic logic that dominated global migrations placed the native-born in a position of dominance. From that standpoint, Luks's painting can be interpreted in two opposing ways: it may reflect the incongruous proximity of the Other "dropped from the sky" into the modern American city, to borrow Ripley's words; or, conversely, it can be interpreted as a distancing of that Other by means of the picturesque. In reality, the two readings coexist, and Luks's painting offers an antimodern image in the sense Lears understands it: it resorts to the picturesque as both a reaction and an adaptation.

Finally, though the urban picturesque attenuated certain contrasts, it also reproduced the most entrenched forms of discrimination in American society. The historians Thomas Bender and Alan Trachtenberg make the same observation: whereas foreign immigrants were more or less integrated into society, African Americans remained marginal.[59] That exclusion was symbolized by the White City, where blacks' participation was suppressed, relegated to a "Colored People Day," and celebrations enlisted the most regressive racist stereotypes.[60] In the years after World War I, African Americans massively migrated toward the metropolises of the Northeast, but their presence was already significant before 1917, which means that the silence with which it was met was probably intentional. The images representing African Americans maintain them in a more than marginal position. The illustrations of Edward Kemble, a specialist on the subject, show African Americans attempting to imitate the white middle class's urban way of life but systematically failing and making fools of themselves; or they confine blacks to stereotypical roles, emphasizing their ignorance and laziness, symbolically excluding them from the modern urban space. Although present in Jacob Riis's photographs, they remain nearly absent from the urban representations of the Ashcan School.[61] It seems that African Americans did not enter the urban imaginary and its illustrations before the end of World War I. It was not until the 1920s and Harlem Renaissance artists such as Jacob Lawrence that a black urban imagery independent of caricature came into being. That rejection, though it reflected political tendencies deep-seated in American society, and though it was in line with what I argued in Part II of this study, also points out, by way of contrast, the value of integration conveyed by picturesque imagery. For the Others whose alterity could be modulated by picturesqueness, the nocturnal urban context could serve as a relatively neutral ground that facilitated their integration into the collective imagination.

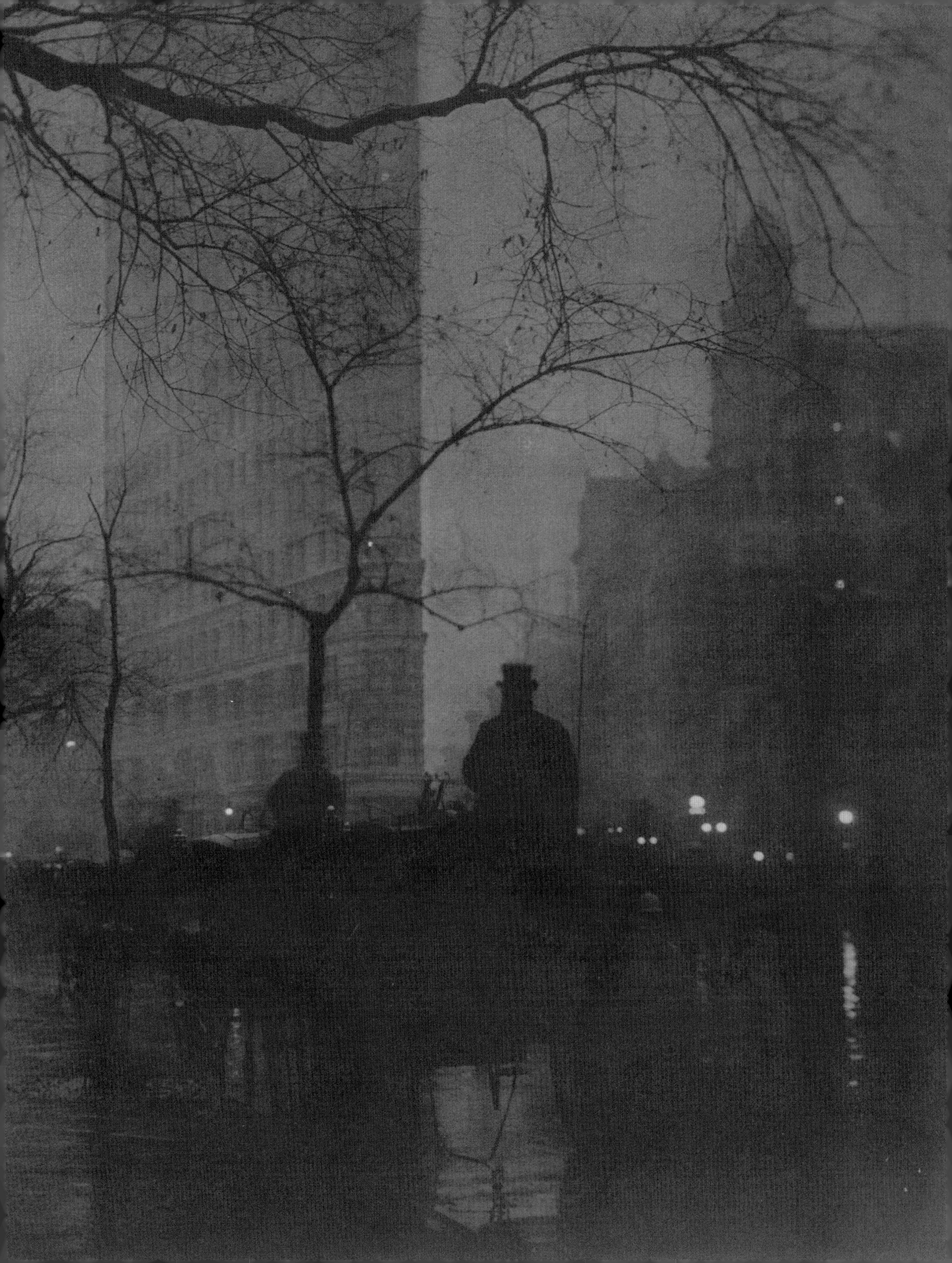

9 Shadow Presences

The Figure in the Urban Landscape

With urban growth, all of society had to revise its image. Traditional manners and conventions were turned on their head by the new living conditions of city dwellers, who had to entirely rethink their social relations. Nocturnal darkness further accentuated the uncertainty that the growth of the big cities and the changes in mores placed on human relationships. One of the changes that most profoundly affected relations between individuals was visual in nature: the urban space made the spectacle, to which it was intimately linked, a mode of sociability in its own right.[1] Big city life, with its novel forms of entertainment, turned all city dwellers into spectators but also into objects of and actors in the spectacle. The exchanges were in the first place optical in nature: city dwellers encountered, judged, and recognized one another primarily through the gaze. The urban night, by virtue of its darkness and because it opened up new social spaces, added an ambiguous dimension to these transformations. In the landscape of the city night, the human presence became difficult to make out, opaque both literally and symbolically. As a result of the darkness, the human form became abstract. For the artists who represented the urban night, that indistinguishable presence emerged in two recurrent figures: the crowd and the shadow, both of which embodied a kind of deterioration of individual identity, or at least a shift to a problematic appearance.

THE PUBLIC SPACE AND THE GAZE

The economic, social, and cultural transformations of the urban environment required to adapt modalities of representation to that new space, but they also gave rise to a reconfiguration of the conditions of vision. Alongside spectacular, sensational, and picturesque images of the city, an entire way of seeing specific to the metropolis developed, detectable in the images themselves. Georg Simmel pointed out the new predominance of vision in human relationships, a situation he linked to such concrete phenomena as the development of mass transport: for the first time, individuals who did not know one another were forced to share the same confined space and exchange looks in silence.[2] Thorstein Veblen also emphasized the visual character of the social exchanges in late nineteenth-century urbanized society, through his concept of "conspicuous consumption": it was through the gaze of others that the social status of the consumer was

Fig. 126 detail

constructed.[3] The experience of the city, that anonymous, overpopulated world saturated with information, caused a profound visual disorientation, to which artists had to adapt. In *Picturing the City,* Rebecca Zurier makes vision and its staging the guiding thread of her analysis of works by the major personalities of the Ashcan School, which appear to have been the first attempts to make the city "legible,"[4] to quote the urbanist Kevin Lynch's reflections on the visual urban environment.[5] But that "legibility," because it was more visual than textual, also reproduced and exaggerated the opacity of the city, exacerbating what John Kasson describes as a "crisis of meanings," a "semiotic breakdown," more than it resolved it.[6]

Nocturnal darkness opened a new field of exploration, where questions of vision were reformulated or became more pressing. In the big cities, governed by the proximity between individuals and the dominance of the gaze, night, the space traditionally associated with intimacy, offered previously unseen visions in which relations between public and private spheres were transformed. Consider this excerpt from William Dean Howells's *A Hazard of New Fortunes,* in which the novel's main characters, the Marches, having recently arrived in New York, discover the domestic and theatrical pleasures of urban voyeurism: "At Third Avenue they took the Elevated for which [Mrs. March] confessed an infatuation. . . . She now said that the night transit was even more interesting than the day, and that the fleeing intimacy you formed with people in second and third floor interiors, while all the usual street life went on underneath, had a domestic intensity mixed with a perfect repose that was the last effect of good society with all its security and exclusiveness. He said it was better than the theatre, of which it reminded him, to see those people through their windows."[7]

The historian Richard Sennett has shown how, in the nineteenth century, the public space was transformed under pressure from urban development, and how these changes affected the very subjectivity of city dwellers, by defining personal identity as a social category in its own right, constructed in relation to the public space and partly in opposition to it.[8] According to Sennett, modern big cities made the individual's involvement in the public sphere, which had been characteristic of the Old Regime, impossible. That new environment condemned city dwellers, wary of those they might encounter in the public space, to a silent isolation and forced them to seek personal fulfillment solely in their private lives. In the public sphere, appearances, considered under the Old Regime to be obstacles to knowledge of an individual, took precedence over speech. During the nineteenth century, they became one of the major axes of social interactions and of ways of defining individual personality.[9]

Many late nineteenth-century cultural products bear out the obsession with appearances and their potential deceptiveness: the novels of Henry James, in which characters spend their time examining the surface of beings and things and wondering about their meaning; the vogue for detective stories, largely sustained by the major magazines of the time;[10] and the phenomenally successful theatrical adaptation of Robert Louis Stevenson's *Strange Case of Dr. Jekyll and Mr. Hyde* in New York in 1887. It became necessary to learn to decipher one's fellows: individuals uninformed about the realities of the city, for example, were encouraged to rely on galleries of types, which, like the guidebooks describing a city's streets and neighborhoods, allowed their users to navigate urban territory. In 1892, no doubt anticipating the flood of tourists that would be unleashed by the World's Columbian Exposition in Chicago, Sigmund Krausz published a gallery of portraits called *Street Types of Chicago,* stereotypical figures that had been recreated in the studio (see fig. 129).[11] Krausz seems to have been inspired by the scientific use of photography in the nineteenth century to catalogue medical or criminal cases,[12] projects that somewhat resembled Riis's and Hine's documentary photography. All these approaches emerged from a will of the ruling classes to classify and discipline by means of the image. Yet the need to scrutinize the Other was so generalized that observers could easily become the observed. A passage from the preface to *Darkness and Daylight* shows that mistrust in appearances was shared by all social classes. In an ironic reversal, it presented the reporter as a potential suspect in the eyes of criminals in the urban slums: "Any one who undertakes to 'see life' in the haunts of vice and crime in New York, especially by night, takes his life in his own hand, and courts danger in many forms. Criminals are a suspicious class. The appearance of a camera in their midst at once suggests to them the Rogues' Gallery, and recalls to their mind crimes known only to themselves. It is not pleasant, in underground dens, where hardened criminals and the vilest outcasts hide from the light of day, to be mistaken for detectives in search of their prey. . . . There are hundreds of places in New York where even the air of respectability is an element of personal danger."[13]

The image, which purported to be an instrument of clarification and legibility, could also introduce doubt. Representations of the human figure in the urban night belonged to that problematic of legibility and opacity and further complicated it. The figures glimpsed in the night assumed an ambiguous form: darkness and presence converged symbolically in the silhouette, the locus for a negotiation of identities. If we adopt Sennett's reflections on the definition of subjective identity in the public space, the silhouette can be seen as a kind of neutralized individual emotionally disengaged from the public space. But the silhouette was also an instrument of definition. The darkness of the crowd enveloped individuals to form an indistinct mass, but silhouettes made it possible to discern identities while restricting them to clearly identifiable types, midway between the familiar and the alien, the anonymous and the legible.

LANDSCAPES BLACK WITH CROWDS

Urban growth produced an unprecedented increase in population density, a spectacular phenomenon in the eyes of observers at the time, who never failed to point out the presence of crowds in the streets of the metropolises.[14] Gerald Stanley Lee, a pastor-turned-journalist, saw the crowd as one of the principal symbols of the modern environment: "The problem of living in this modern world is the problem of finding room in it. The crowd principle is so universally at work through modern life that the geography of the world has been changed to conform to it. We live in crowds. We get our living in crowds. We are amused in herds. Civilization is a list of cities. Cities are the huge central dynamos of all being. The power of a man can be measured to-day by the mile, the number of miles between him and the city; that is, between him and what the city stands for—the centre of mass." Lee declared the need to control the urban crowd by means of charismatic leaders, but he was relatively optimistic about the multitudes, advancing the idea that the crowd can be morally "good" and can prove to be a source of inspiration for artists.[15] That positive vision stands in contrast to other works on the subject that captured the American public's attention, including the English translation of Gustave Le Bon's *Psychologie des foules*, published in the United States in 1896 under the title *The Crowd: A Study of the Popular Mind.* Le Bon conveyed the idea that the crowd constitutes an entity distinct from the individuals that form it,[16] with an autonomous but weak psychology particularly sensitive to suggestion, especially from images: "Crowds are to some extent in the position of the sleeper whose reason, suspended for the time being, allows the arousing in his mind of images of extreme intensity which would quickly be dissipated could they be submitted to the action of reflection. . . . Crowds being only capable of thinking in images are only to be impressed by images. It is only images that terrify or attract them and become motives of action."[17] Conversely, the image of that crowd so easily captivated exerted an undeniable fascination of its own. In fact, the press reveled in representations of the multitude, where the amalgam of bodies was made even more striking by the homogeneity of colors that resulted from the medium used, usually photography or engraving. Mariana Griswold Van Rensselaer commented on the spectacle of the streets in the metropolis, which seemed literally black with crowds, because of the uniformity of urban dwellers' dress: "Our downtown streets, in their busy hours, show crowds that are unusually black, not only because they are very dense, but because black is the customary wear of men."[18] In the big cities, the crowd was in reality a daily spectacle, sometimes brought out by regularly occurring celebrations such as election nights, but also quite simply by the logistical structure of the city, where certain neighborhoods saw heavy traffic at certain hours (figs. 118, 119). The nocturnal context, privileged by illustrators who depicted these urban crowds, produced a dual indetermination: the intermingling of all or nearly all social classes favored by the darkness was in fact accentuated by the blurriness of the image, in which the figures were clustered together in dark masses. These visions, whether looking down from high above or closer to street level, emphasized the density of the crowd, even while raising the question of its fluidity. The illustration that *Harper's Weekly* devoted to the presidential election of 1892 shows, for example, rows of illuminated streetcars motionless amidst the crowd. Meanwhile, W. H. Crane's illustration, as if observing a hierarchy of modes of transportation, juxtaposes pedestrian traffic and horse-drawn carriages, which are themselves flanked by railroad traffic. John Sloan's *Six O'Clock, Winter,* takes up that traffic iconography but adopts a twofold point of

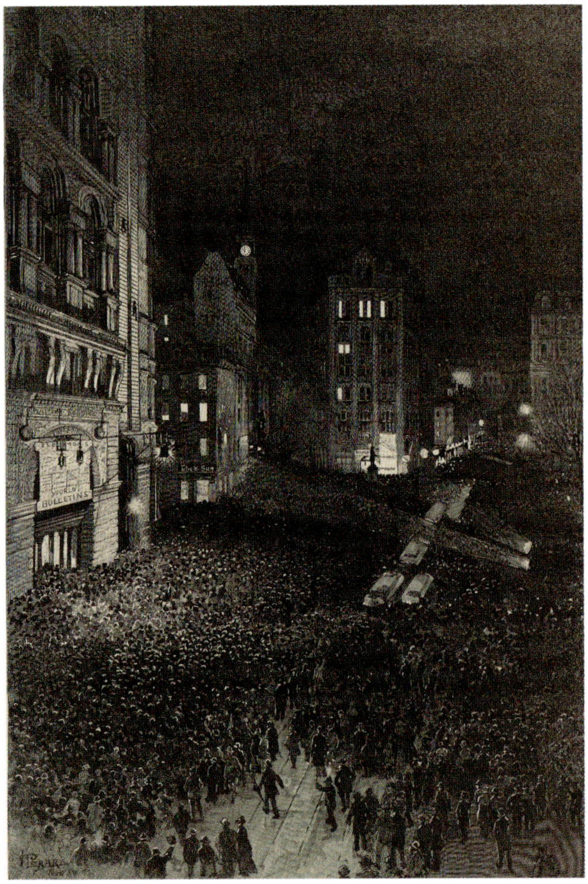

FIG. 118. V. Perard, "Newspaper Row, New York, on Election Night," *Harper's Weekly* 36, no. 1874 (November 19, 1892). Beinecke Rare Book and Manuscript Library, Yale University.

view (fig. 120). The scene, conspicuously captured at the level of the faces of passersby, nevertheless presents a wide enough viewing angle (wider, one may surmise, than that of the pedestrians) to encompass New York's famous "El," a feature characteristic of the landscape of Greenwich Village, where Sloan lived and where he painted most of his subjects. On the platform, Sloan showed a second crowd, above and in addition to the first. The perspective of the elevated tracks, further accentuated by the arrival of a train, creates a dynamic and controlled impression of the image as a whole, compensating for the static and chaotic aspect of the crowd below. Zurier notes that Sloan replicated the imagery of the flow of traffic used by H. G. Wells, for example, in *The Future in America:* "Thence, if it is late afternoon, one may walk back to City Hall Park and encounter and experience the convergent stream of clerks and workers making for the bridge, mark it grow denser and denser, until at last they come near choking even the broad approaches of the giant duct, until the congested multitudes jostle and fight for a way. They arrive marching afoot by every street in endless procession; crammed trolley-cars disgorge them; the Subway pours them out. . . . The distinctive effect is the mass, the black torrent, rippled with unmeaning faces, the great, the unprecedented multitudinousness of the thing, the

FIG. 119. W. H. Crane, "Junction of Broadway and Sixth Avenue," *Harper's Weekly* 35, no. 1787 (March 21, 1891). Beinecke Rare Book and Manuscript Library, Yale University.

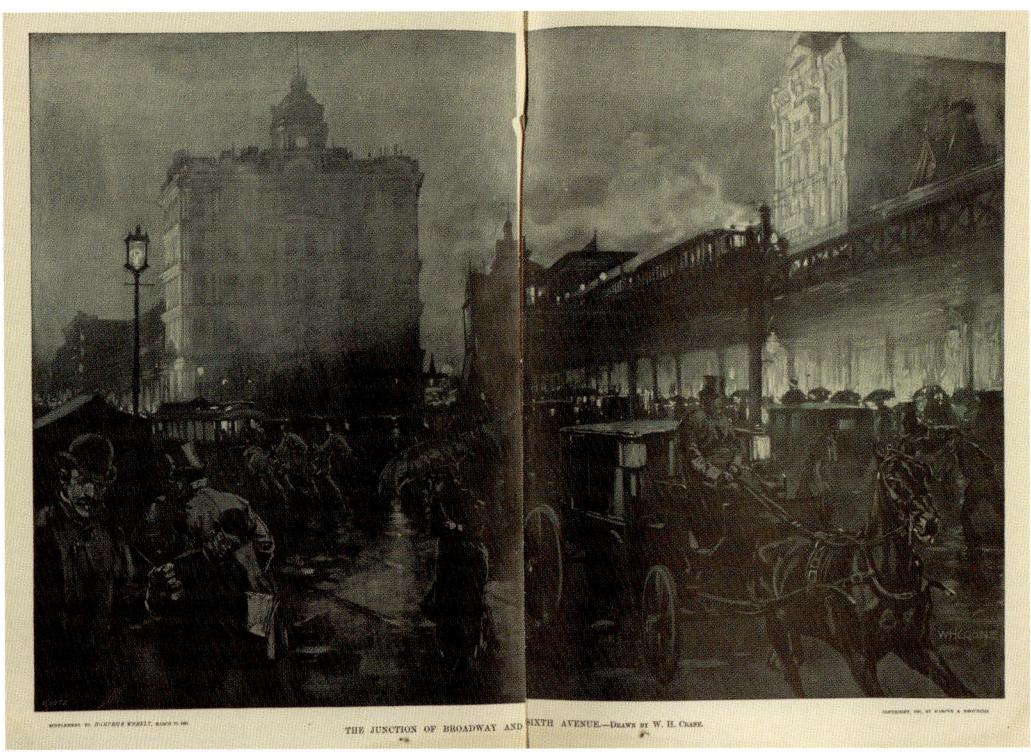

inhuman force of it all."[19] This imagery can be linked to the vocabulary used in an article from the *Literary Digest*, which described the crowd as a dynamic force of its own, to be managed following the principles of engineering: "The similarity between the flow of a liquid and the movement of a dense crowd of people must have struck many an observer. The principal difference is that motion is transmitted through a fluid chiefly by pressure and cohesion, whereas in a crowd each human particle has a motor of its own. When a ripple runs through a crowded ferry-boat as it approaches the slip it is due not to gravity or surface friction but to the desire of each constituent of the crowd to get home to his dinner. It is possible, however, to deal with and control a crowd in much the same way as a mass of liquid particles, and such a problem of control is thus approximated to one of hydraulic engineering."[20] The insistence on crowd control is significant: the emphasis in the images evoked above on the movement of individuals may in fact reveal a certain uneasiness about the potential disorder of the masses. At a time when news of recent discoveries and theories in the field of physics, such as the law of entropy, were reaching the general public, the metaphor of "human particles" used in the *Literary Digest* article was potentially unstable, since it suggested, beyond the model of a channeled and controlled fluid, a movement of chaos and decomposition. *Six O'Clock*, with its two levels of crowd traffic, can thus be read as a dual vision of the multitude: controlled and disciplined by the regularity of mechanized transportation in the top part of the image; freer and more disorderly in the bottom part, where the "other half" is depicted. The painting can also be compared to a second work by Sloan with an almost identical format and composition. In *Election Night*, painted five years before *Six O'Clock*, the crowd surrenders to a chaotic and carnivalesque movement (fig. 121).[21]

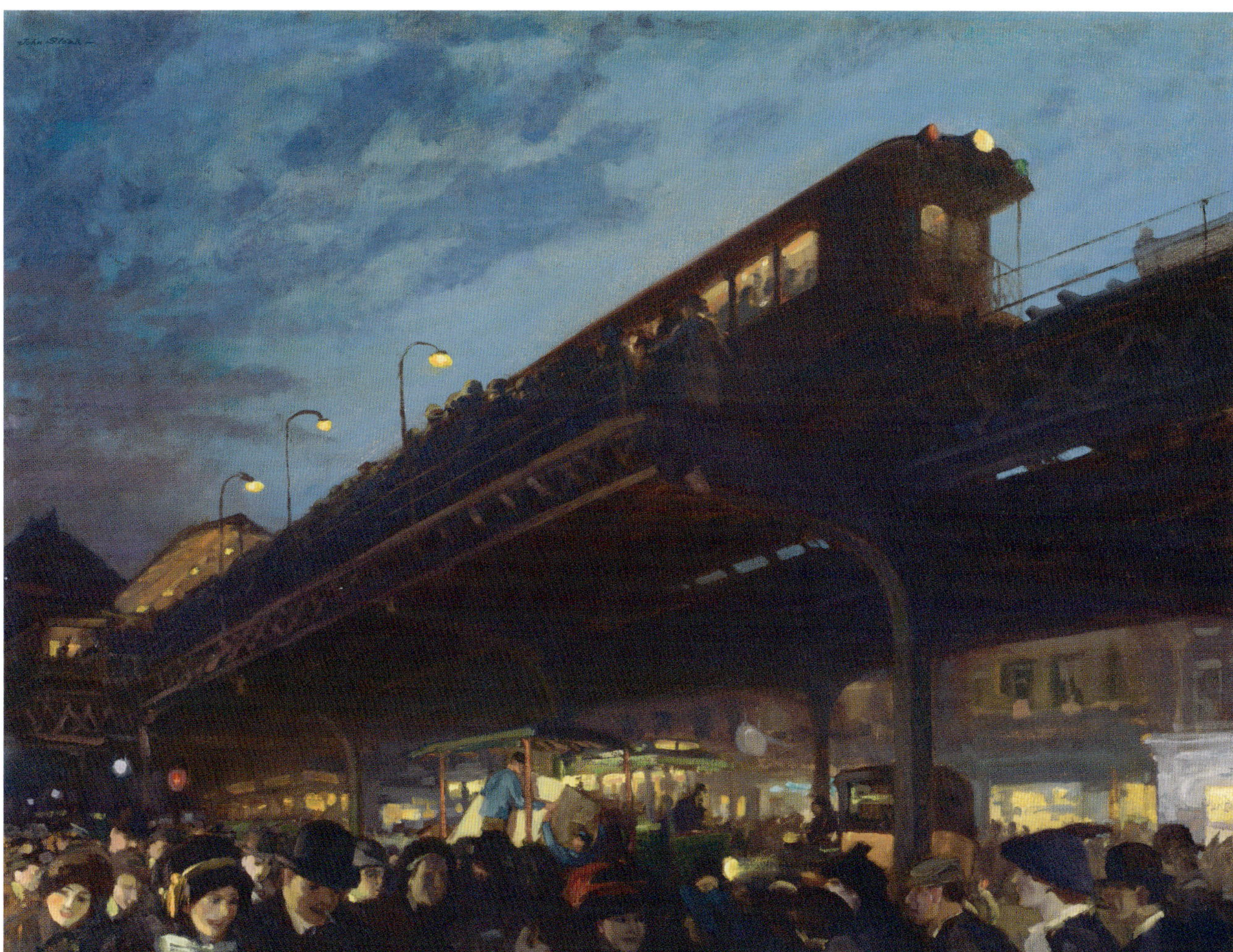

FIG. 120. John Sloan, *Six O'Clock, Winter*, 1912. Oil on canvas, 66.4 × 81.3 cm (26 1/8 × 32 in.). Phillips Collection, Washington, D.C.

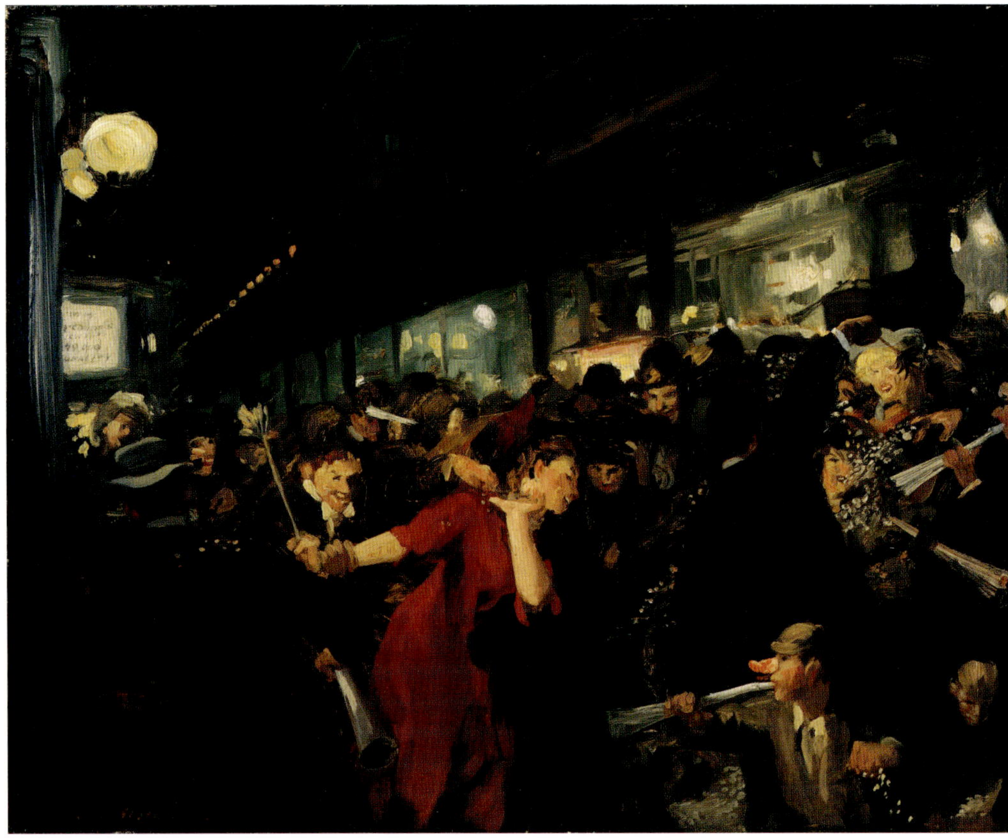

FIG. 121. John Sloan, *Election Night*, 1907. Oil on canvas, 67 × 81.9 cm (26 3/8 × 32 1/4 in.). Memorial Art Gallery of the University of Rochester: Marion Stratton Gould Fund.

The painting shows a tangle of bodies dressed in bright colors; the faces are sometimes masked. The grotesque atmosphere is reminiscent of James Ensor's paintings or, earlier in the pictorial tradition, Pieter Breughel the Elder's representations of festive gatherings or Hieronymus Bosch's scenes of grotesque outbursts. Whereas in *Six O'Clock* the El line cuts the image in two, here it runs along the upper edge of the painting, leaving almost the entire field to popular revelry. The artist himself related his experience of that evening, when the crowd was, in his words, "so dense in places that it [was] impossible to control one's movement."[22]

The festive night depicted by Sloan, though its referent was a national democratic ritual that reinforced the crowd's symbolic unity, gives a glimpse of the possibility of another type of commotion, another way the crowd might occupy the public and political space. The multitude, described by Le Bon as irrational and impulsive, subject to manipulation by images and feelings, could indeed appear worrisome. With the rise of powerful workers' unions and the violence of their repression, the threat of social unrest was a palpable menace to many observers. To name but a few examples of the social violence that marked the turn of the twentieth century, the Haymarket Square Riot in Chicago in 1886, the Homestead Riots at the Carnegie Steel works in 1892, the nationwide railroad strikes in 1893–1894, the coal miners' strike in Pennsylvania in 1902, and the assassination of President William McKinley by the anarchist Leon Czolgosz in 1901 all led the elites to believe in the dangers of anarchism and to look suspiciously at massive popular gatherings.[23] The *Literary Digest*'s proposal that the circulation of city dwellers be controlled through a system based on a scientific approach (which brings to mind the labor rationalization methods introduced by Frederick Winslow Taylor in his *Principles of Scientific Management*) appeared as the reaction of an anxious ruling elite striving to impose a rational order on the perceived chaos of the masses.[24]

In contrast to the indeterminate black torrent of the working-class multitude, gatherings composed of people from wealthier social milieus were portrayed as distinguished, in all the senses of the word. For example, an illustration in *Harper's Magazine* for an article titled "When the City Amuses Itself" depicts, in front of a very Whistleresque landscape, a crowd dressed primarily in white: women, men, and children mingle in lively but civil companionship, each individual clearly distinct

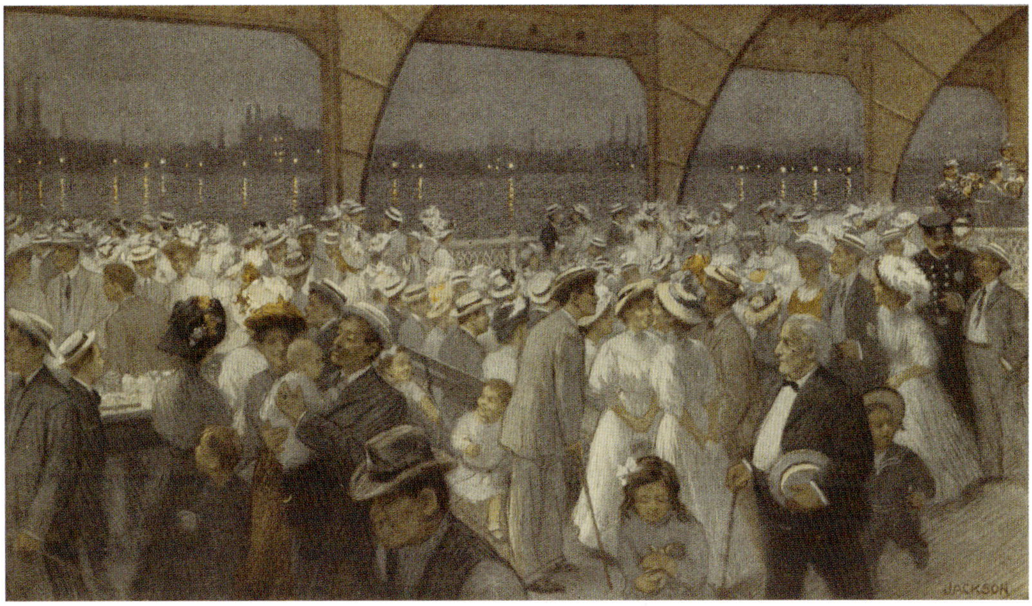

FIG. 122. John Edwin Jackson, "Day and Night the Recreation Piers Are Full of Life," 1909, *Harper's Weekly* 53, no. 2733 (May 15, 1909). Art and Picture Collection, New York Public Library, Astor, Lenox and Tilden Foundations.

FIG. 123. John Sloan, *The Coffee Line*, 1905. Oil on canvas, 54.6 × 80.3 cm (21 ½ × 31 ⅝ in.). Carnegie Museum of Art, Pittsburgh, Fellows of the Museum of Art Fund, 83.29.

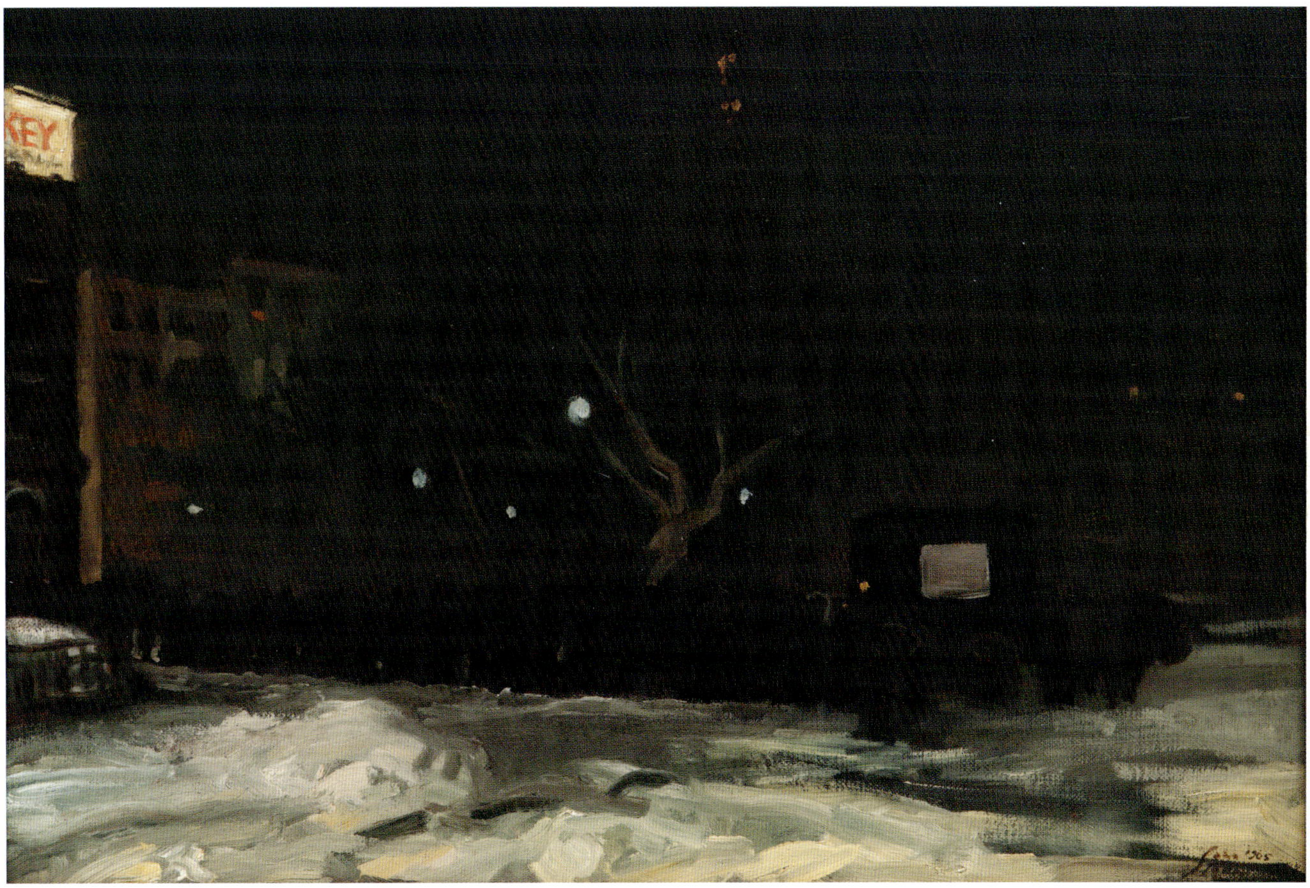

from the group (fig. 122).[25] The opposition between darkness and light was thus transposed onto the depiction of crowds, with blackness and indetermination reserved for the working classes, brightness for the elites. The division was even more striking in representations of one last type of popular gathering in the urban context: that of poor people waiting in line outside for material assistance, often food, to be dispensed to them. Sloan, for example, painted *The Coffee Line* in 1905 (fig. 123), and in 1900 Shinn created *Fleischmann's Bread Line*,[26] a reference to the charitable works of the yeast manufacturer Louis Fleischmann, who had bread distributed to the

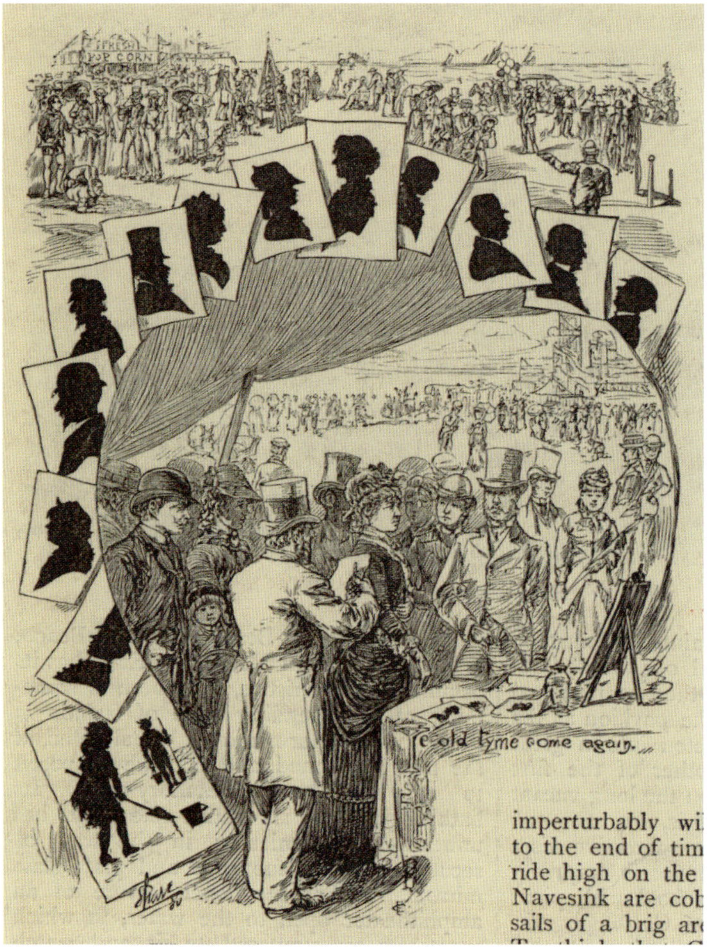

FIG. 124. Henry Pruett Share, "The Silhouette Artist," *Scribner's* 20, no. 3 (July 1880), Art and Picture Collection, New York Public Library, Astor, Lenox and Tilden Foundations.

poor every night at midnight outside his bakery.[27] The two works express ambivalence in several ways: through them, the artists demonstrated their compassion for these marginalized men suffering from hunger in midwinter, the black line of people contrasting in both cases to the snow on the ground, which underscores the dire fate they face. In fact, however, the emphasis placed on form, as in *Fire on 24th Street* (see fig. 113), undercuts the social consciousness to which these paintings might have borne witness. In both works, the indistinction characteristic of Whistler's art also contributes to keeping the poor at a distance: they now form only a compact mass, barely visible against the dark background, in which the individuals remain anonymous, unable to elicit any sympathy in the beholder. Their bodies subjected to the discipline of standing in a queue, they incarnate a crowd whose energies have been channeled, even disciplined into a "line" more than a group of free individuals. *The Coffee Line* and *Fleischmann's Bread Line* are the antithesis of the chaos of *Election Night*. In these images, darkness and urban poverty are carefully contained within a remote and abstract form.

DISCERNING IDENTITIES: TYPOLOGIES OF SHADOW

Conversely, the darkness that blurred the bodies of the poorest people into a single mass also served to isolate individuals who populated the urban landscape. When they did not repress individuality in a collective anonymity, artists questioned identity through the recurrent use of silhouettes. The pictorial genre of the silhouette, very much in vogue in the late eighteenth and early nineteenth centuries, experienced a nostalgic revival at the turn of the twentieth century. This is indicated by an illustration depicting one of the amusements offered visitors to Coney Island, the booth of an artist who specialized in silhouette portraits (fig. 124). Late nineteenth-century artists appropriated not only the silhouette form but also the values with which it had been vested in the previous century. In Johann Kaspar Lavater's *Essais sur la physiognomie* (*Essays on Physiognomy*), published in 1775–1778, the author speculated on the capacity of shadow and silhouette to reveal the personality of the subject depicted, and he used it to establish a classification system.[28] The silhouette was reclaimed a century later in a large variety of visual works, from magazine illustrations to advertising playing cards. Like Krausz's *Street Types of Chicago*, these series of illustrations functioned as a typology of individuals in the urban space.

In representations of the city at night, one of the most visible types almost always appeared in silhouette. This was the hackney cab driver, dressed in his characteristic top hat and perched on his carriage (figs. 125, 126). Alfred Stieglitz touted his *Reflections: Night—New York* (see fig. 49) as the first example of a night photograph to include a living subject: the shot captured the presence of a horse-drawn cab and its driver in the background. The same figures reappeared more clearly a few months later in *The Glow of Night—New York* (see fig. 48).[29] The silhouette of the coachman seemed generic enough to adapt to a vision of the city that ordinarily excluded human presence. That type became an element of the urban landscape, a public and depersonalized figure, sufficiently motionless for his silhouette to be imprinted on a negative even during the long exposure time required by the darkness. Distance was marked by the effacement of

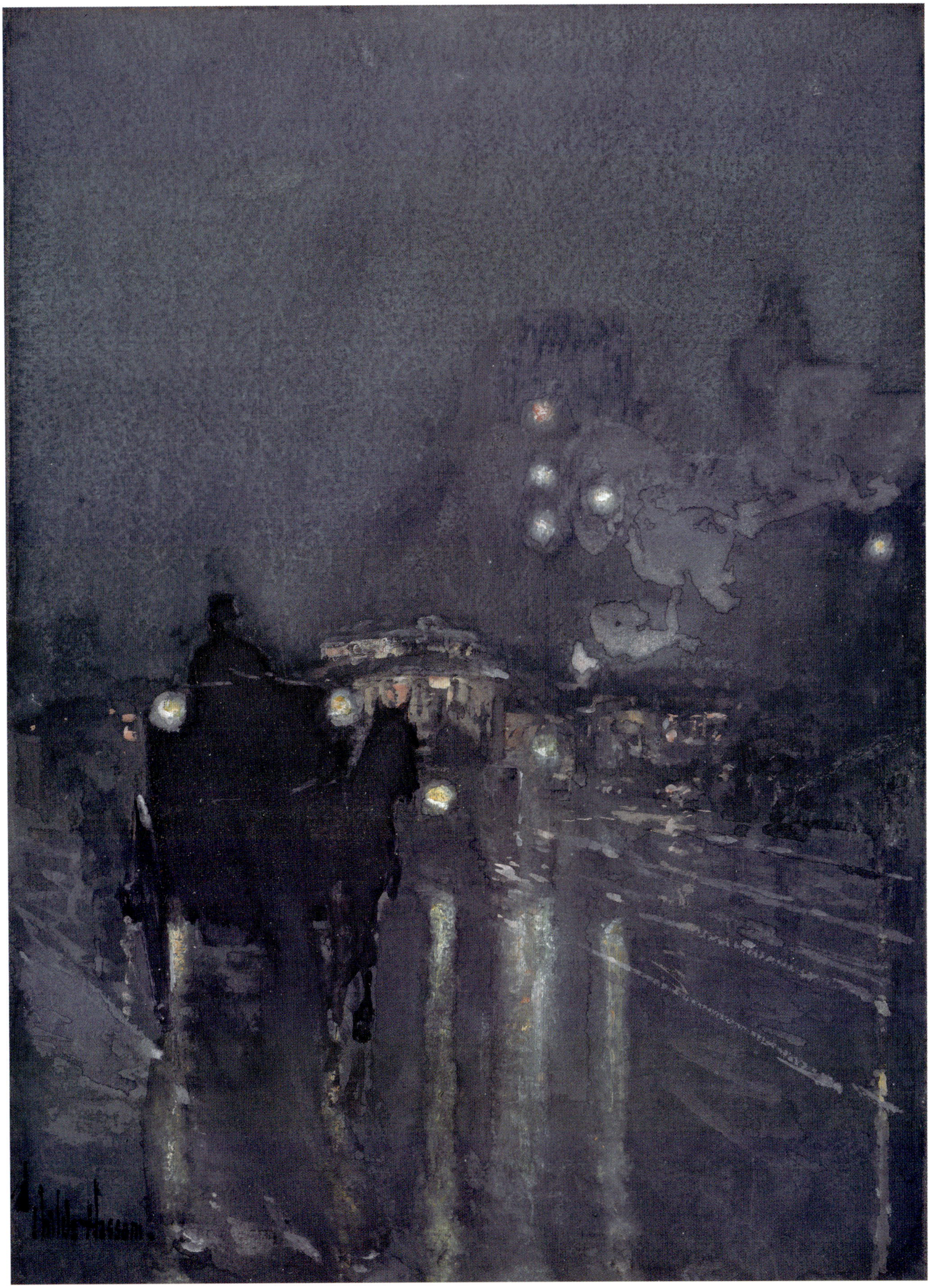

FIG. 125. Childe Hassam, *Nocturne, Railway Crossing, Chicago*, 1893. Opaque watercolor on paper, sheet, 40.6 × 29.8 cm (16 × 11 ¾ in.). Museum of Fine Arts, Boston. Hayden Collection—Charles Henry Hayden Fund (62.986).

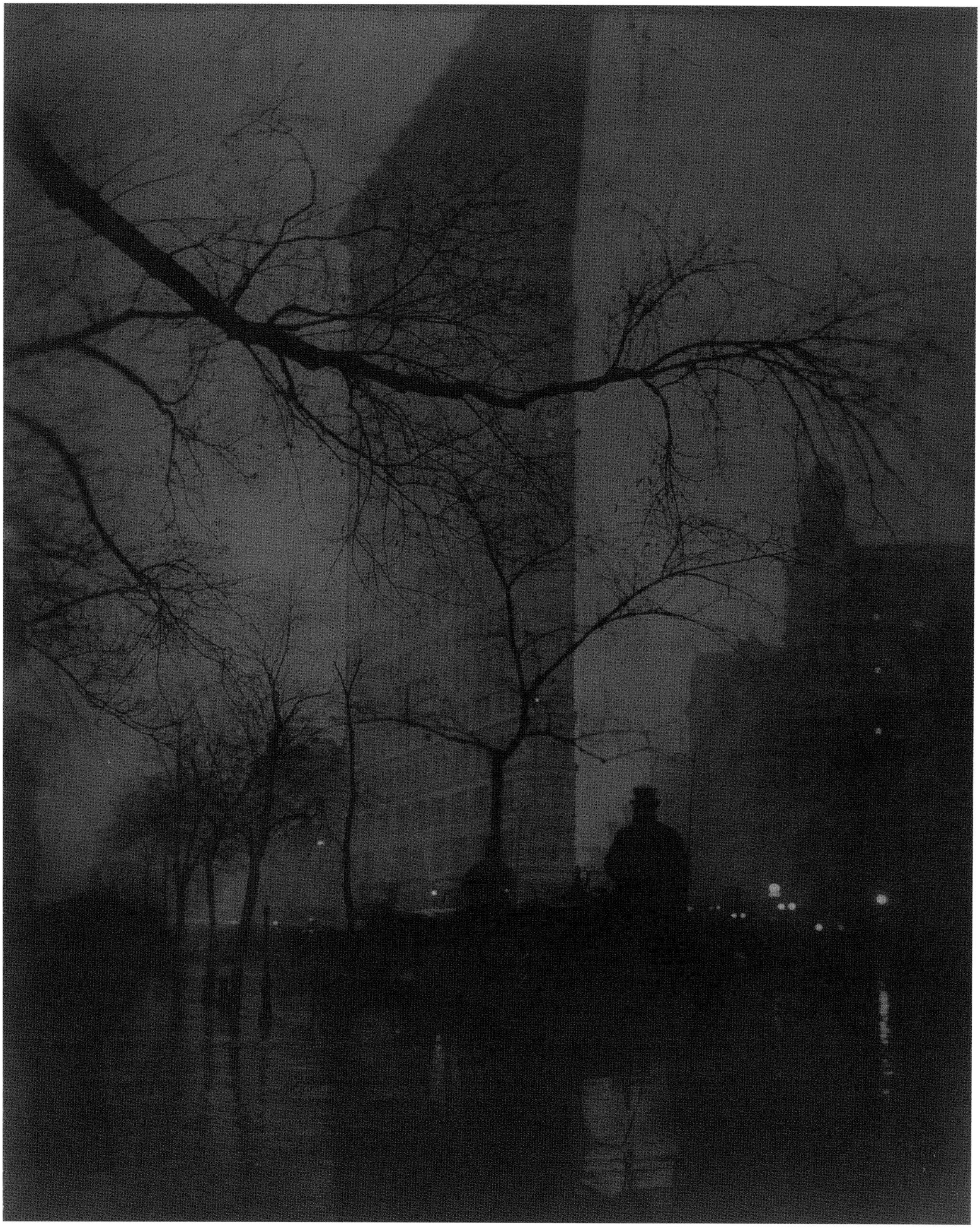

FIG. 126. Edward Steichen, *The Flatiron*, 1904, printed 1909. Gum bichromate over platinum print, 47.8 × 38.4 cm (18 13⁄16 × 15 1⁄8 in.). Metropolitan Museum of Art, Alfred Stieglitz Collection, 1933 (33.43.39).

individual features and an emphasis on a few recognizable characteristics: the hat, the carriage, the dark mass formed by the cab and its driver. Through the artist's use of shadow and abstraction, the silhouette made the urban space more legible. The beholder, whom the artist clearly expected to be familiar with this figure, was encouraged to look at the painting as he did objects in the street: he had to decode the forms that stood out against the darkness, just as, in the street, he had to identify the cab he would be able to hire.

In the urban setting, the hackney cab's figure was not neutral or devoid of connotations. Guidebooks for visitors to the big cities alerted their readers about the dishonesty of "hackmen." For example, *Chicago by Day and Night* warned: "There is a well-grounded suspicion in some quarters that only the hackmen of Niagara can compete with the hackmen of Chicago in their fondness for extortion and their success in practicing it."[30] Cab drivers also earned their shady reputation from providing one of the first means by which city dwellers could carry on illicit sexual relationships. A study on prostitution from that time mentioned in its first pages the role they played in the operation of brothels: "Chauffeurs and cabmen also do a thriving business in soliciting customers for vice resorts, a service for which they receive an ample commission. Standing at street corners or in front of hotels and restaurants, they urge men in low tones to go to houses or to 'ladies' clubs' as they are sometimes called."[31] The silhouettes present in the nocturne artists' works would have easily been read in these terms by contemporary beholders. The figure of the cabman thus essentialized the play of distances and the equivocal social relationships in the urban landscape: devoid of individual characteristics, they made him disappear behind his job, but at the same time they turned him into an emblem of a shady promiscuity.

The female equivalent, or rather complement, of that figure was the silhouette of the solitary woman, which suggested prostitution. Cabmen and prostitutes frequented the same neighborhoods, in search of the same clients. In the panoramic view that introduces the next-to-last chapter of *Maggie, a Girl of the Streets,* Stephen Crane mentions a long row of cabs parked along the street, before coming to focus on the figure of Maggie, who has become a mere "girl of the painted cohorts."[32] In *Cab Stand at Night, Madison Square* and *Fifth Avenue Nocturne,* Childe Hassam formed a similar visual link between the cabs and the isolated streetwalkers, equally dividing the space of the canvas between the two (figs. 127, 128). The historian Timothy Gilfoyle explains that the new spaces of sociability created by urbanization and the changes that restructured American society in the nineteenth century opened new possibilities for a multitude of sexual practices. Several of them can be categorized as prostitution, though he, along with several other historians of the subject, emphasizes their fluidity: seduction, like all other social relations, tended to migrate from the traditional sphere to that of overtly

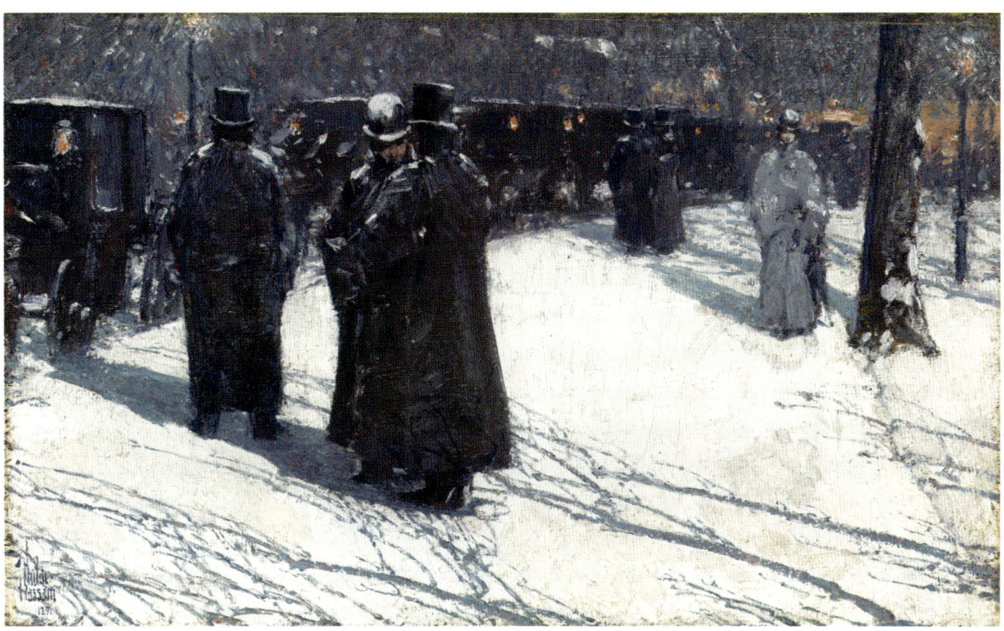

FIG. 127. Childe Hassam, *Cab Stand at Night, Madison Square,* 1891. Oil on panel, 22.7 × 36.6 cm (8 15/16 × 14 3/8 in.). Bequest of Annie Swan Coburn (Mrs. Lewis Larned Coburn), Smith College Museum of Art, Northampton, Massachusetts.

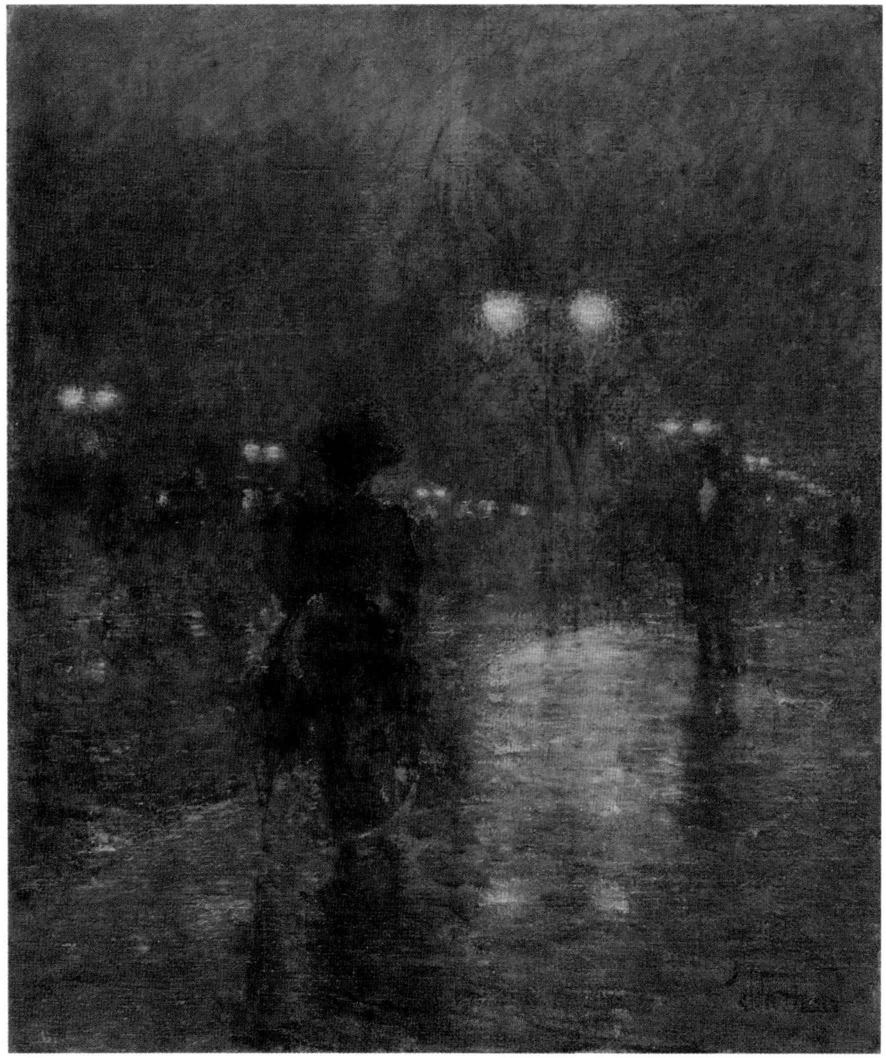

FIG. 128. Childe Hassam, *Fifth Avenue Nocturne,* c. 1895. Oil on canvas, 61.2 × 51 cm (24 1/16 × 20 1/16 in.). Cleveland Museum of Art, Anonymous gift (1952.538).

pecuniary exchanges. It became increasingly common, for example, for young single women of the middle class to trade the pleasure of their company for dinner at a restaurant or an outing. New professional categories, such as erotic dancer and stripper, developed on the fringes of prostitution, obscuring the boundaries between acceptable interactions and outright immorality.[33] In the general transformation of social relations, even as the distinction between licit and illicit, moral and immoral sexual relations was becoming increasingly blurred, the silhouette of the solitary woman, which recurs often in Childe Hassam's works, embodied both the necessity of resorting to stereotypes and the uncertainty that reigned in the realm of social appearances. Gilfoyle shows that the transformations of the urban space and the emergence of new places of pleasure in the city contributed to the decline of brothels and made prostitution less visible. It spread more discreetly over the urban territory, no longer resulting systematically from professional specialization. Prostitution, now occasional or informal, became increasingly difficult to recognize. Books of the time that examined the question of prostitution were the first to point out the difficulty of pinning down the subject. In *Metropolitan Life Unveiled,* J. W. Buel acknowledged the impossibility of an exact and exhaustive assessment: "By recent estimate, based on reports submitted from various charitable and municipal officers, Gotham has fifteen thousand registered prostitutes, and perhaps four times that number of women who are secret followers of the destructive vice."[34] This multiplicity of practices was further complicated by the great variety of appearances within the category of prostitute itself, as indicated in Rupert Hughes's description of prostitution around

Broadway: "Here and there women of various stages of prosperity wandered erratically, ogling every detached man, yet rarely showing more than a passive solicitude for attention. It is only in the minor streets that a 'Good evening, dear,' is ventured, for the police in uniform or in plain clothes insist on that outward respectability which is so pleasant in Paris and so odiously absent in London. Some of the willing sisters were somewhat tawdry, but the poorer members of the ancient sorority prefer the darker streets. To Broadway flock those chiefly of the finer ware, and the wayfarer need not walk far or wait long to see a dozen beauties, who would grace any company and who go gowned like duchesses adrift."[35] Hughes detailed the identifiable techniques of the prostitutes and the diversity of their modes of dress, and showed them moving in a primarily visually oriented environment: potential clients were singled out by the prostitutes' gaze, even as police officers imposed respect for proprieties. The differentiation of the women based on their looks corresponded to different degrees of light: the ugliest prostitutes took refuge in the darkest streets, while the most beautiful exposed themselves to the brightness of Broadway. Above all, their elegant appearance raised a fundamental problem for the observer, who sometimes had trouble determining the social status of the women he was observing. By way of response, that confusion required the development of an increased capacity for discernment. The type who appears under the label "Out for a Stroll" in Krausz's portrait gallery (fig. 129) can thus be read on two different levels: the young woman represented seems at first sight to be simply a young, elegant woman, but her gesture of lifting the pleats of her skirt with her hand, her posture, and her come-hither look directed at the beholder suggest to a more seasoned observer that she could be a prostitute. The image, whose title remains conspicuously neutral, plays on the same ambiguities as those that governed the dynamic of the gaze in the street.

The silhouettes of solitary women participated in that problematic of the gaze: darkness made the identity of these women at once conspicuous and ambiguous, underscoring their isolation in a public place at night but masking almost all the signs that would otherwise have made it possible to identify them precisely. As Kathy Peiss shows, beginning in the late nineteenth century, a growing number of women were employed in occupations that led them to move around the city alone at night. Dreiser's heroine Carrie can again serve as an example: although her relations with the men she meets take place outside social norms, the young woman does not exactly have the status of a prostitute. Having failed at occupations commonly practiced by single women living in the city (she is first employed in a factory, then in a department store), she finally manages to lead an independent life by making a name for herself in the theater. Her career demonstrates all the nuances of the various options available to young women who migrated to the city at the turn of the twentieth century. She achieves independence and professional success, but at the cost of a few compromises with the moral conventions of her time. In the same way, Everett Shinn's painting *Girl on Stage*[36] places a female figure in an ambiguous situation: though brightly lit by the footlights, from the artist's point of view she is in great part obscured. Her right hand, immersed in darkness, and the two patches of light—suggesting grotesque

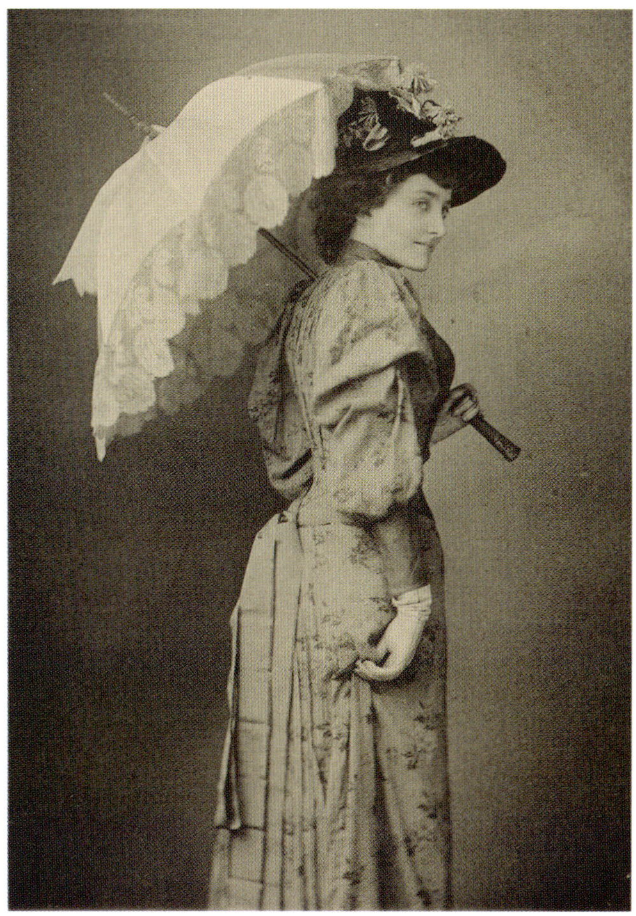

FIG. 129. Sigmund Krausz, "Out for a Stroll," in *Street Types of Chicago: Character Studies*, Chicago, Max Stern and Co., 1892. Beinecke Rare Book and Manuscript Library, Yale University.

masks—that form in the darkness before her seem to indicate the effacement of her individual identity behind the artificiality of her theatrical character. The shape of her body, particularly her corseted waist, is emphasized by the light, whereas her face is reduced to a vague *profil perdu.* The young woman is exposed and concealed in the same gesture: having become a public woman, she loses by the same token what distinguishes her as an individual.

Although female silhouettes were revealing shadows that fixed the figures thus represented in the identifiable role of women of loose morals, they also obliterated other information about these individuals. As in the case of silhouettes of hackney cabs, the beholder (particularly if he was male) found himself placed in a situation vis-à-vis the painting that he may have experienced in the street. He was obliged to scrutinize the female form standing out against the darkness and do his best to read its details: shape of the body, cut of the clothing, accessories, gestures, bearing. These silhouettes, considered from the point of view of a potential client, frustrated the gaze, in that they deprived the observer of information necessary to determine whether the transaction seemed desirable. For example, he found it impossible to make a distinction, as Hughes did, between the ugliest and prettiest women. Ethnic identity was another criterion that the darkness concealed in the urban landscape, and which almost all the images considered here leave ambiguous. A 1913 survey of the population of Bedford Hills, one of the main reformatories for New York City, estimated the proportion there of white women born in the United States at about 63 percent, that of foreign-born women at 24 percent, and that of African American women at 13 percent. The same study also pointed out that, in the illicit bars and back rooms of cabarets, individuals involved in prostitution were more likely than their contemporaries to transgress the rule of racial segregation.[37] Adding to the possibility of racial mixing was a symbolic confusion that attributed an ambiguous ethnic identity to prostitutes. In the late nineteenth century, organized prostitution was considered a "white slave trade." Jane Addams, for example, proposed an analogy between prostitution and black slavery in the South before the Civil War.[38] That comparison illustrates that women engaged in prostitution tended to fall into a special category, a gray zone analogous to nighttime, inasmuch as it concealed identities. This brings us back to the discussion of Tanner's *Salomé* introduced in Part I (see fig. 62): the prostitute personified a combination of alterity and taboo promiscuity, which was conveyed through the ambiguous opacity of darkness.

Even so, blackness is more revealing of the attitude of the artist toward the reality of sexual relations in the urban space than of the type to which these women may have belonged. In *Painted Love,* Hollis Clayson analyzes the fascination with prostitution manifested by the impressionists through their many representations—often very crude—of prostitutes.[39] Although Hassam claimed to belong to the American impressionist school, his approach was much more moderate than those of his French predecessors. His use of nocturnal darkness can be seen as a strategy that Clayson elsewhere describes as characteristic of late nineteenth-century American art, once again in contrast to the practices of the French impressionist artists. In an article on paintings of nocturnal Paris by American artists, Clayson demonstrates that these artists functioned as "outsiders" and used the nocturne to create an image of the French capital that was both modern and welcoming.[40] Her conclusions could be extended further: when Hassam returned to the United States, the darkness he had employed during his youth in Paris to reenchant a city that remained unwelcoming to him served to cover with a modest veil the prostitution depicted so vividly by the impressionists, even while showing that the artist was privy to the modern pictorial practices they had established.

The silhouette thus performed a multiplicity of sometimes contradictory functions. It singled out the type, but at the same time disrupted identity on several levels, emphasizing the ambiguities more than it dispelled them. In so doing, it engaged the beholder in a mode of vision in which, as in the actual urban night, he had to examine appearances, relying somewhat on the artist's complicity. But in this way the artist, in treating the question of prostitution obliquely, seemed to allow simultaneously a certain dose of prudery and a confusion about the impossibility of determining female identities on the streets at night. One last dimension of the silhouette arose from that oscillation between attraction and repulsion, between a knowing proximity and the powerlessness to decode anonymity: for Hassam and for his beholders—in principle male—there was no doubt an erotic pleasure to be had simply by maintaining the state of indetermination. The female silhouette emerging from the darkness

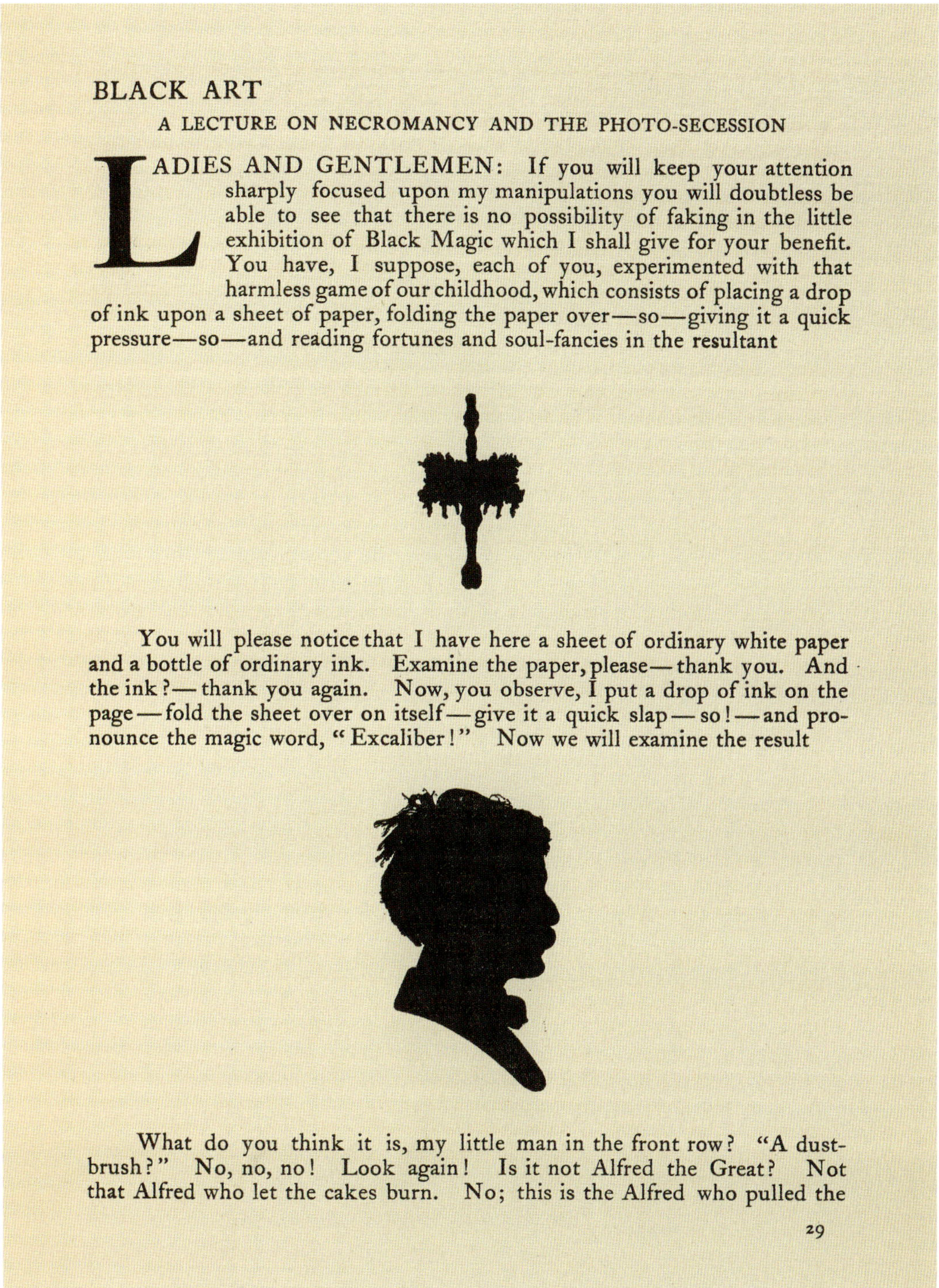

BLACK ART

A LECTURE ON NECROMANCY AND THE PHOTO-SECESSION

LADIES AND GENTLEMEN: If you will keep your attention sharply focused upon my manipulations you will doubtless be able to see that there is no possibility of faking in the little exhibition of Black Magic which I shall give for your benefit. You have, I suppose, each of you, experimented with that harmless game of our childhood, which consists of placing a drop of ink upon a sheet of paper, folding the paper over—so—giving it a quick pressure—so—and reading fortunes and soul-fancies in the resultant

You will please notice that I have here a sheet of ordinary white paper and a bottle of ordinary ink. Examine the paper, please— thank you. And the ink?— thank you again. Now, you observe, I put a drop of ink on the page — fold the sheet over on itself — give it a quick slap — so! — and pronounce the magic word, "Excaliber!" Now we will examine the result

What do you think it is, my little man in the front row? "A dust-brush?" No, no, no! Look again! Is it not Alfred the Great? Not that Alfred who let the cakes burn. No; this is the Alfred who pulled the

29

FIG. 130. John Barrett Kerfoot, "Black Art," *Camera Work* 8 (October 1904). Beinecke Rare Book and Manuscript Library, Yale University.

of *Fifth Avenue Nocturne,* neither too close nor too far away, sufficiently vague without being completely formless, allowed the beholder to project his desires and fantasies onto her. Rather than containing and restricting meanings, that silhouette seemed to embody an openness in which a certain creativity could find free expression.

A last series of examples will serve to complement these reflections on silhouettes and urban identities: those that depict the artists themselves, beginning with a series of silhouette portraits by John Barrett Kerfoot, published in *Camera Work* in 1904 (fig. 130). They represent five of the most important personalities in the

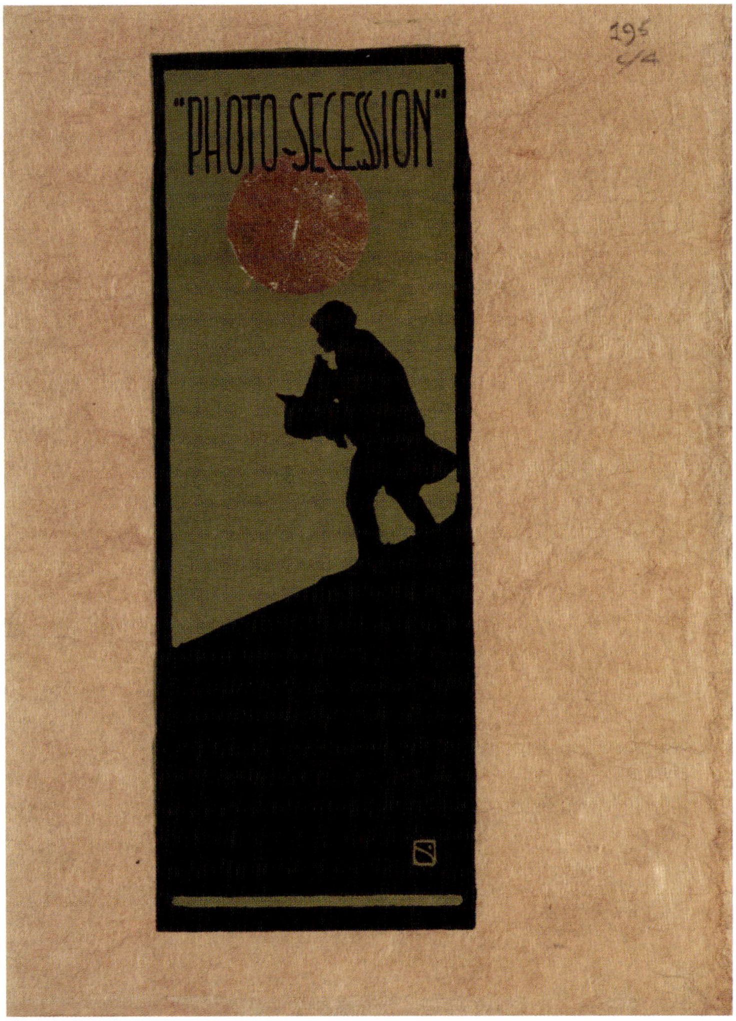

FIG. 131. Edward Steichen, Front cover of Photo-Secession catalogue, 1906. Royal Photographic Society.

Photo-Secession movement: Alfred Stieglitz, Edward Steichen, Alvin Langdon Coburn, Gertrude Käsebier, and Kerfoot himself. The silhouettes, Kerfoot announced, took shape on the paper as a result of a "black art," almost an art of divination, a kind of Rorschach test *avant la lettre,* in which a drop of ink set down on a folded sheet of paper revealed the observer's fate and the soul's imagination.[41] The procedure adopted (the reverse of photography because it reveals by means of darkness, calling nostalgically to an older, pre-technological form of portrayal) and the elitist complicity with the readers of *Camera Work* it assumed (they were supposed to be able to recognize the profiles of the personalities represented), linked that negative art to the pictorialist aesthetic. Two years later, the silhouette technique was taken up by Edward Steichen for his creation of the poster advertising the Photo-Secession exhibition of 1906 (fig. 131). Stieglitz, recognizable by his mustache, is represented equipped with a camera and in moonlight, on what could be the roof of a building. The depiction confers on the photographer the appearance of an adventurer, even a villain operating under cover of darkness. Unlike the previous examples, in this illustration the silhouette is not passive, it is not simply a cliché or a space for the beholder's projections: it also points to the active source of other images. Rather than distancing the figure considered, it serves as a mediation for the beholder's gaze, opening onto other potential images.

In John Sloan's engraving *Night Windows* (1910), the artist's silhouette is difficult to make out at first glance. Perched on the roof of a building and with his back turned to the beholder, he introduces an additional level of complexity (fig. 132). The artist represented here, completely engrossed as he is in the spectacle of a young woman in a sensual pose illuminated in the window frame, does not see what is happening just below him. In that much more prosaic scene, a second woman is busy hanging laundry outside her bedroom window, while a mustached man reclines on her bed. The clothesline forms a diagonal symbolically linking the housewife to the space of the beholder outside the picture's frame. The person contemplating the engraving is doubly, even triply, a voyeur, since he can observe the intimate lives of the two women as well as the artist's own voyeurism.[42]

The setting for the scene, which suggests a powerful but invisible light source behind the building the artist is watching, and which emphasizes the intricate architecture that weaves all the elements together, seems to be a commentary on the potentialities and difficulties of vision occasioned by the nocturnal urban space. From his elevated point of view, the artist is portrayed as a somewhat ironic replica of the heroes in William Dean Howells's *A Hazard of New Fortunes:* the voyeur does not see everything and may also find himself the object of the other's gaze. His opaque and yet sharply delineated silhouette gives the lie to his apparent simplicity. It recapitulates all the ambiguities of a vision deployed on several levels and encompassing multiple meanings. It contributed toward modulating the distance between individuals, serving by turns—or simultaneously—as an opaque screen, an interpretive grid, a visual relay point, and a space of projection. It marked presences in the urban landscape, but it indicated at the same time

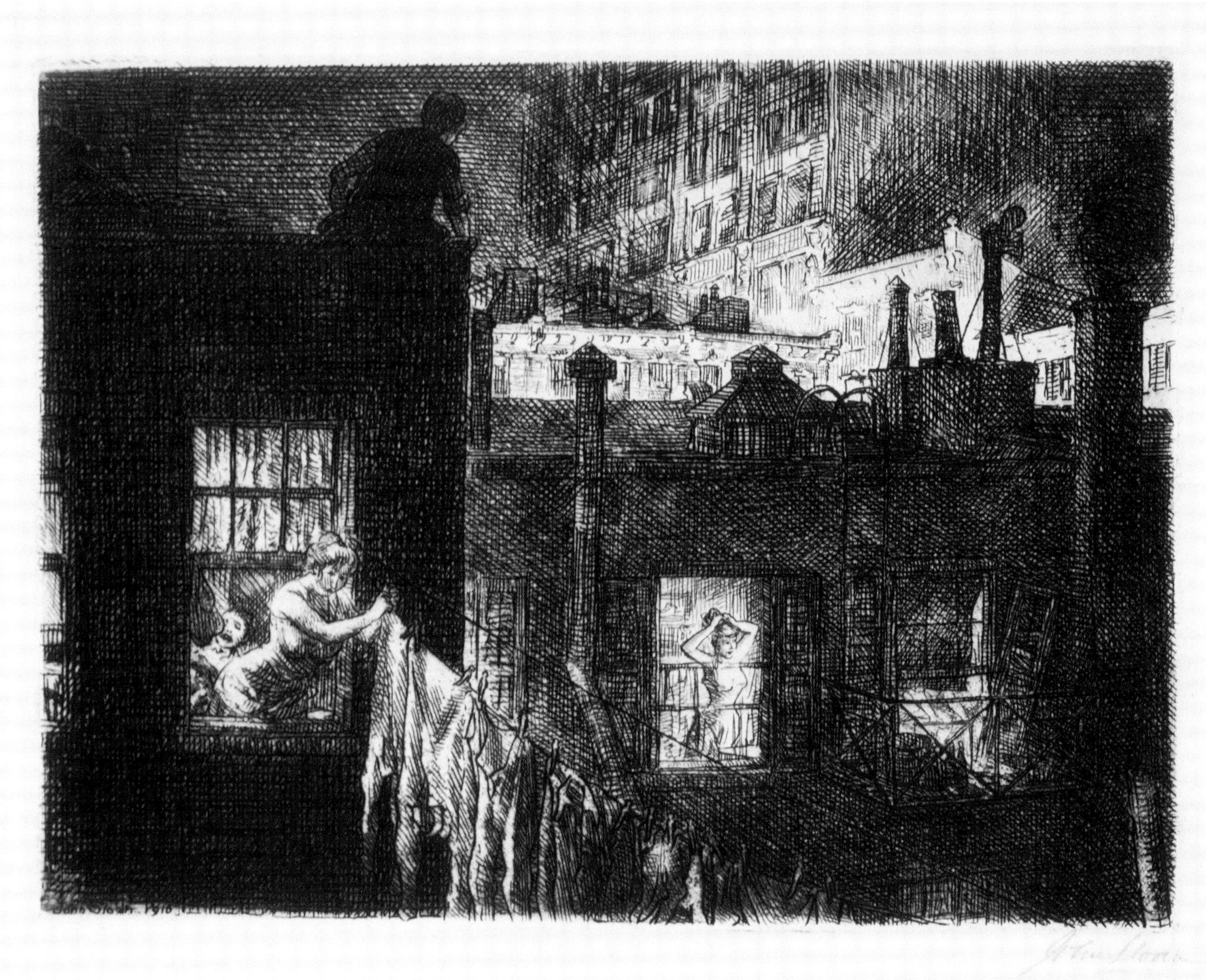

FIG. 132. John Sloan, *Night Windows*, 1910. Etching on paper, 13.3 × 17.1 cm (5 1/4 × 6 3/4 in.). Phillips Collection, Washington, D.C.

the impossibility of fixing fluctuating identities. *Night Windows* can serve as a paradigm for nocturnal urban vision, showing that, though the gaze was liberated in the urban space, it did not provide an all-powerful vision. The dominant, objective, and unique point of view disappeared in favor of a pluralistic notion of the gaze. The nocturnal urban landscape is here reduced to a series of windows, each providing an ambiguous interface between the inside and the outside, and through which one has to constantly rethink one's relation to the Other.

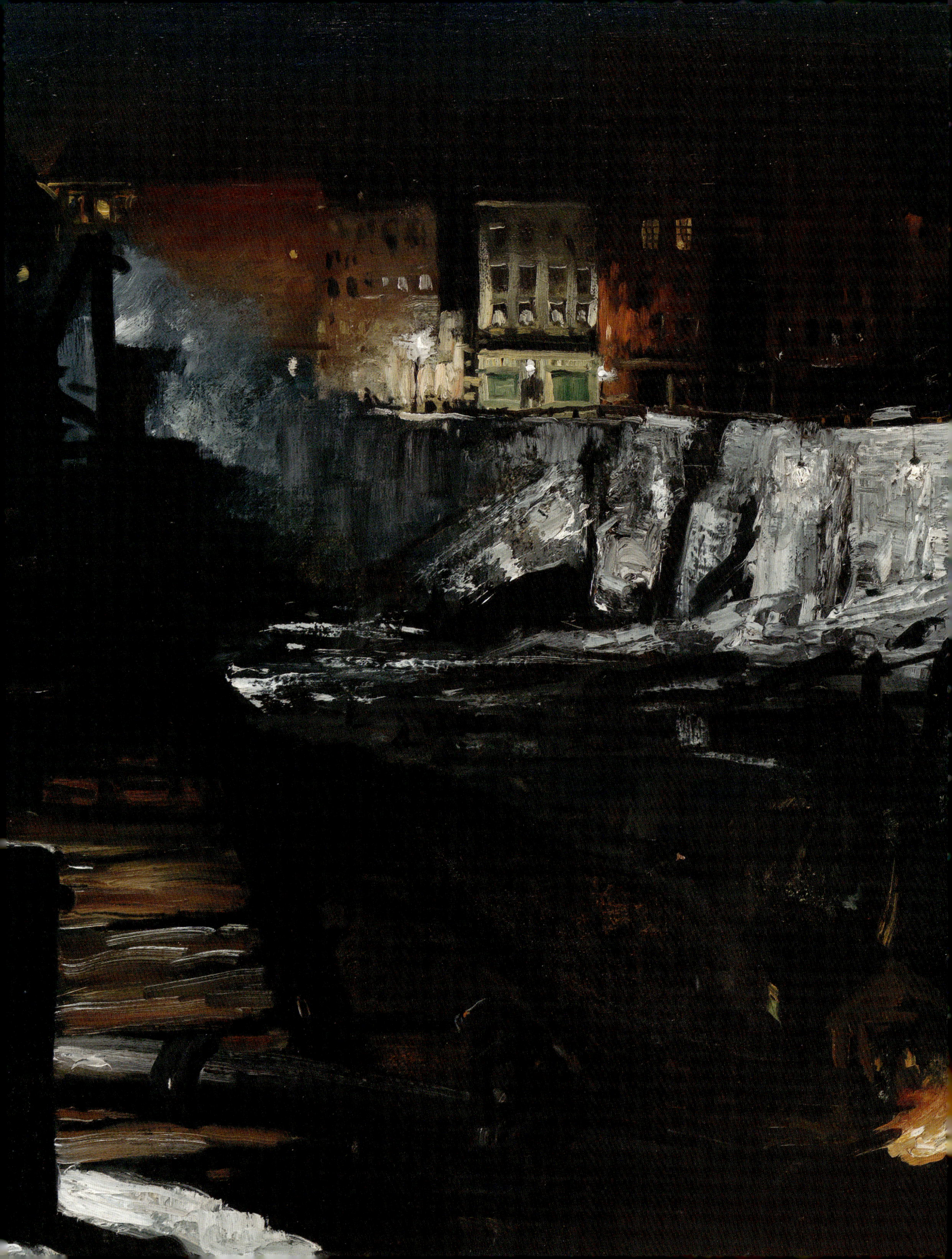

10 The Urban Nocturne and the Redefinition of the American Landscape

Some representations of the urban night accommodated the presence of the Other one way or another, using contrast or the picturesque to keep it at a distance, or immersing it in an ambiguous darkness. In a good number of images, however, artists attempted to depict the urban environment in and of itself, neglecting or effacing the marks of human presence. They signaled out architectural innovations, particularly the skyscraper, as emblems for the uniqueness of the American urban landscape. Here, as in the cases previously studied, adaptation to the radical novelty of the metropolis did not occur without conflicts and ambivalence. The constitution of a visual urban culture ultimately culminated in a revision of the notion of landscape, to which the nocturne made an essential contribution. At a time when the majority of city dwellers came from rural areas or small towns, the nocturne eased the transition toward acceptance of a landscape entirely transformed by urbanization. Furthermore, the nocturne aesthetic, more than a process of adaptation, highlighted certain fundamental characteristics of the urban environment. Through the nocturnal imagery of the city, a series of visual codes was set in place, inaugurating a reading of the sublime and of modernity that in large measure still dominates the perception and appreciation of the urban landscape.

"TOWARD AN URBAN VISION": GIVING UP THE RURAL LANDSCAPE

Many artists, especially tonalist painters such as Herman Murphy, Dwight Tryon, and Léon Dabo, were at first reluctant to represent the city and preferred nostalgic landscapes in the style of Jean-Charles Cazin's peaceful rural scenes (see figs. 17, 20, 21). In *Toward an Urban Vision: Ideas and Institutions in Nineteenth-Century America,* Thomas Bender analyzes cultural responses to the transformations of the urban environment in the nineteenth century and shows the important role played by the vision of the landscape developed by Frederick Law Olmsted in particular.[1] Efforts to think about and redefine the urban landscape and to supplant the model of the rural landscape deeply engrained in many city dwellers' minds played a crucial role in Americans' adaptation to urban realities: "Feeling the multiplicity of the city's stimulation, the artifice of its organization,

Fig. 149 detail

the complexity and intensity of its demands, the oppressive monotony of its streets and buildings, Americans who were moving from the country into the city longed for the occasional relief provided by the more familiar natural landscape of their rural past."[2] The transition from landscape to cityscape occurred partly through the nocturnal landscape, which contributed in the first place toward naturalizing urban forms. In the dialectical relationship between city and country, night offered a sort of transitional ground that drew from both at once. In that way, it performed visually a function similar to that which Olmsted sought to orchestrate with parks placed in the very center of large cities. New York's Central Park, which Olmsted designed with Calvert Vaux in 1858, was supposed to offer relief to individuals suffering from the psychological pressures of the big city and to open up an orderly space of contact for the various strata of society, one that favored social harmony and democracy.

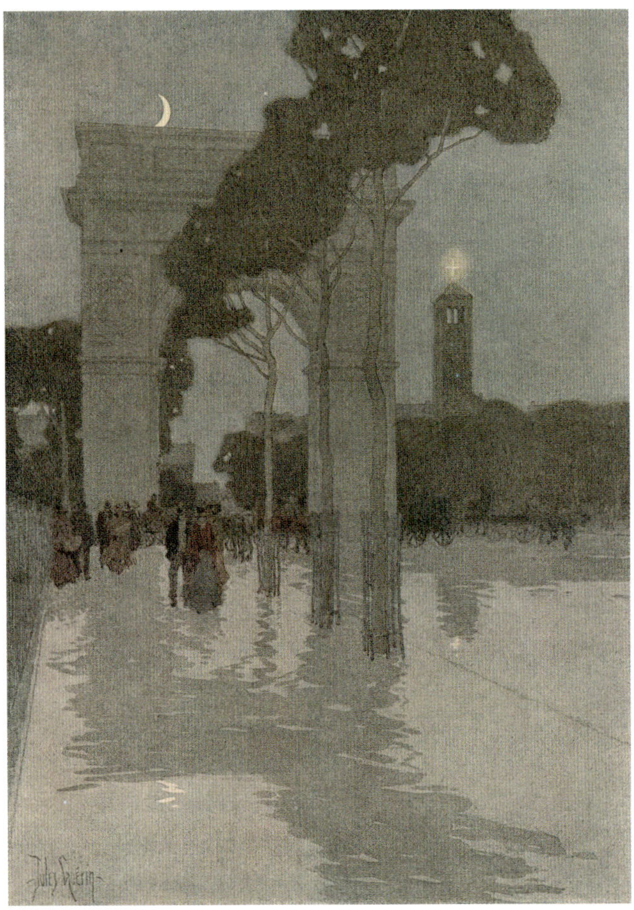

FIG. 133. Jules Vallée Guérin, *The Washington Arch in Washington Square (Stanford White, Architect), Century Magazine* 6, no. 4 (1905). Art and Picture Collection, New York Public Library, Astor, Lenox and Tilden Foundations.

Lewis Mumford acknowledges the transformative power of Olmsted's project, which, through the use of antimodern pastoral forms, in reality promoted an adaptation to the modern vision of the city: "By making nature urbane he naturalized the city."[3] Some thirty or forty years after the creation of Central Park, night in some sense came to replace green spaces, offering a harmonized version of the urban landscape. In "A Plea for the Picturesqueness of New York," published in *Camera Notes* in 1900, Sadakichi Hartmann evoked a series of picturesque views of the city that he judged beneficial to an artist photographer: among them, night views held a preponderant place. Hartmann emphasized the harmonizing function of the night. He suggested, for example, that his readers visit Madison Square Park, located at the foot of the Flatiron Building in the heart of Manhattan: "Place yourself at one of its corners on a rainy night and you will see a picture of peculiar fascination. Dark silhouettes of buildings and trees, surrounded by numerous light reflections, are mirrored in the wet pavement as in a sheet of water."[4] The views of Washington Park proposed by Jules Guérin (fig. 133), and Steichen's *Flatiron* (see fig. 126), a shot taken from Madison Square Park, precisely, seem to follow Hartmann's recipe to the letter, combining nocturnal darkness and other natural elements (trees, rain, snow, or fog) with the silhouettes of skyscrapers, which can be made out behind the branches. For Guérin as for Steichen, natural elements act as screens that mask the architecture, while at the same time tempering its straight lines and luminous appearance. According to William Sharpe, Steichen's photograph reflects the vision of a young man newly arrived in New York, still imprinted with the rural landscapes of Michigan, where he grew up. The lacelike mesh of branches in the foreground moderates and ruralizes the striking form of the skyscraper.[5] This intertwined vegetation is one of the features which, with obscurity and atmospheric conditions, greatly contributes to the blurred, filtered aesthetics of pictorialist photography. The photographer James B. Carrington, who in 1900 published a series of nocturnal photographs of New York in *Scribner's Magazine*, interpreted meteorological variations as embellishing factors: "On stormy nights when the rain makes the asphalt and the cobble-stones shine with long reflections from the lamps and windows, the seeker after the picturesque finds most satisfaction. Where a pool has collected there is a spot of liquid gold relieved against the blackness of

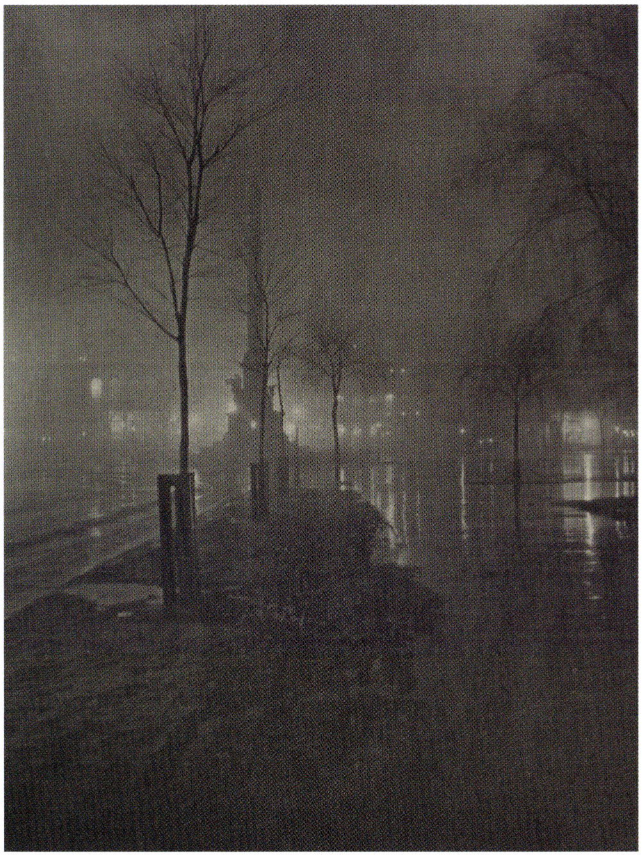

FIG. 134. William A. Fraser, *Wet Night, Columbus Circle, New York,* 1899. Photogravure on chine collé mounted on cream wove paper, sheet: 18.4 × 13.5 cm (7 1/4 × 5 5/16 in.); image: 16.3 × 12.2 cm (6 7/16 × 4 13/16 in.). National Gallery of Art, Washington, D.C. Anonymous gift (2002.120.23).

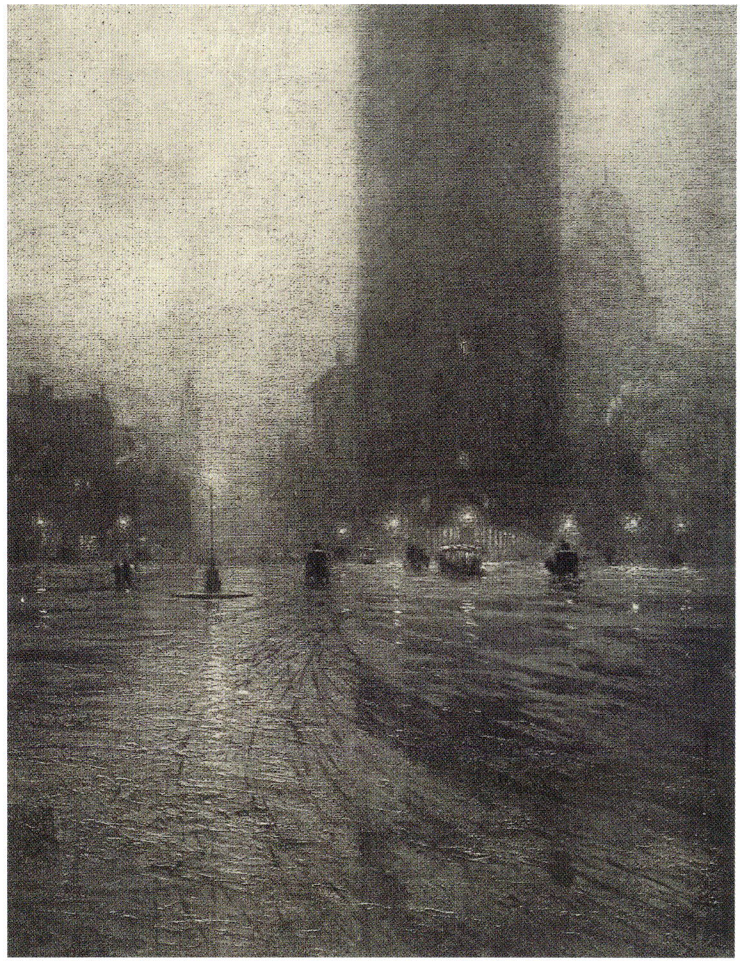

FIG. 135. Birge Harrison, *The Flatiron Building on a Rainy Night,* 1908, after a photograph by H. S. Bennett, *The Craftsman* 13, no. 4 (January 1908).

the surrounding asphalt. The snow, too, when it falls adds an indescribable air of unreality to the streets, accentuated by the muffling effect it has upon the sharp clatter of hoof-beats."[6] That muffling of both sight and sound is also found in William Fraser's *Wet Night, Columbus Circle, New York,* where the city vanishes completely in the night and mist and is summed up by a few glimmers of electric light that punctuate a hazy horizon line (fig. 134). In Fraser's photograph, the rostral column at Columbus Circle is aligned with the trees, merging with them to assume the appearance of a natural form.

These visions, which mask the city behind nature, seem to have resulted from an elitist and rather reactionary point of view. An article in *The Craftsman,* illustrated by reproductions of paintings by the tonalist Birge Harrison, defined his urban aesthetic in terms very similar to the exclusive "antivision" described in the first part of this study: "The insensitive to New York's fascinatingly ugly ways feel a sense of bewilderment at this vogue," the author explained, but true artists like Harrison knew how to find beauty in the city. The description accompanying another nocturnal view, which depicts the Judson Tower (fig. 135), reiterated the rhetoric of blurriness and the diversion of the gaze toward a sentimental interiority: "It is a winter night scene, with the foreground of barren trees and long grotesque shadows of branches slanting over the shining pavements. The light from 'The Judson' tower glows softly, timidly through the glare of electricity—a kindly gleam fraught with reminiscent sentiment to many of the older dwellers about the Square. The Flatiron Building is handled with a full understanding of the strange poetical possibility of this three-cornered ugly structure. Mr. Harrison has given it a mellow charm in the drip of a soft spring storm. The outlines of the building and the cars and cabs are softened with the blur of rain, and as you face the picture the faint ineffable stirring of the heart that comes with the early April shower is yours."[7] Here, again, the strategy adopted aims to gain distinction and refinement through a negative aesthetic based on the rejection of ordinary ugliness. But that aesthetic was also part and parcel of the dialectic of antimodernity: these screens, which ward off the urban landmarks, simultaneously integrate them into a dynamic vision. In Guérin's views of Washington Park, this vision is marked by the diagonals traced by the walkway and the reflection of trees on the wet pavement, while in Fraser's work, spindly trees guide the beholder's eyes toward the electric lights. Beyond that first, obscured plane, the discreet sources of light inserted into the background create a tension that intensifies the contrast between natural and built forms.

A comparison between two images published in *The Pittsburgh Survey* a few years apart allows us to evaluate the transition towards a fully urban aesthetic. Pittsburgh, cradle of the American steel industry, was the exact opposite of a rural landscape. The first image, a 1908 charcoal drawing by Joseph Stella (fig. 136), provides what Didier Aubert sees as an "almost mortuary interpretation" of the cityscape: "Immersed in black smoke, the power of Pittsburgh is represented by the delicate, spectral silhouettes of long smokestacks. . . . The spectacular dimension of industrial visions simultaneously reveals a sometimes ominous blackness."[8] Stella seems to have been inspired by the misty veils Whistler superimposed on the industrial smokestacks bordering the Thames, as indicated in a passage from the autobiography Stella wrote (in the third person) at the end of his life: "Besides, he discovered for himself the aesthetic beauty of Pittsburgh and surroundings as a landscape, beauty lying in the arabesque forms given by the structures of those huge volcano-like steel mills, emerging from the fluctuating waves of smoke and fog, with an eloquent mystery."[9] Although such a reinterpretation, at a distance of several decades, necessarily entailed certain distortions and revisions, these words suggest the extent to which Stella shared the attitudes of his time. To understand Pittsburgh as a "landscape" in its own right, the artist had to project onto it a picturesque frame adorned

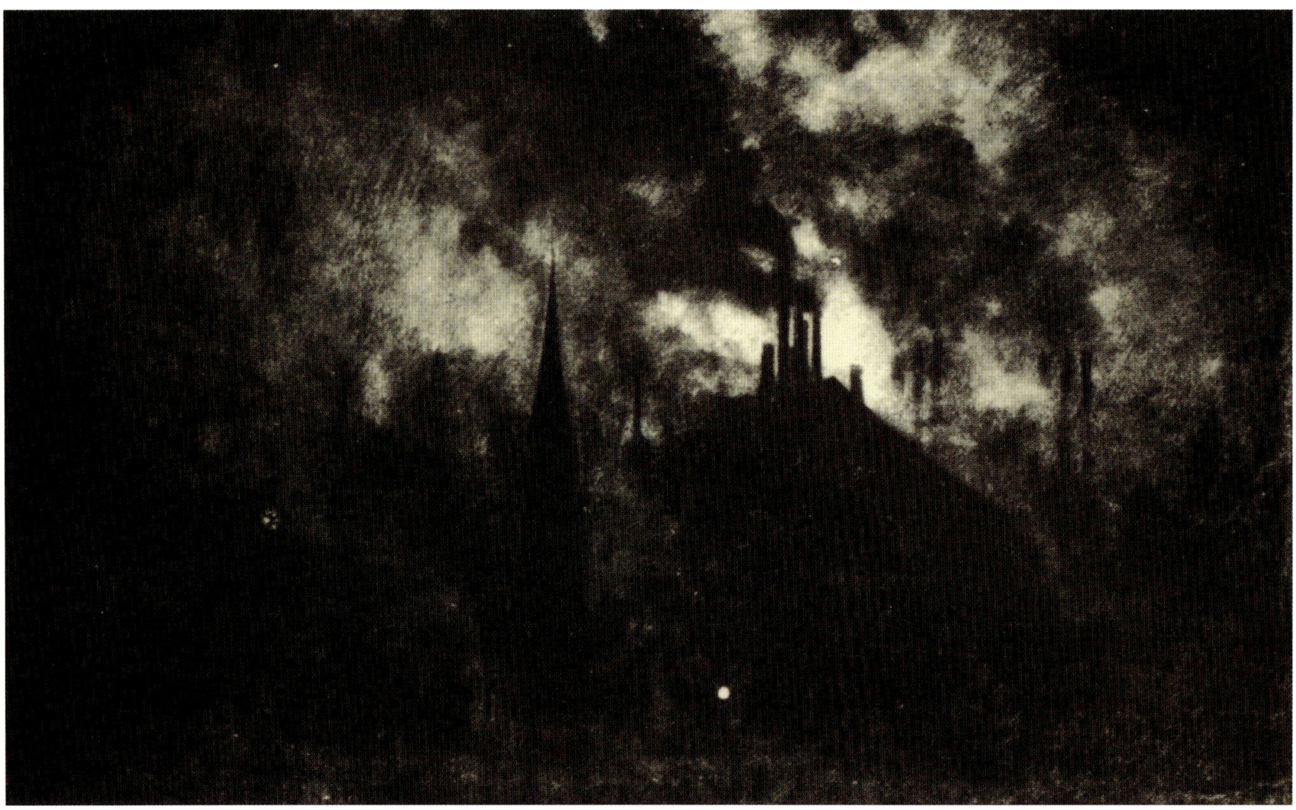

FIG. 136. Joseph Stella, *Pittsburgh*, 1908. Charcoal on paper, 55.9 × 71.1 cm (23 × 28 in.). Carnegie Library of Pittsburgh.

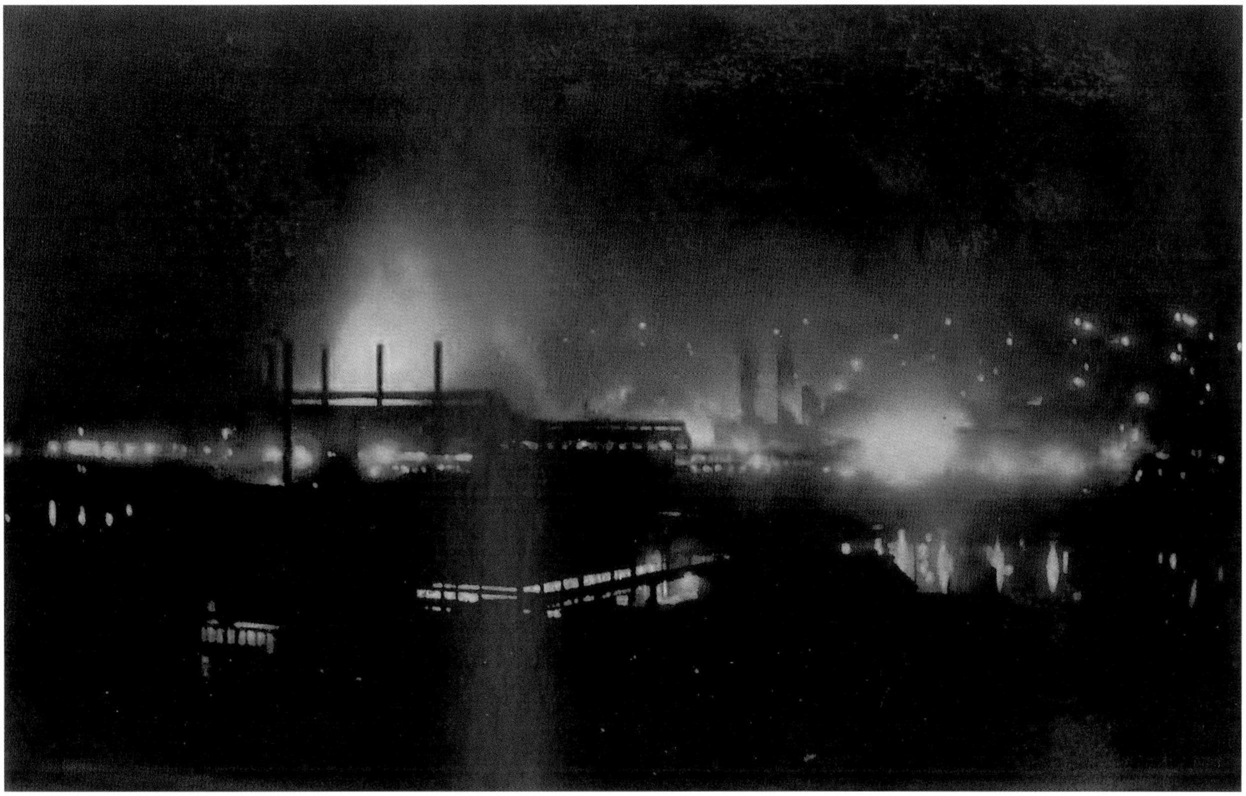

FIG. 137. Lewis Wickes Hine (attributed), "River at Night: Looking down on the Jones and Laughlin Mills from the Pittsburgh Side," 1914, in Paul Underwood Kellogg (ed.), *The Pittsburgh Survey* (New York: Charity Organization Society of the City of New York, 1914), vol. 6, frontispiece.

with "arabesques," while attempting to naturalize the industrial structure to make it look like a "volcano." Here, the fog and smoke of Pittsburgh play an essential role, enveloping the landscape in an "eloquent mystery." Stella's formulation makes evident the inversion of the process that many producers of nocturnal urban views shared: to make the landscape "emerge" as such, they first had to cover it, envelop it in darkness, make it a blur. The second view of Pittsburgh, a photograph published a few years later in a subsequent volume of *The Pittsburgh Survey,* also depicts the blast furnaces of the steel industry; but, unlike in the scene by Stella, who immerses the landscape in smoke, the industrial buildings appear as distinct masses illuminated by bright electric lights (fig. 137). The image is in a different medium and its ambition is less explicitly aesthetic than Stella's drawing, but the photograph, which serves as the frontispiece to the survey, also attests to a perception of the industrial city as landscape. This was a remarkable evolution: in 1914 it became possible to represent the urban and industrial space directly, in a pictorial space from which the fog has dissipated. But though it does without the veil of mist with which Whistler covered the details of the banks of the Thames, this photograph has not completely abandoned the visual principles of the Whistleresque nocturne. The nocturnal view remains distant, and the river still separates the beholder from the scene. The electric lights, reflected on the surface of the water, surround with their halo the dark silhouettes of the buildings and confer on them a mysterious and poetic dimension.

In Stella's work, the dark mist covers the Pittsburgh landscape, the better to make the scene emerge from it. In the photograph, by contrast, it is technology that, in a radical reversal of point of view, brings the landscape into being: Aubert remarks that the river would not be visible without the reflection of the electric lights, which traces the outlines of that new landscape.[10] Night operates as the neutral ground between the origin and the culmination of these two opposing movements. It is undeniable, however, that by the 1910s the orientations indicated by the *Pittsburgh Survey* image had come to predominate. In the last phase of the nocturne vogue, night became the frame for new aesthetic explorations in works—including Joseph Stella's most famous paintings—that seemingly no longer

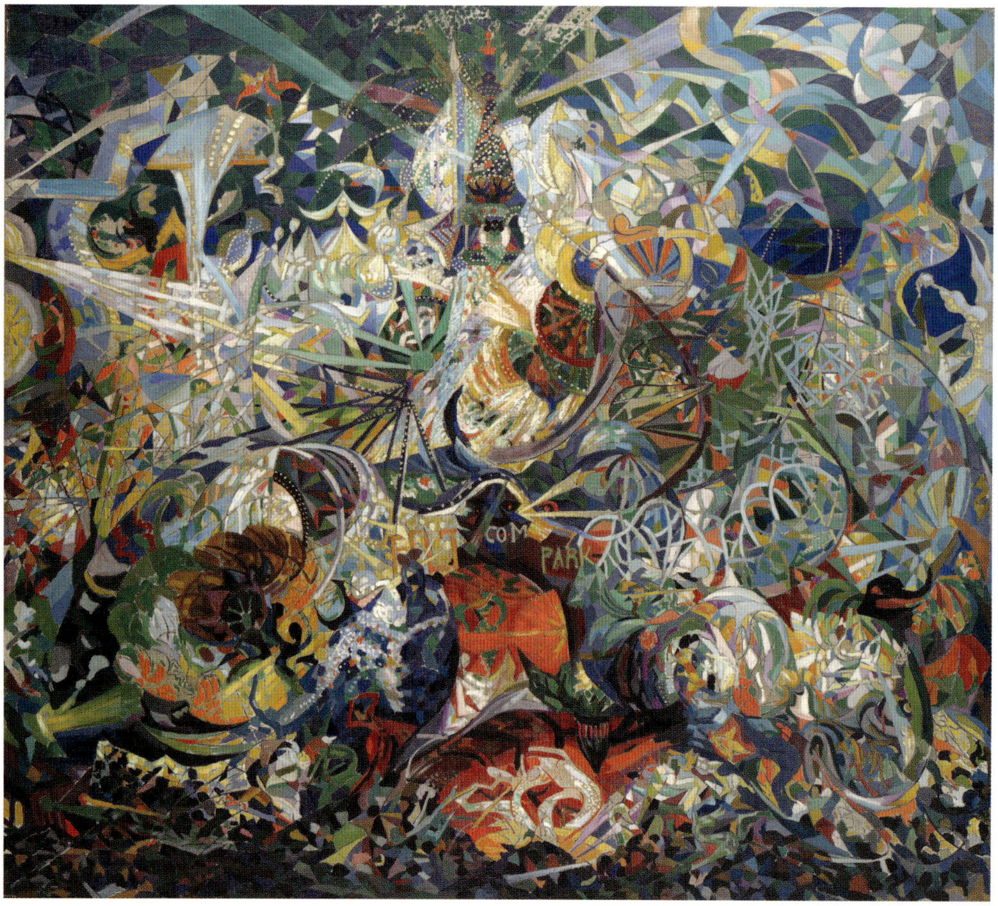

FIG. 138. Joseph Stella, *Battle of Lights, Coney Island,* Mardi Gras, 1913–14. Oil on canvas, 195.6 × 215.3 cm (77 × 84 3/4 in.). Yale University Art Gallery, New Haven, Connecticut. Gift of Collection Société Anonyme (1941.689).

FIG. 139. Charles Sheeler, *American Landscape,* 1930. Oil on canvas, 61 × 78.8 cm (24 × 31 in.). Museum of Modern Art, Gift of Abby Aldrich Rockefeller.

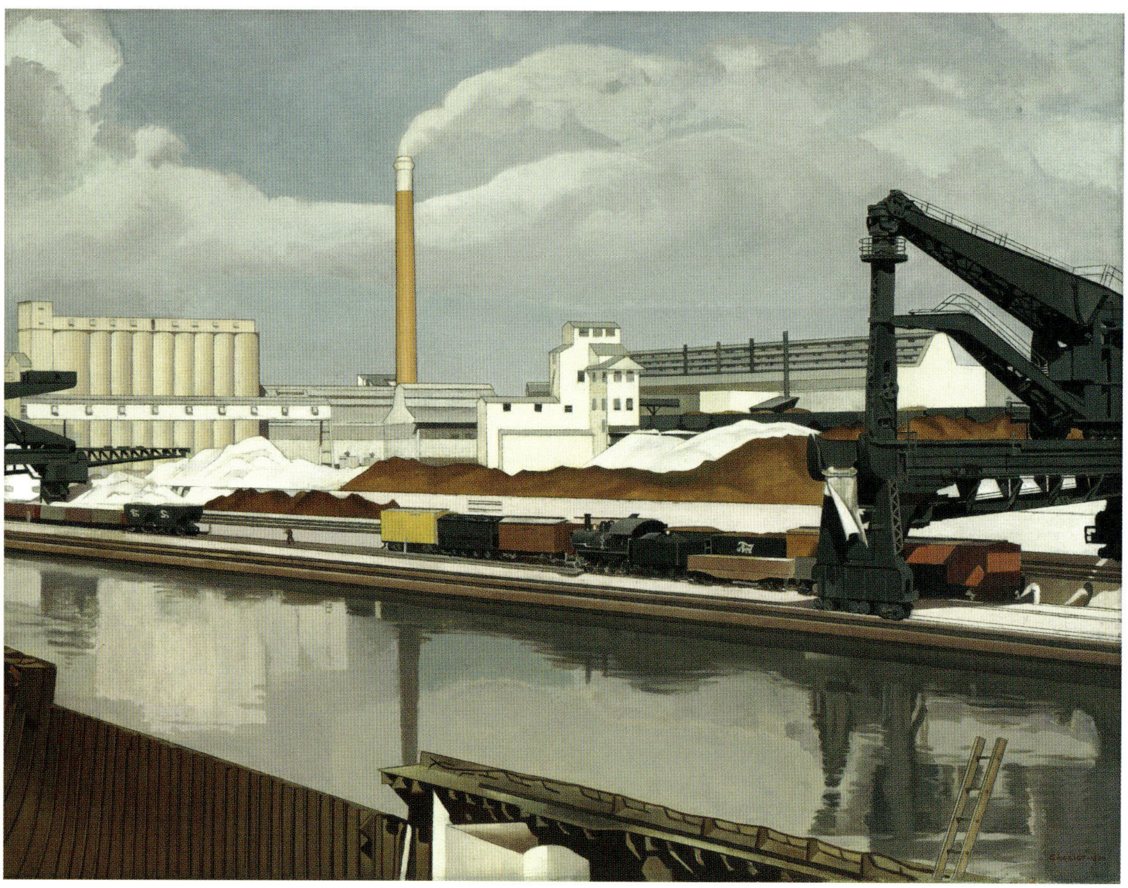

felt the need to depict the urban and industrial landscape at a remove (fig. 138). Soon, the cityscape would become easily imaginable outside the nocturnal context: in 1930, when Charles Sheeler titled his depiction of the Ford factory at River Rouge *American Landscape*, the gesture was certainly somewhat provocative, but he was articulating a truth to which most of his beholders had now become accustomed (fig. 139). From that standpoint, the tonalists' deserted rural landscapes can be reinterpreted as the very sign of the metropolis's triumph: these melancholy views of an abandoned countryside, rather than simply standing in contrast to urban landscapes, constitute their logical counterpart. The spectacular growth of the big cities was only the most visible phase of the "incorporation" of the United States, and the decline of the countryside was an integral part of a global system of development.[11] Nostalgic pastoral nocturnes, which continued to be created by artists living primarily in the country's major urban centers, repeated symbolically the marginalization of the rural landscape, a marginalization already suggested in my analysis of N. C. Wyeth's Cream of Wheat illustration of 1906 (see fig. 85). Here, the countryside was relegated to the fringes of a system of exchange (of both communications and commercial goods) now dominated by the metropolis. Night allowed artists to adapt their vision to the novelty of the urban environment, and at the same time it conveyed a wistful deference toward a landscape whose loss they were grieving.

THE TECHNOLOGICAL SUBLIME AND THE TRANSFORMATION OF URBAN PERSPECTIVES

Before the advent of a truly modernist aesthetic, the two decades prior to World War I saw the development of a specifically urban aesthetic in American art. Yet, rather than imagine the evolution that was initially formal in nature, marked by the radical ruptures of the artistic avant-garde and "progressing" toward modernism, it is more interesting to read the images of the nocturnal city in relation to tendencies rooted in a larger culture than in an exclusively art historical perspective. Behind the natural forms used to screen the city, a landscape came into view that was marked by what David Nye calls the "technological sublime."[12] In representations of the nocturnal city, this sublime was most often expressed through three recurring figures: the bridge, the skyscraper, and electric lighting. From these three elements, all intimately linked to recent technological innovations (the mastery of metal architecture, the advance of electricity, and the invention of the elevator) and to broader socioeconomic transformations (urbanization and capitalist development), a modern sublime emerged, reorienting vision and rendering the landscape as abstract, purified forms.[13] Darkness reinforced the sublime. William Dean Howells, for instance, shows his heroes in raptures at the novelty of the urban spectacle, in which night obliterated details and allowed modern infrastructures to redefine the vanishing points: "The architectural shapes of houses and churches and towers, rescued by the obscurity from all that was ignoble in them, and the coming and going of the trains marking the stations with vivider or fainter plumes of flame-shot steam—formed an incomparable perspective."[14] Nighttime obscurity not only transcended the ugliness of daily life; in isolating and underscoring the presence of artificial structuring elements, it also played a role in redrawing the urban environment.

The skyscraper, the most characteristic and most conspicuously artificial form in the American urban landscape, was the first element of the new urban sublime, celebrated in painting, photography, popular illustrations, and postcards (fig. 140). One of the most famous examples in this regard, the Flatiron Building, towering over the intersection of Broadway, Fifth Avenue, and Twenty-Second Street in New York City, appears in the works of various artists, from Steichen to Sloan. Sharpe analyzes the striking contrast, in Steichen's photograph, between the silhouette of the Flatiron and that of the cabman, interpreting it as one of the sources of the image's power: the man is dwarfed by the sublime immensity of the building.[15] Sloan's *Throbbing Fountain, Night*, in which the Flatiron is seen through the tree branches of Madison Square Park, a powerful spray of water spurting up at its center, can also be read as the first moment in a revision of the codes of the sublime (fig. 141). Sloan highlighted the verticality of the building, while disguising it behind the trees in the park. At the same time, he symbolically reiterated its presence at the center of the image, in the form of the spurting fountain, which could be interpreted as a diminished, urban version of the geysers in U.S. national parks. On one hand, the fountain suggests a still-present but domesticated nature; on the other, it—like the maze of branches—contributes toward naturalizing the Flatiron. The paradigm that serves as a filter through which urban architecture is perceived here is not so much the pastoral as the natural sublime. Henry James, for

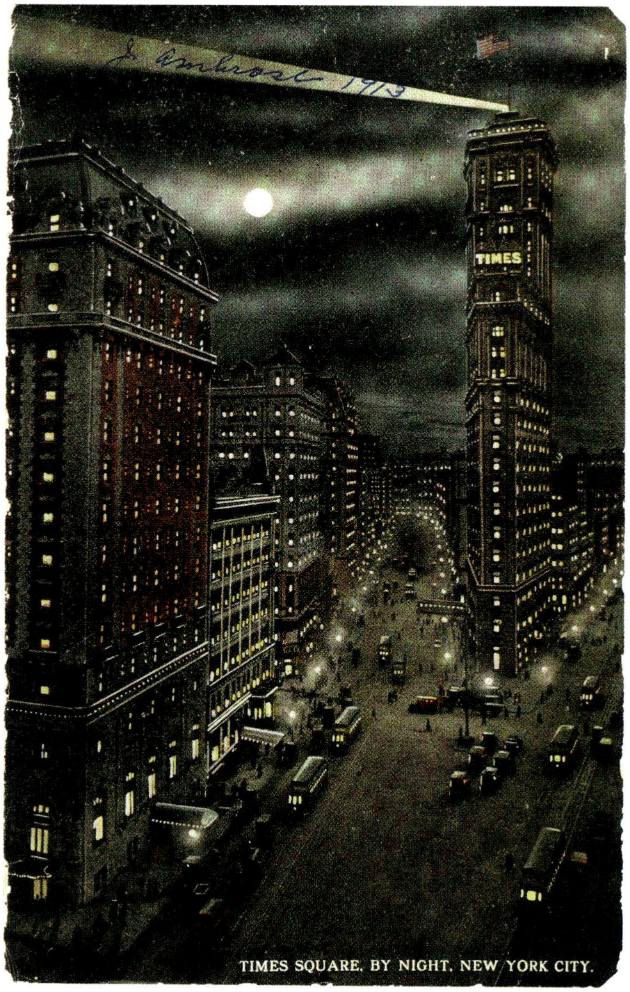

FIG. 140. American Art Company, *Times Square at Night, New York City*, 1913. Postcard, 8.8 × 14 cm (3 ½ × 5 ½ in.). Collection of the author.

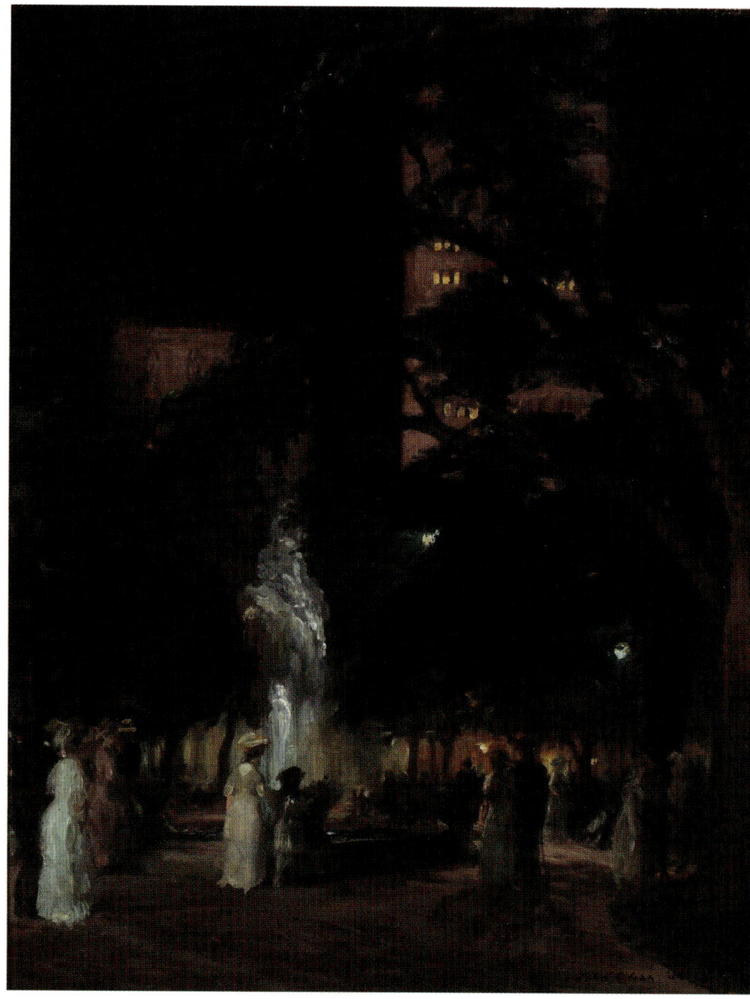

FIG. 141. John Sloan, *Throbbing Fountain, Night*, 1908. Oil on canvas, 81.6 × 66.4 cm (32 ⅛ × 26 ⅛ in.). Delaware Art Museum, Gift of the John Sloan Memorial Foundation, 1997.

example, considered the spectacle of skyscrapers in relation to the sublime landscapes of America's wide-open spaces, describing the façade of one high-rise as "high and wide as the mountain-wall that drops the Alpine avalanche" and discerning in another a "cliff-like sublimity."[16] The comparison of streets bordered by skyscrapers to canyons quickly became a cliché. It was repeated by James B. Carrington, for example, in his article on the New York night: "Downtown most of the streets have become black cañons, here and there lined with rows of gleaming, sputtering, electric lights."[17] In 1912 the pictorialist photographer Alvin Langdon Coburn held an exhibition titled "New York from Its Pinnacles," in which he gave a literal interpretation of the comparison, juxtaposing high-angle shots of streets in the metropolis and landscapes of the Grand Canyon and Yosemite (see fig. 146).[18]

The skyscraper thus lent itself to an aestheticized and spiritualized vision in the sublime mode. When, for example, Henry James described the "white towers" of Manhattan perceived through the veil of local meteorological variations, he ultimately granted them a certain beauty: "The weather, such as it was, worked wonders for the upper reaches of the buildings, round which it drifted and hung very much as about the flanks and summits of emergent mountain-masses."[19] The skyscrapers that had invaded the urban landscape, having become the bearers of a "message for the eyes," also came to compete with the spiritual message of a mode of architecture they dwarfed: that of church steeples. Many newspaper articles lamented the domination of these "crude and commercial" buildings in the cityscape, a physically and visually overwhelming presence that seems also to have extended to the city's religious life, where the almighty dollar replaced the Christian God (fig. 142). Modern skyscrapers, symbols of triumphant capitalism, were the antithesis of church steeples, which were spurned as ridiculously obsolescent by comparison.[20] Before 1916, the year municipal regulations were adopted,[21] urban territory was divided into lots and was not subject to any building codes. Nothing prevented private entrepreneurs from increasing the returns on their real estate investments by building their towers ever higher. Ascent toward the heavens thus became a symbol more of an aggressive ambition aimed at profit than of a metaphysical aspiration. One reporter, for example, denounced the ascendancy of modern architecture, which made churches invisible in the cityscape, and at the same time evoked the spiritual change that accompanied it: "Now the spirit of the enterprise is showing its proudest attainment by the invasion of high buildings into that sky which, to our ancestors, was the great type of the unknown and mysterious."[22] Like twilight, which for James conferred on skyscrapers an ephemeral distinction, night tempered that vision, reinvesting the landscape with a mysterious aura and drawing skyscrapers toward a sublime that gave rise to both admiration for technological achievement and religious contemplation. Carrington noted the atmosphere of Wall Street, transformed once night had fallen: "Among the great towers of silence in the business district there is an impressive contrast with the day's feverish activity. They seem to be resting and waiting in dignified quiet for another day to have renewed within their walls the eternal struggle for gain that they were built to provide for."[23] In Carrington's eyes, night transformed the image of mechanical force characteristic of skyscrapers, but it also increased that force tenfold and gave it a sublime dimension: "By day the city has limits. It is a measurable quantity with definite bounds, but with the coming down of night it seems to spread out into space that only the imagination can take hold of. It is a thing of apparent power in the brilliant light of day, and the spirit that animates and drives its infinite activities is as irresistible as some mighty engine. But the impression of potential energy that you get after dark is even stronger. The mere passivity of the city by night is full of thrill. You feel with a keener sense the littleness and the relative powerlessness of the individual unit, and are conscious that unknown tendencies and influences, of which you can have no knowledge and no control, are being stored up against you."[24]

The technological sublime, inspired by the architectural achievement of the skyscraper, also encompassed other structures that increasingly dotted the urban landscape, such as bridges and elevated railroad tracks. Here as well, adaptation did not occur without contradictions and conflicts. The urban planner Sylvester Baxter considered the metal architecture used in most of these structures an aesthetic "nightmare" that destroyed the landscape, while Hartmann embraced it as the reflection

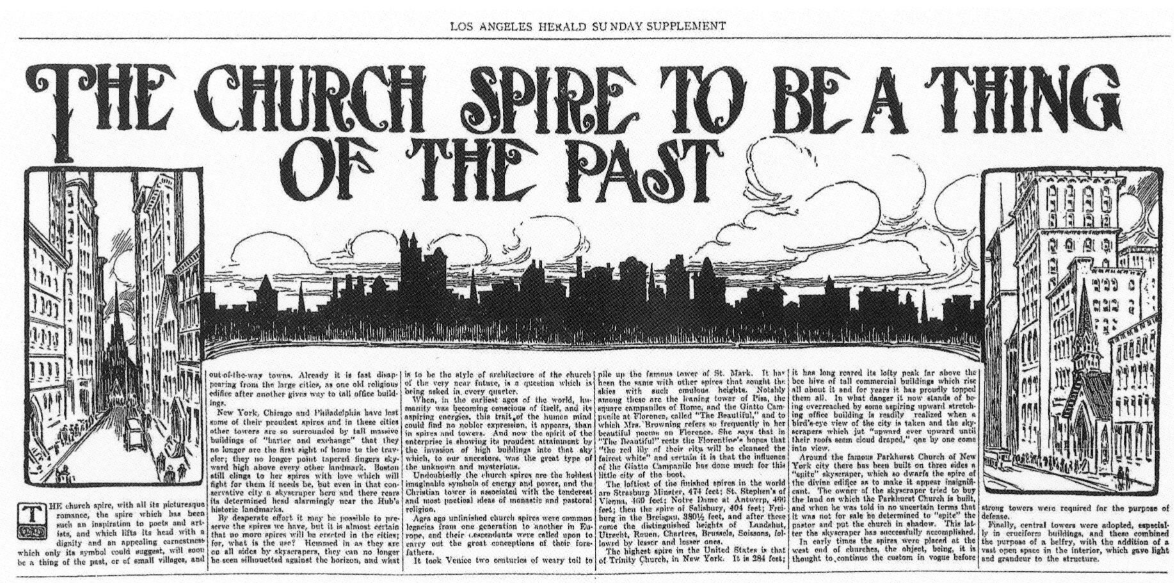

LOS ANGELES HERALD SUNDAY SUPPLEMENT

THE CHURCH SPIRE TO BE A THING OF THE PAST

THE church spire, with all its picturesque romance, the spire which has been such an inspiration to poets and artists, and which lifts its head with a dignity and an appealing earnestness which only its symbol could suggest, will soon be a thing of the past, or of small villages, and out-of-the-way towns. Already it is fast disappearing from the large cities, as one old religious edifice after another gives way to tall office buildings.

New York, Chicago and Philadelphia have lost some of their proudest spires and in these cities other towers are so surrounded by tall massive buildings of "barter and exchange" that they no longer are the first sight of home to the traveler; they no longer point tapered fingers skyward high above every other landmark. Boston still clings to her spires with love which will fight for them if needs be, but even in that conservative city a skyscraper here and there rears its determined head alarmingly near the Hub's historic landmarks.

By desperate effort it may be possible to preserve the spires we have, but it is almost certain that no more spires will be erected in the cities; for, what is the use? Hemmed in as they are on all sides by skyscrapers, they can no longer be seen silhouetted against the horizon, and what is to be the style of architecture of the church of the very near future, is a question which is being asked in every quarter.

When, in the earliest ages of the world, humanity was becoming conscious of itself, and its aspiring energies, this trait of the human mind could find no nobler expression, it appears, than in spires and towers. And now the spirit of the enterprise is showing its proudest attainment by the invasion of high buildings into that sky which, to our ancestors, was the great type of the unknown and mysterious.

Undoubtedly the church spires are the boldest imaginable symbols of energy and power, and the Christian tower is associated with the tenderest and most poetical ideas of monastic and pastoral religion.

Ages ago unfinished church spires were common legacies from one generation to another in Europe, and their descendants were called upon to carry out the great conceptions of their forefathers.

It took Venice two centuries of weary toil to pile up the famous tower of St. Mark. It has been the same with other spires that sought the skies with such emulous heights. Notably among these are the leaning tower of Pisa, the square campaniles of Rome, and the Giatto Campanile at Florence, called "The Beautiful," and to which Mrs. Browning refers so frequently in her beautiful poems on Florence. She says that in "The Beautiful" rests the Florentine's hopes that "the red lily of their city will be cleansed the fairest white" and certain it is that the influence of the Giatto Campanile has done much for this little city of the boot.

The loftiest of the finished spires in the world are Strasburg Minster, 474 feet; St. Stephen's of Vienna, 460 feet; Notre Dame at Antwerp, 406 feet; then the spire of Salisbury, 404 feet; Freiburg in the Breisgau, 380½ feet, and after these come the distinguished heights of Landshut, Utrecht, Rouen, Chartres, Brussels, Soissons, followed by lesser and lesser ones.

The highest spire in the United States is that of Trinity Church, in New York. It is 284 feet; it has long reared its lofty peak far above the bee hive of tall commercial buildings which rise all about it and for years it has proudly topped them all. In what danger it now stands of being overreached by some aspiring upward stretching office building is readily realized when a bird's-eye view of the city is taken and the skyscrapers which jut "upward ever upward until their roofs seem cloud draped," one by one come into view.

Around the famous Parkhurst Church of New York city there has been built on three sides a "spite" skyscraper, which so dwarfs the spire of the divine edifice as to make it appear insignificant. The owner of the skyscraper tried to buy the land on which the Parkhurst Church is built, and when he was told in no uncertain terms that it was not for sale he determined to "spite" the pastor and put the church in shadow. This latter the skyscraper has successfully accomplished.

In early times the spires were placed at the west end of churches, the object, being, it is thought to continue the custom in vogue before strong towers were required for the purpose of defense.

Finally, central towers were adopted, especially in cruciform buildings, and these combined the purpose of a belfry, with the addition of a vast open space in the interior, which gave light and grandeur to the structure.

FIG. 142. "The Church Spire to Be a Thing of the Past," *Los Angeles Herald,* April 29, 1909.

of American identity.[25] As in the case of the skyscraper, it was often by emphasizing the elevation of these structures that artists managed to integrate them into an aestheticized landscape, preferably perceived in the dark of night: "A peculiar sight can be enjoyed standing on a starlit night at the block house near the northwest entrance of the Park. One sees in the distance the illumined windows of the West Side and the Elevated, which rises at the double curve at One Hundred and Tenth Street to dizzy heights, and whose construction is hardly visible in the dimness of night. A train passes by, like a fantastic fire-worm from some giant fairyland, crawling in mid-air."[26] That view, highly prized by observers of the time, was replicated, for example, in the picture in the background behind Charles G. D. Roberts's poem "New York Nocturne" (fig. 143). It puts the accent on a sinuous and graceful line, which, according to an article in the *Saint Paul Globe,* might dominate the urban landscape of the future (fig. 144).[27] In these two illustrations, the page layout reinforces the impression of verticality, while turning the structure into a decorative frame for the text. The metal frameworks were transformed from a "nightmare" into an ornament, their idealized arabesque silhouettes dematerialized in the darkness, acquiring, in the *Saint Paul Globe* illustration, the consistency of billows of smoke exhaled by the architects. But whereas that image leans resolutely in the direction of the decorative, the illustration accompanying Roberts's poem, which more clearly opts for darkness, tends toward sublimity, which is also expressed in Steichen's astonishing 1903 photograph of the Brooklyn Bridge (fig. 145). The latter image illustrates to what extent these new structures, in their unprecedented forms and dimensions, prompted artists to adopt innovative approaches. Viewed from a slight

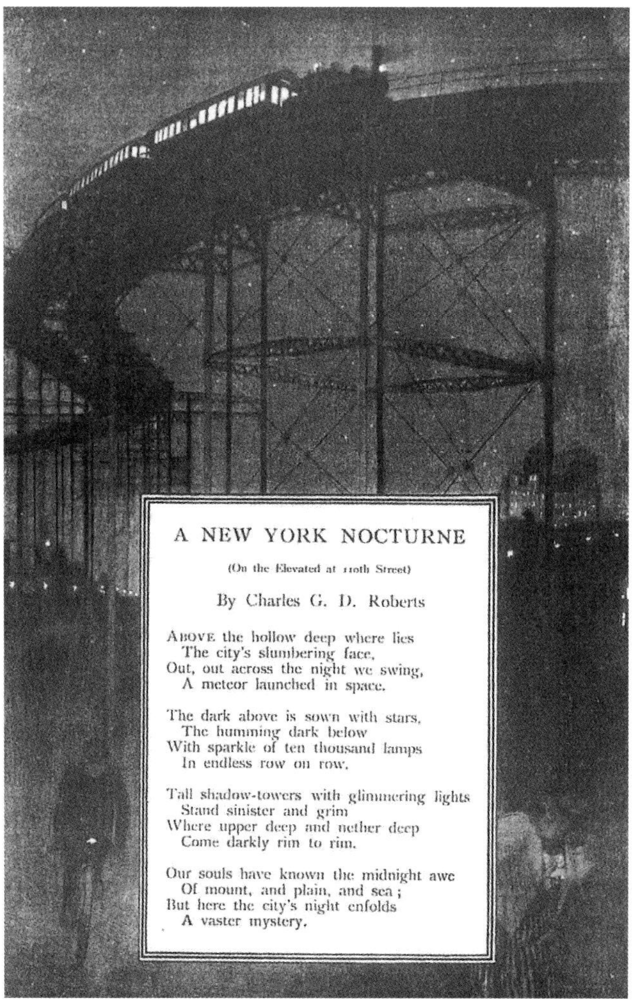

A NEW YORK NOCTURNE

(On the Elevated at 110th Street)

By Charles G. D. Roberts

ABOVE the hollow deep where lies
The city's slumbering face,
Out, out across the night we swing,
A meteor launched in space.

The dark above is sown with stars,
The humming dark below
With sparkle of ten thousand lamps
In endless row on row.

Tall shadow-towers with glimmering lights
Stand sinister and grim
Where upper deep and nether deep
Come darkly rim to rim.

Our souls have known the midnight awe
Of mount, and plain, and sea;
But here the city's night enfolds
A vaster mystery.

FIG. 143. "A New York Nocturne," *Scribner's Magazine* 24, no. 4 (October 1898).

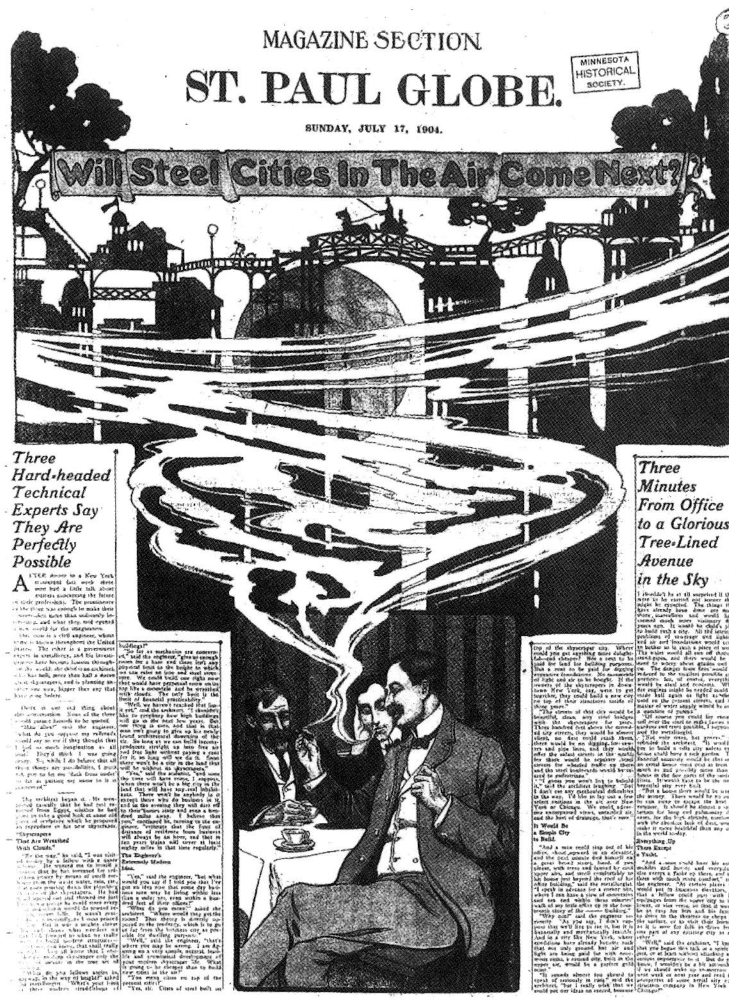

MAGAZINE SECTION

ST. PAUL GLOBE.

SUNDAY, JULY 17, 1904.

Will Steel Cities In The Air Come Next?

Three Hard-headed Technical Experts Say They Are Perfectly Possible

Three Minutes From Office to a Glorious Tree-Lined Avenue in the Sky

FIG. 144. "Will Steel Cities in the Air Come Next?" *Saint Paul Globe,* July 17, 1904.

angle and from below, the bridge is rendered as a horizontal as much as a vertical structure. The pylon, whose Gothic arches can be made out, occupies the center of the image, the anchor point for the deck of the bridge, which, in a dynamic effect, runs toward the upper right-hand corner of the image. The image's verticality marks an inversion of the conventions of landscape painting, somewhat reminiscent of the Japanese-inspired composition of Whistler's *Nocturne: Blue and Gold—Old Battersea Bridge* (see fig. 13). The structures rising out of the night thus seem to metamorphose from "fact" to "symbol," to borrow Alan Trachtenberg's terminology concerning the Brooklyn Bridge.[28]

These sublime views of the city's architecture, compared to the bare landscapes of the tonalists who contented themselves with representing expanses of water, open country, or simply the night sky, reintroduced into the nocturne a strong sense of perspective. But they were by no means a return to a traditionally structured composition—on the contrary. Rather, they reflected a radical revision of space in the cityscape. The architect Montgomery Schuyler complained about the disproportionate reconfiguration of the urban landscape that, according to him, skyscrapers caused: "Everybody will admit that if we had a city of 'magnificent distances,' a city of which the great avenues bore the same relation to a ten-story cornice line of bordering buildings that our actual streets bear to the three-story buildings with which those who laid them out expected them to be lined, there would be no hardship at all and no grievance in fixing a ten-story cornice line for such streets. In fact, in order to domesticate the sky-scraper and bring it within the reign of law, we need to revise the municipal arrangements which were made without prevision of its

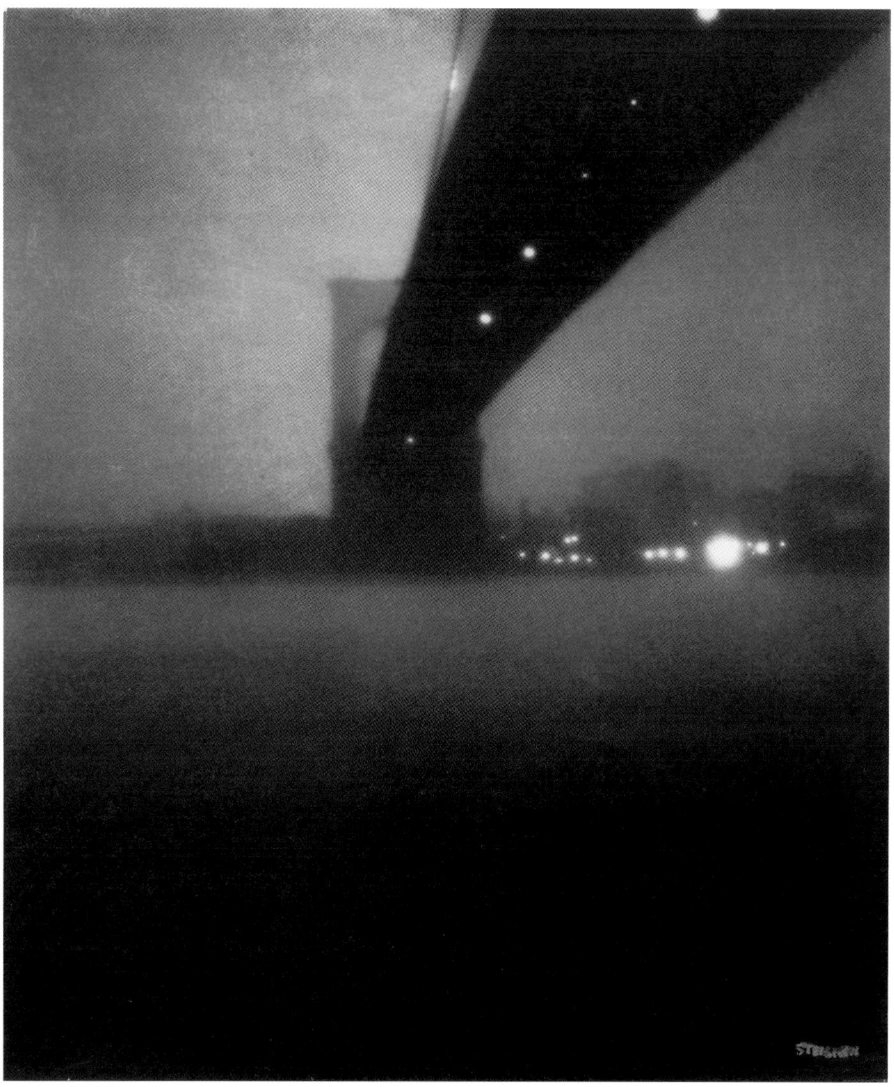

FIG. 145. Edward Steichen, *Brooklyn Bridge*, 1903. Gelatin silver print, 43.8 × 36.2 cm (17¼ × 14¼ in.). Bank of America Collection.

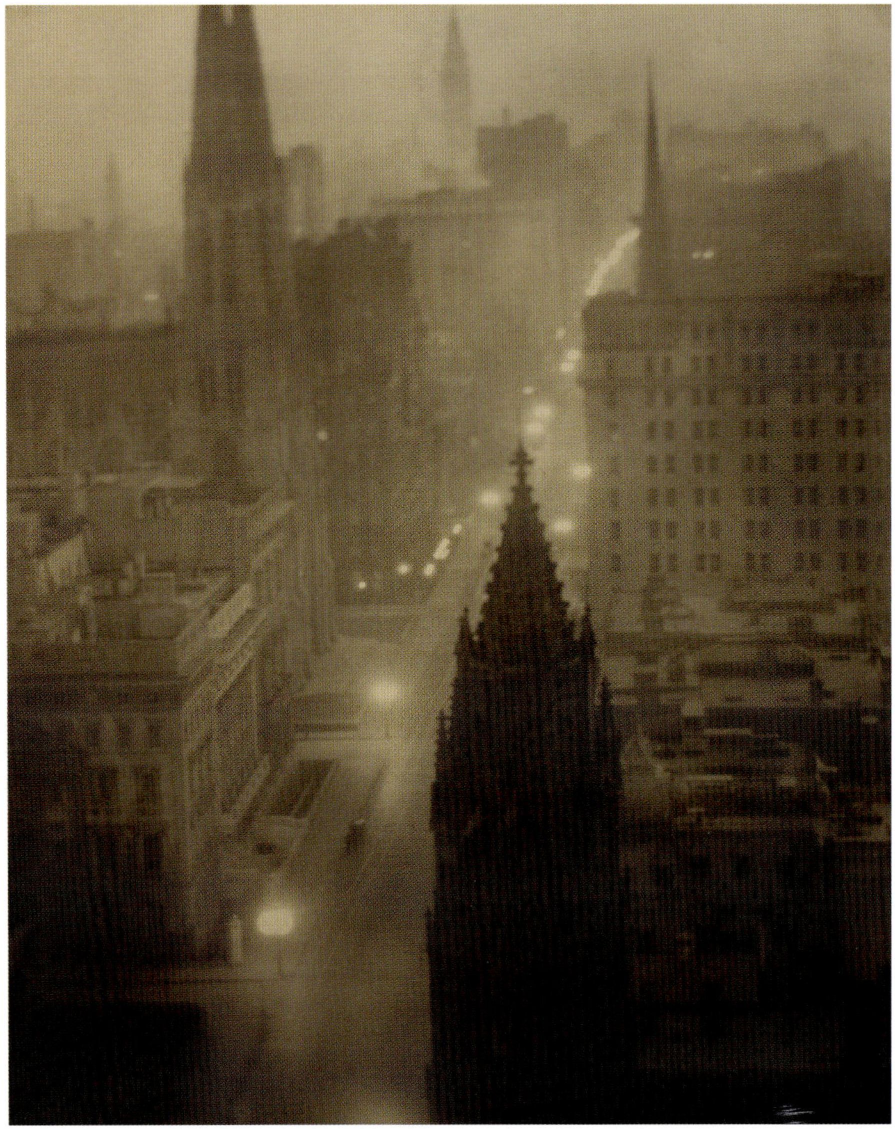

FIG. 146. Alvin Langdon Coburn, *Fifth Avenue from the St. Regis*, c. 1905. Platinum print, image: 40 × 31.6 cm (15 3/4 × 12 1/2 in.). George Eastman Museum, Rochester, NY. Bequest of the photographer (1967.0144.0247).

advent."[29] Schuyler seemed ready to accept the gigantic scale of the skyscrapers only on the condition that their oversized proportions be extended to the entire urban landscape. His blueprint for a rational urban architecture brings to mind the White City's broad avenues lined with enormous buildings. The writer Edgar Saltus, for his part, did not share that hesitancy. On the contrary, he envisioned the American city with its skyscrapers as a "colossal city" with "giant hotels," "gigantic office buildings," and "Gargantuan department stores," much more than a larger version of Schuyler's city with its well-ordered proportions: "Without effort you may foresee the day when Fifth Avenue will be a dark lane, flanked on either side by sheer white heights, with, above, a slender stretch of tender blue."[30] The urban "landscape," turned on its end, compressed, and expanded to inconceivable proportions, had reached its limit, underscored by the thin streak of blue that was supposed to signify the sky. The sublime technological vision thus disrupted proportions, distances, and perspectives. Like Steichen, producers of images were often forced to adopt original and extreme points of view. The Manhattan skyline, to be grasped in its entirety, had to be viewed from the banks of the Hudson River in New Jersey or from Brooklyn. The tall skyscrapers generated views from below and street canyon perspectives, but they also gave rise to spectacular high-angle views of the city, as in Coburn's explorations (fig. 146). And in general, the bridges and towers that occupied the cityscape were regularly reused by artists to structure their compositions and guide the beholder's gaze, as is evident in views of the El painted by Sloan (see figs. 120, 121).

"ALL THAT IS SOLID MELTS INTO AIR": THE DISINTEGRATION OF FORMS IN THE DARKNESS

The restructuring of the landscape in the urban space was underscored by one last form of the technological sublime, that of electric lighting. Nye grants a special place to the electrical sublime in his analysis of the cultural meanings of technology. Electric lighting, more than merely one innovation among others, in fact functioned as a "double," not sublime but sublimating, for technology. In the indistinct space of the misty night, electricity literally traced out the landscape and made volumes emerge and distances fluctuate. Nye points out electricity's capacity to "edit" and unify the landscape, concealing some features while accentuating others, turning the city into a "purified world of light, simplified into a spectacular pattern."[31] Urban nocturnes, putting into play glints of light against the dark background of the night, proposed an analytic view of the landscape, transforming it into an abstract vision. That visual metamorphosis gave rise to contradictory readings from observers at the time. The electrical sublime obviously transcended the city's materiality, particularly its visible affiliation with the development of an aggressive capitalism, and turned it into an idealized vision. But paradoxically, electricity, which brought about that transformation, was the result of that very development, a combination of industrialization and wild capitalism. Because electricity introduced a vision dominated by detachment, where connections and networks were concealed behind a spectacular result, it provided the visual paradigm for the entire economic and social infrastructure that formed around the big cities in the late nineteenth and early twentieth centuries.

An illustrated article published in the Sunday edition of the *Saint Paul Globe* in 1904 described for Midwestern readers the "lighted wonder" New York was becoming at night, contrasting the coldness of financiers' calculations to the unintentionally sublime spectacle they produced at night: "They built to save cent per cent; they upreared a city of stars," the enthusiastic reporter proclaimed (fig. 147).[32] The article summoned forth the commonplace imagery of Oriental magic and splendor, comparing the night city to Babylon and Nineveh, but only to better define a phenomenon whose modernity contrasted with the mythological nature of those cities. The author pointed out several times that light rendered the forms of the landscape abstract: "The colossii [*sic*] change as if the clear, darkening air had transmuted them at a touch into something of its own fabric; the vast stiff masses, that but now shouldered each other in uncompromising rigidity, melt into one mighty sweep of heights, that has become still more vast, but is stiff and rigid no more. Angles and straight lines dissolve. The outlines of trusses and beam and granite become nebulous; the very skylights turn to flame; and every chimney is a triumphal tower."[33] Skyscrapers, similarly dissolved in the night air, seemed to have no ground to stand on. Here electricity imitated nothing less than the sky, radically reversing natural perspectives and inspiring Ezra Pound with this image of a Promethean New York: "And New York is the most beautiful city in the world? It is not far from it. No urban night is like the night there. . . . Squares after squares of flame, set up and cut into the aether. Here is our poetry, for we have pulled down the stars to our will."[34] When the lights went out, the spectacle vanished before one's eyes. But, in an apotheosis of idealization, the reporter for the *Saint Paul Globe* asserted that the vision persisted in a form even more ethereal than electricity, that of memory: "New York is dark—but its spell will never free the soul of him who has seen it."[35] The illustrations accompanying the article documented that abstraction produced by the combined effects of night and electricity: the images show a rhythmic juxtaposition of façades punctuated by the brightly lit openings of the windows. In the illustration at the bottom of the page, the Gothic arches of the Brooklyn Bridge and the reflections of the East River create an effect of distance. By contrast, in the central image, the city seems to dissolve into a flat, abstract motif. While the first illustration adopts the codes of the Whistleresque nocturne, complementing them with a distant view of the city composed of reflections and smoke, the second, in plunging the gaze directly into the urban landscape, paradoxically produces a result almost more faithful to the precepts of art for art's sake, a picture detached from any external reference and purely decorative.

That conspicuous dematerialization of the city and its commercial buildings seems to have been the result of a materialistic process, originating in a capitalist regime where, to borrow the words of Karl Marx and Friedrich Engels, "all that is solid melts into air."[36] Trachtenberg shows that the growing invisibility of economic relations was becoming institutionalized, especially with the development of a system based on the principle of "limited-liability" capital. According to him, at the

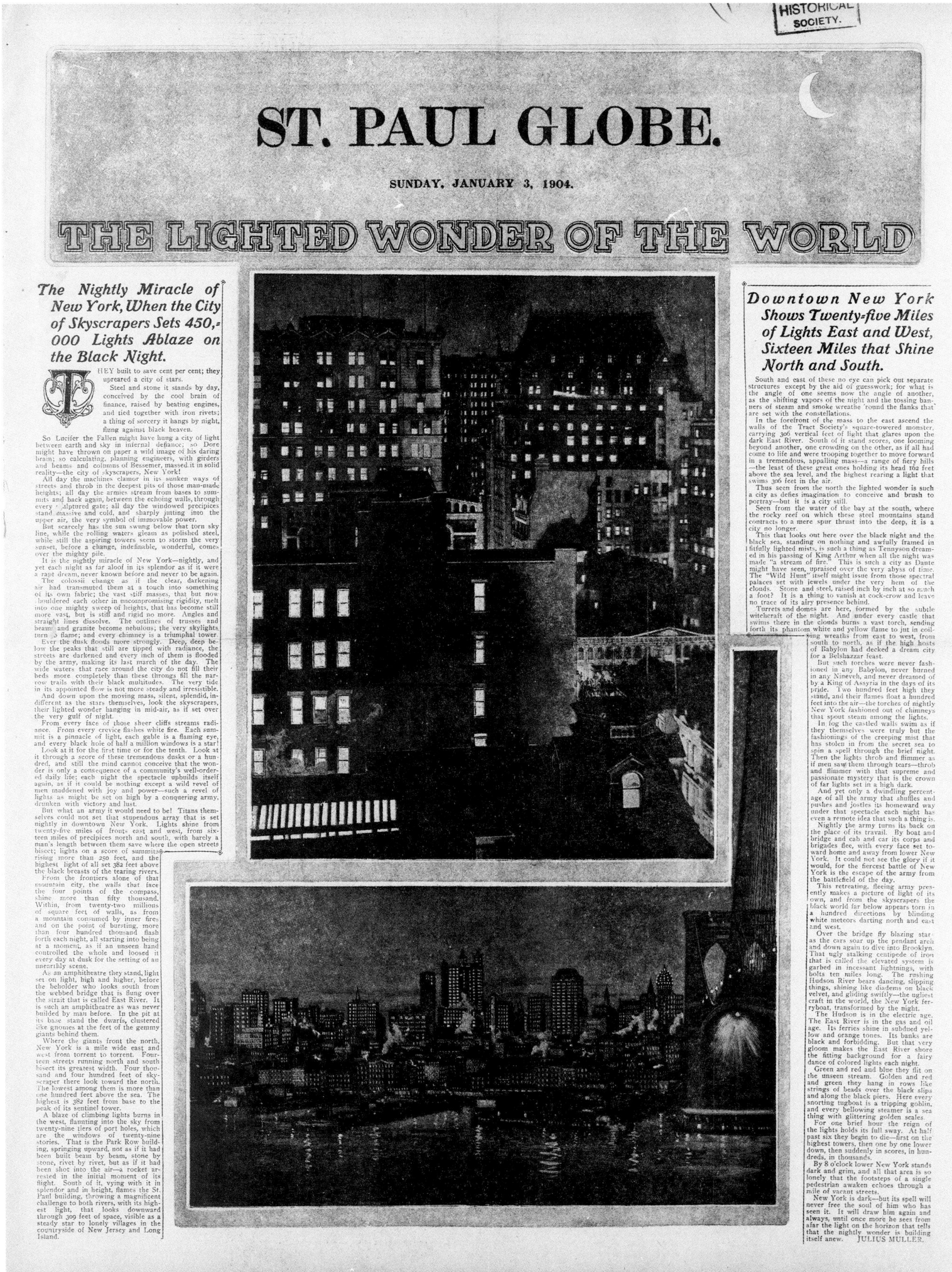

ST. PAUL GLOBE.

SUNDAY, JANUARY 3, 1904.

THE LIGHTED WONDER OF THE WORLD

The Nightly Miracle of New York, When the City of Skyscrapers Sets 450,000 Lights Ablaze on the Black Night.

THEY built to save cent per cent; they upreared a city of stars.

Steel and stone it stands by day, conceived by the cool brain of finance, raised by beating engines, and tied together with iron rivets; a thing of sorcery it hangs by night, flung against black heaven.

So Lucifer the Fallen might have hung a city of light between earth and sky in infernal defiance; so Dore might have thrown on paper a wild image of his daring brain; so calculating, planning engineers, with girders and beams and columns of Bessemer, massed it in solid reality—the city of skyscrapers, New York!

All day the machines clamor in its sunken ways of streets and throb in the deepest pits of those man-made heights; all day the armies stream from bases to summits and back again, between the echoing walls, through every sculptured gate; all day the windowed precipices stand massive and cold, and sharply jutting into the upper air, the very symbol of immovable power.

But scarcely has the sun swung below that torn sky line, while the rolling waters gleam as polished steel, while still the aspiring towers seem to storm the very sunset, before a change, indefinable, wonderful, comes over the mighty pile.

It is the nightly miracle of New York—nightly, and yet each night as far aloof in its splendor as if it were a rapt dream, never known before and never to be again.

The colossii change as if the clear, darkening air had transmuted them at a touch into something of its own fabric; the vast stiff masses, that but now shouldered each other in uncompromising rigidity, melt into one mighty sweep of heights, that has become still more vast, but is stiff and rigid no more. Angles and straight lines dissolve. The outlines of trusses and beams and granite become nebulous; the very skylights turn to flame; and every chimney is a triumphal tower.

Ever the dusk floods more strongly. Deep, deep below the peaks that still are tipped with radiance, the streets are darkened and every inch of them is flooded by the army, making its last march of the day. The wide waters that race around the city do not fill their beds more completely than these throngs fill the narrow trails with their black multitudes. The very tide in its appointed flow is not more steady and irresistible.

And down upon the moving mass, silent, splendid, indifferent as the stars themselves, look the skyscrapers, their lighted wonder hanging in mid-air, as if set over the very gulf of night.

From every face of those sheer cliffs streams radiance. From every crevice flashes white fire. Each summit is a pinnacle of light, each gable is a flaming eye, and every black hole of half a million windows is a star!

Look at it for the first time or for the tenth. Look at it through a score of these tremendous dusks or a hundred, and still the mind cannot conceive that the wonder is only a consequence of a community's well-ordered daily life; each night the spectacle upbuilds itself again, as if it could be nothing except a wild revel of men maddened with joy and power—such a revel of lights as might be set on high by a conquering army, drunken with victory and lust.

But what an army it would need to be! Titans themselves could not set that stupendous array that is set nightly in downtown New York. Lights shine from twenty-five miles of fronts east and west, from sixteen miles of precipices north and south, with barely a man's length between them save where the open streets bisect; lights on a score of summits rising more than 250 feet, and the highest light of all set 382 feet above the black breasts of the tearing rivers.

From the frontiers alone of that mountain city, the walls that face the four points of the compass, shine more than fifty thousand. Within, from twenty-two millions of square feet of walls, as from a mountain consumed by inner fires and on the point of bursting, more than four hundred thousand flash forth each night, all starting into being at a moment, as if an unseen hand controlled the whole and loosed it every day at dusk for the setting of an unearthly scene.

As an amphitheatre they stand, light set on light, high and higher, before the beholder who looks south from the webbed bridge that is flung over the strait that is called East River. It is such an amphitheatre as was never builded by man before. In the pit at its base stand the dwarfs, clustered like gnomes at the feet of the gemmy giants behind them.

Where the giants front the north, New York is a mile wide east and west from torrent to torrent. Fourteen streets running north and south bisect its greatest width. Four thousand and four hundred feet of skyscraper there look toward the north. The lowest among them is more than one hundred feet above the sea. The highest is 382 feet from base to the peak of its sentinel tower.

A blaze of climbing lights burns in the west, flaunting into the sky from twenty-nine tiers of port holes, which are the windows of twenty-nine stories. That is the Park Row building, springing upward, not as if it had been built beam by beam, stone by stone, rivet by rivet, but as if it had been shot into the air—a rocket arrested in the initial moment of its flight. South of it, vying with it in splendor and in height, flames the St. Paul building, throwing a magnificent challenge to both rivers, with its highest light, that looks downward through 309 feet of space, visible as a steady star to lonely villages in the countryside of New Jersey and Long Island.

Downtown New York Shows Twenty-five Miles of Lights East and West, Sixteen Miles that Shine North and South.

South and east of these no eye can pick out separate structures except by the aid of guesswork; for what is the angle of one seems now the angle of another, as the shifting vapors of the night and the tossing banners of steam and smoke wreathe 'round the flanks that are set with the constellations.

In the forefront of the mass to the east ascend the walls of the Tract Society's square-towered monster, carrying 306 vertical feet of light that glares upon the dark East River. South of it stand scores, one looming beyond another, one crowding on the other, as if all had come to life and were trooping together to move forward in a tremendous, appalling mass—a range of fiery hills—the least of these great ones holding its head 162 feet above the sea level, and the highest rearing a light that swims 306 feet in the air.

Thus seen from the north the lighted wonder is such a city as defies imagination to conceive and brush to portray—but it is a city still.

Seen from the water of the bay at the south, where the rocky reef on which these steel mountains stand contracts to a mere spur thrust into the deep, it is a city no longer.

This that looks out here over the black night and the black sea, standing on nothing and awfully framed in fitfully lighted mists, is such a thing as Tennyson dreamed in his passing of King Arthur when all the night was made "a stream of fire." This is such a city as Dante might have seen, upraised over the very abyss of time. The "Wild Hunt" itself might issue from those spectral palaces set with jewels under the very hem of the clouds. Stone and steel, raised inch by inch at so much a foot? It is a thing to vanish at cock-crow and leave no trace of its airy presence behind.

Turrets and domes are here, formed by the subtle witchcraft of the night. And under every castle that swims there in the clouds burns a vast torch, sending forth its phantom white and yellow flame to jut in coiling wreaths from east to west, from south to north, as if the high hosts of Babylon had decked a dream city for a Belshazzar feast.

But such torches were never fashioned in any Babylon, never burned in any Nineveh, and never dreamed of by a King of Assyria in the days of its pride. Two hundred feet high they stand, and their flames float a hundred feet into the air—the torches of nightly New York fashioned out of chimneys that spout steam among the lights.

In fog the castled walls swim as if they themselves were truly but the fashionings of the creeping mist that has stolen in from the secret sea to spin a spell through the brief night. Then the lights throb and flimmer as if men saw them through tears—throb and flimmer with that supreme and passionate mystery that is the crown of far lights set in a high dark.

And yet only a dwindling percentage of all the army that shuffles and pushes and jostles its homeward way under that spectacle each night has even a remote idea that such a thing is.

Nightly the army turns its back on the place of its travail. By boat and bridge and cab and car its corps and brigades flee, with every face set toward home and away from lower New York. It could not see the glory if it would, for the fiercest battle of New York is the escape of the army from the battlefield of the day.

This retreating, fleeing army presently makes a picture of light of its own, and from the skyscrapers the black world far below appears torn in a hundred directions by blinding white meteors darting north and east and west.

Over the bridge fly blazing stars as the cars soar up the pendant arch and down again to dive into Brooklyn. That ugly stalking centipede of iron that is called the elevated system is garbed in incessant lightnings, with bolts ten miles long. The rushing Hudson River bears dancing, slipping things, shining like diadems on black velvet, and gliding swiftly—the ugliest craft in the world, the New York ferryboat, transformed by the night.

The Hudson is in the electric age. The East River is in the gas and oil age. Its ferries shine in subdued yellow and orange tones. Its banks are black and forbidding. But that very gloom makes the East River shore the fitting background for a fairy dance of colored lights each night.

Green and red and blue they flit on the unseen stream. Golden and red and green they hang in rows like strings of beads over the black slips and along the black piers. Here every snorting tugboat is a tripping goblin, and every bellowing steamer is a sea thing with glittering golden scales.

For one brief hour the reign of the lights holds its full sway. At half past six they begin to die—first on the highest towers, then one by one lower down, then suddenly in scores, in hundreds, in thousands.

By 8 o'clock lower New York stands dark and grim, and all that area is so lonely that the footsteps of a single pedestrian awaken echoes through a mile of vacant streets.

New York is dark—but its spell will never free the soul of him who has seen it. It will draw him again and always, until once more he sees from afar the light on the horizon that tells that the nightly wonder is building itself anew. JULIUS MULLER.

FIG. 147. "The Lighted Wonder of the World," *Saint Paul Globe,* January 3, 1904.

turn of the twentieth century the American metropolis became emblematic of the advance of capitalism and corporations. The hold exerted by the capitalist system grew in tandem with its invisibility: as the sources of production moved farther and farther from the places of consumption, consumers were increasingly dependent on distribution networks, which usually remained invisible to them and were part of a system of transactions that was more and more abstract.[37] Trachtenberg sees the spectacular disconnection between the façade and the interior of skyscrapers as the symbol for that growing abstraction: "As buildings stretched upward, too high to be taken in by the eye at once, their inner work as corporate headquarters or clearing houses of arcane transactions receded from view, from intelligibility, and from criticism."[38] The effect of visual fragmentation produced by electric lights projected onto the façades of skyscrapers reinforced that dissimulation. In an interpretation that references Jean Baudrillard's reflections, Nye considers electricity a "sign" of capitalism, but he rather quickly returns to an aesthetic notion of the electrical sublime. His analysis could no doubt be expanded, on the basis of Trachtenberg's argument: the force of that aesthetic seemingly lay precisely in its proximity to capitalism's modes of operation, which were infiltrating Americans' daily lives at the time. Because electricity, a mysterious energy both material and immaterial, was produced beyond the sight of city dwellers and was distributed through hidden networks, it was itself emblematic of that general occultation of exchanges.[39] Abstraction and sublimation seem to have been merely the visual side of "incorporation."

In that sense, works that move in the direction of formal sparsity can also be construed as participating in the increasingly abstracted capitalistic system. They waver between an aesthetic appreciation of a sublimated vision and a consciousness of the grip that the new environment was exerting on subjective perception. In Alfred Stieglitz's photograph *From the Back Window, 291* (fig. 148), for instance, the largest zone of visible light turns out to be an advertising billboard. Although the contrast in the photograph is so sharp that the billboard is barely legible, its presence is still suggestive. When Stieglitz took the shot, he was in the process of publishing a special issue of *Camera Work,* in which he invited a series of personalities from the art world to answer the question: "What is 291?" referring to the gallery he opened ten years earlier at 291 Broadway in New York City. That gesture scarcely concealed his promotional ambition. A few of the responses portray the gallery as a space particularly attuned to the abstraction represented in the photograph. John W. Breyfogle proposes this definition: "An Arena for disembodied souls; for stardust, molecules, animalcula. . . . An upside-down house . . . builded [*sic*] upon empty space between existences."[40] The painter Arthur Dove suggests a parallel between the gallery and the art exhibited there: "The question, 'What is 291?' leaves one in the same position in explaining it as the modern painter is in explaining his painting. The modern painting does not present any definite object. Neither does '291' represent any definite movement in one direction."[41] Although these commentaries evince an elitist desire for distinction through indetermination, they also suggest a vision close to what the nocturnal urban environment showed modern city dwellers. While these responses, through more or less obscure games, eliminated the possibility of an actual definition, page after page the same sign reappears with the force of a logo: the articles are of different lengths and their content varies, but each bears the same title, which repeats the emblematic number of the gallery, 291. In that sense, the photograph itself, whose title also includes the name of the gallery, can be read as a kind of indirect advertising. From his "back window," Stieglitz, in an ironic twist, showed and at the same time obscured the commercial relationship by aestheticizing it.

One last example of a nocturnal urban landscape pushed the dissolution of forms even further: George Bellows's *Excavation at Night* represents a limit case in which darkness threatens to engulf the subject of the painting completely (fig. 149).[42] But it was precisely the formless, the chasm, that Bellows was trying to represent: rather than the spectacle of skyscrapers vanishing in the darkness, leaving only the trace of their illuminated windows, he chose to show the work preliminary to the construction of a new landmark in New York, Penn Station, which opened two years after the painting was created. If the electrical sublime is the visual translation of the abstraction of relationships in the capitalist metropolis, Bellows's *Excavation,* by contrast, is akin to what Joseph Schumpeter calls "creative destruction," the paradoxical process inherent to the development of capitalism.[43] Many commentators were in fact astonished by the speed at which the landscape of American

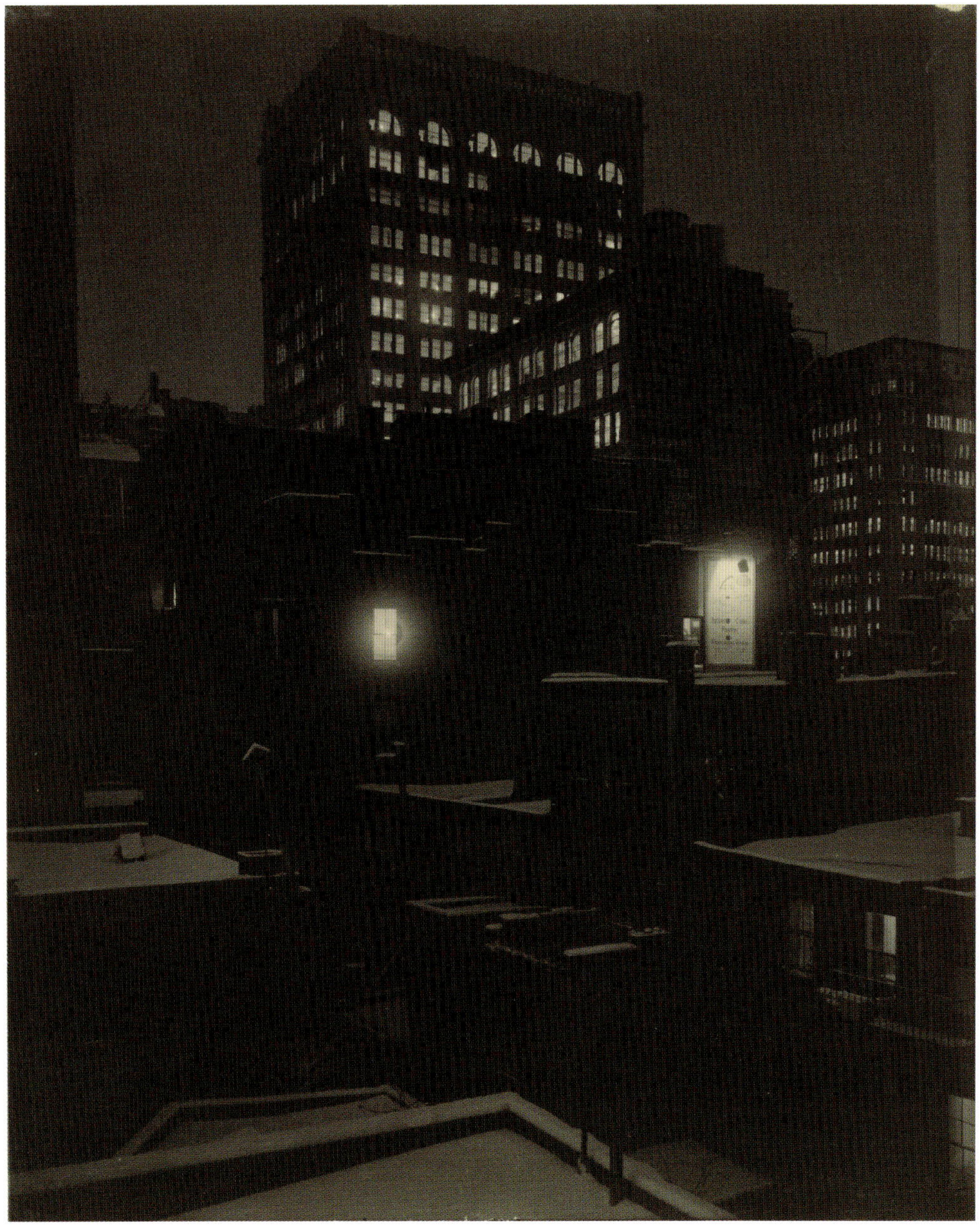

FIG. 148. Alfred Stieglitz, *From the Back Window, 291*, 1915. Platinum print, 47.8 × 38.4 cm (9 7/8 × 7 15/16 in.). Metropolitan Museum of Art, Alfred Stieglitz Collection, 1949 (49.55.35).

metropolises passed through the various phases of demolition and reconstruction, which made the city impossible to recognize after a few years. Consider this joke from the time about Chicago: "'When were you in Chicago?' 'Last week.' 'Oh, well! Then you know nothing about it. The city has entirely changed since then.'"[44] Henry James saw skyscrapers as the symbols of that essentially ephemeral city: "Crowned not only with no history, but with no credible possibility of time for history, and consecrated by no uses save the commercial at any cost, they are simply the most piercing notes in that concert of the expensively provisional into which your supreme sense of New York resolves itself."[45] The idea of the city's constant transformation fascinated the crowds that flocked to Coney Island and the concessions of the world's fairs, to sample carnivalesque spectacles in which urban architecture was inverted, dismantled, annihilated. Curiosity seekers could thus visit Henry Roltair's famous "upside-down house" and witness, in addition to the reconstitution of urban fires, stagings of the floods that had swept through the city of Galveston in 1900, or the 1906 earthquake and fire of San Francisco.[46] When the remains of the World's Columbian Exposition vanished in a fire as immense as the White City, Chicago residents rushed to the surrounding hills to make the most of the spectacle.[47] The destruction—particularly in

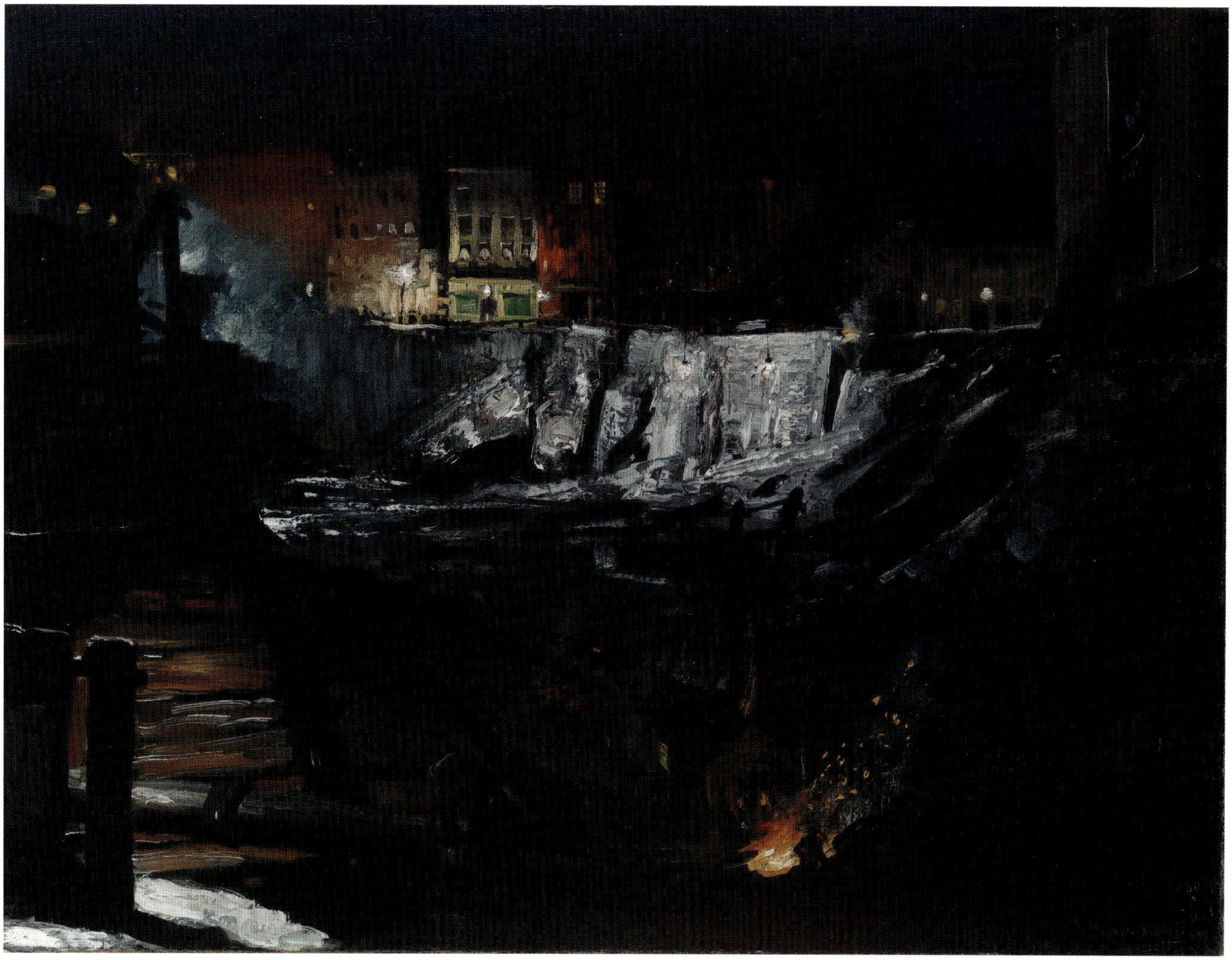

FIG. 149. George Bellows, *Excavation at Night*, 1908. Oil on canvas, 86.4 × 111.8 cm (34 × 44 in.). Crystal Bridges Museum of American Art, Bentonville, Arkansas, 2010.77.

Chicago, whose innovative architecture is considered one of the indirect consequences of the 1871 fire—seemed to give rise to a redesign of the urban landscape. Conversely, that redesign occasioned further destruction, all in an endless cycle.

Bellows's *Excavation at Night* leaves the beholder suspended between creation and destruction. Here, night no longer serves simply to keep the elements of the landscape at a distance; it also reveals a hole in the landscape, the potential for a profound transformation. *Excavation* seems to be, more than a landscape, the vision of a permanently mutating environment. Forged in the darkness of the torn-up ground are not only a new city but also the forms used to envision it in the future. In that sense, the darkness of night and Bellows's chasm seem to function in the same way: *Excavation at Night* shows simultaneously the formless chaos of destruction and the propagation of a potential creativity. But it suspends the beholder's gaze between these two extremes, above a gaping void. Bellows's painting, then, embodies the paradigm of an anti-landscape oscillating between circumspect contemplation of the modern city's disorder and fascination with the infinite renovation behind it. In the face of the gigantic and constantly changing construction site constituted by the spectacle of the urban environment, night allowed the artist to deploy new visual modalities and to give a new meaning to indetermination. Restraint and uncertainty, attraction and admiration are here maintained in equilibrium, in a darkness that could be called, to borrow Henry James's term, purely "provisional."

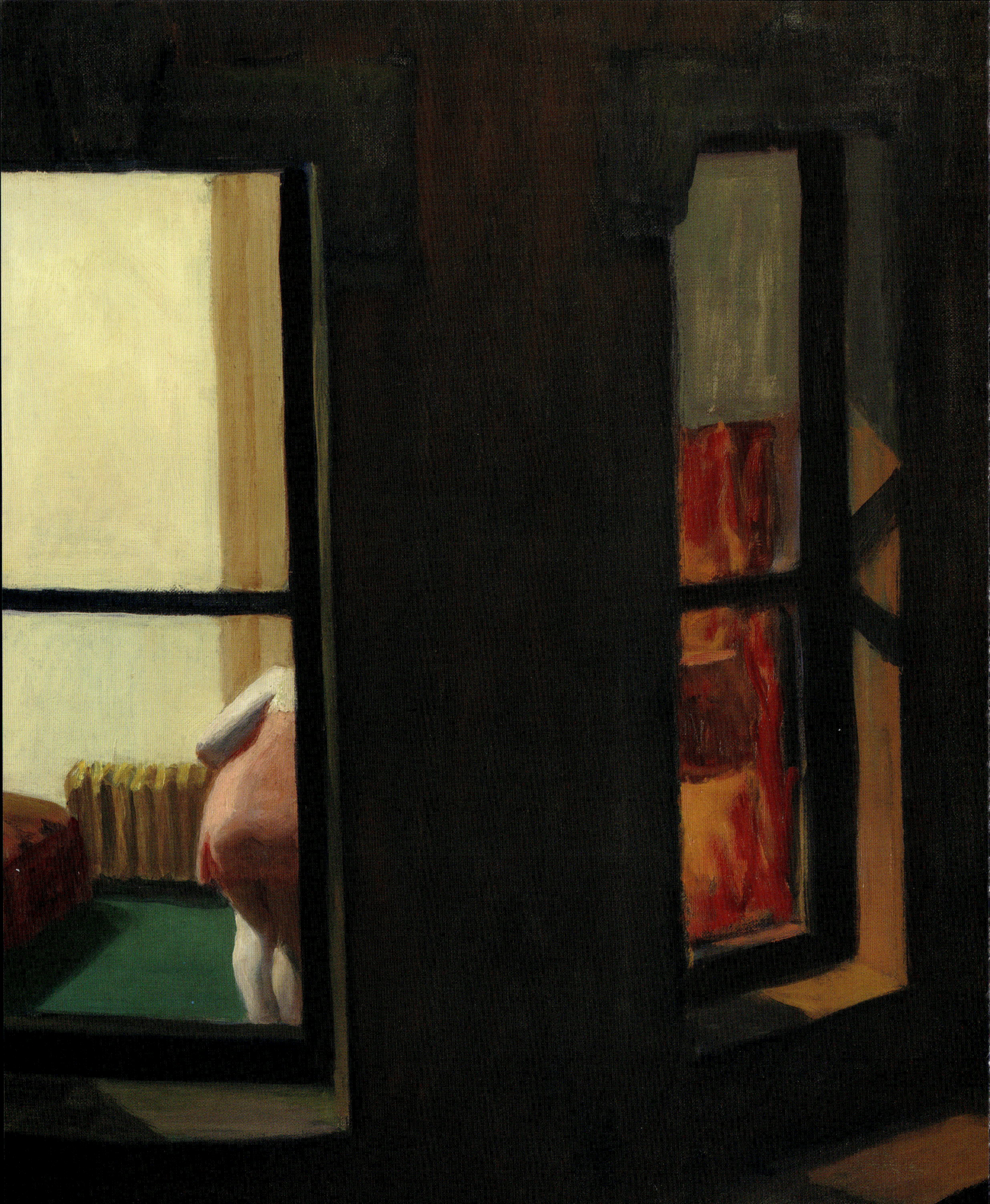

Conclusion

In 1907 the *New York Herald* published an installment of Winsor McCay's comic strip *Little Nemo,* in which the young hero dreams he is lost among skyscrapers in the company of Imp, a recurring secondary character (fig. 150). Both of them have reached gigantic Alice in Wonderland proportions that comparatively dwarf the city to the size of a playground. The chaotic collision of disparate elements, amusing by its very absurdity, is also so because, in the end, it is only a distorted and exaggerated reflection of a spectacle McCay's readers confronted on a daily basis. In and of itself, the image encapsulates the themes I have addressed in this book. This early comic strip, the product of a rapidly expanding visual culture, thematizes Nemo's ever-surprised take on a world in which the limits of the visible and the invisible, the rational and irrational, seem to be constantly called into question. It is, moreover, an inward-looking take, the staging of a dream that repeats episode after episode. His companion, a black child dressed only in a loincloth, like the individuals exhibited in the anthropological sections of the world's fairs, personifies the archetype of the Other. A hybrid of sorts between caricatures of the "native," as seen by white imperialism, and the minstrel show stereotype of blacks with protruding lips and inordinately white eyes, he is also the dark double of the little boy in his white nightshirt. Finally, the diminished environment in which they move inverts the sense of disorientation imposed on the daily lives of American urban dwellers by the colossal architecture of the big city. Nemo's adventures remained within the lighthearted register of popular entertainment, but, like them, the art of the nocturne made use of symbolic displacement to lend expression to a series of meanings more or less latent in the culture of its time.

Night, more than simply a pictorial theme, was a mode of vision, a filter through which reality was reordered in accordance with criteria more easily acceptable to the nocturne's audience. But the manipulations of the genre were laden with ambivalence and paradox: the nocturne concealed as much as it showed and denied as much as it confessed. Nocturne artists attempted to distinguish their works from their visual environment, but they adopted a strategy that was bound to fail, and which, moreover, betrayed the ambiguity of their own position. In choosing an aesthetic of blurriness and darkness, in a context where images were improving in quality and

Fig. 151 detail

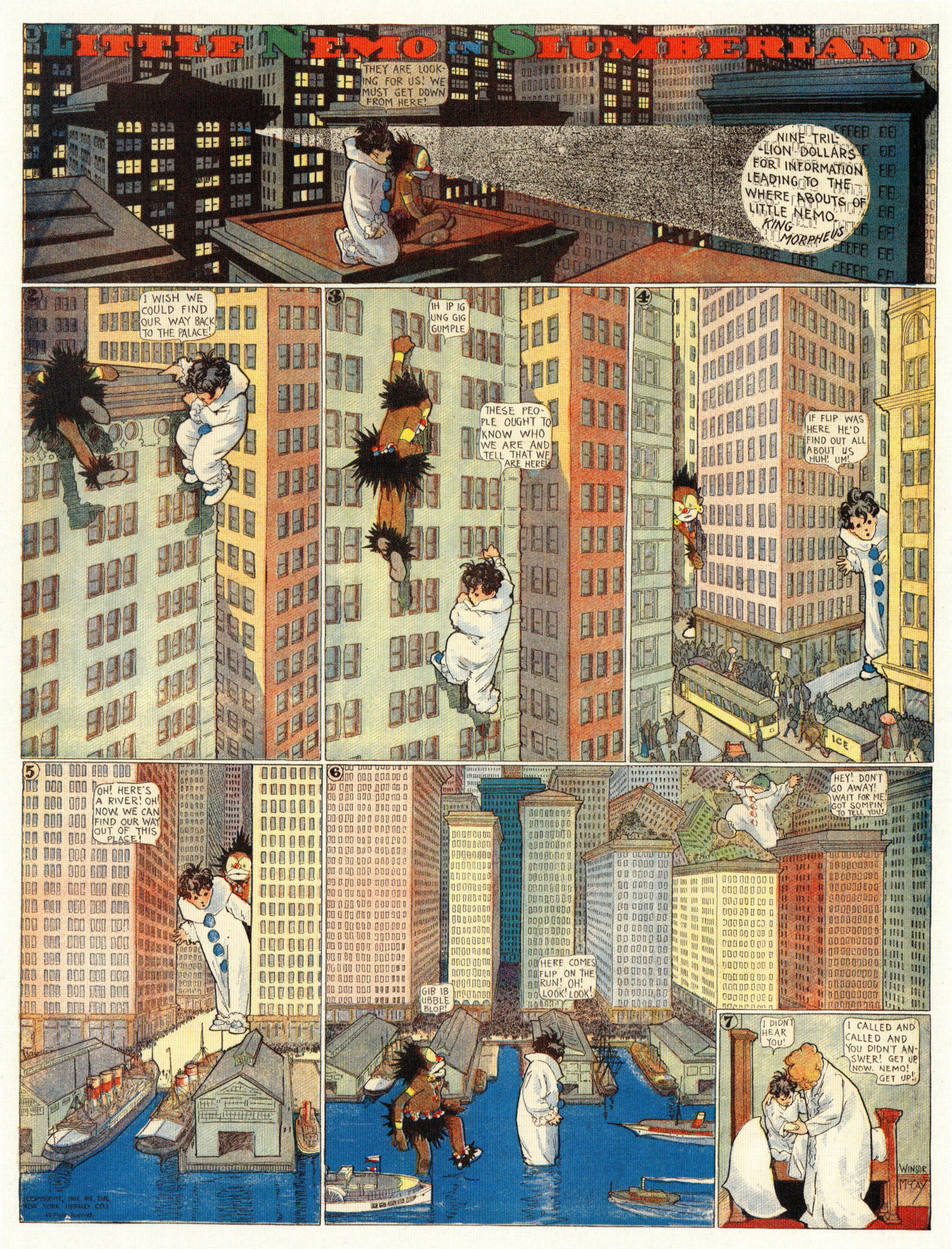
LITTLE NEMO IN SLUMBERLAND
THEY ARE LOOKING FOR US! WE MUST GET DOWN FROM HERE!
NINE TRILLION DOLLARS FOR INFORMATION LEADING TO THE WHEREABOUTS OF LITTLE NEMO. KING MORPHEUS
I WISH WE COULD FIND OUR WAY BACK TO THE PALACE!
IH IP IG UNG GIG GUMPLE
THESE PEOPLE OUGHT TO KNOW WHO WE ARE AND TELL THAT WE ARE HERE!
IF FLIP WAS HERE HE'D FIND OUT ALL ABOUT US HUH! UM!
ICE
OH! HERE'S A RIVER! OH! NOW, WE CAN FIND OUR WAY OUT OF THIS PLACE!
HEY! DON'T GO AWAY! WAIT FOR ME! GOT SOMPIN TO TELL YOU!
HERE COMES FLIP ON THE RUN! OH! LOOK! LOOK!
GIB IB UBBLE BLOP!
I DIDN'T HEAR YOU!
I CALLED AND CALLED AND YOU DIDN'T ANSWER! GET UP NOW, NEMO! GET UP!
WINSOR McCAY

FIG. 150. Winsor McCay, "Little Nemo in Slumberland," *New York Herald,* September 29, 1907. San Francisco Academy of Comic Art Collection, Ohio State University, Billy Ireland Cartoon Library and Museum.

increasing in quantity, they acknowledged that they were deliberately taking the losing side; and though they pretended not to belong to the sphere of image production and exchange, they could not help but play by the rules of the market. The nocturne also turned out to be an effective medium for treating the question of racial difference in an environment where light and darkness were already being broadly exploited by racist and imperialist rhetoric. Placed in the service of an equivocal game of contrasts and erasures, it absorbed the Other into the night. That art of darkness was supposed to epitomize the superiority of white civilization. And yet, though it adopted the simplified oppositions of popular culture, it revealed as well the fragility of the clichés, by suggesting possible inversions and the blurring of boundaries. The visible presence of the Other persisted in the nocturne, where the white man could find himself symbolically supplanted by his own shadow. Finally, in representations of the urban night, the filter of the nocturne allowed artists to temper the spectacle of alterity by varying distances. In the metropolises, at a time when American city dwellers were witness to a permanent reconfiguration of economic and social relations, the darkness of the nocturne made it possible both to moderate the change by giving it a blurry form and to create a visual space where, precisely, indetermination predominated. The various modalities of the nocturne—negative promotional strategy, effacement, visual distancing of alterity—were marked by a contradictory dynamic. That was both its strength and its weakness. The nocturne was effective because it opened an ambiguous visual space, but the artists, even while putting into play ambiguities and slippages of meaning, did not control all its significations. To borrow the musical terminology of which Whistler was so fond, though in a certain way the nocturne made it possible to harmonize the American landscape at the turn of the twentieth century, dissonances persisted.

The remaking of the visible landscape in the nocturne should be understood on several different levels. Even as the nocturne reflected changes that affected Americans' visual environment, it also attested to an evolution in how they *imagined* their landscape. The antimodern function of the nocturne, which allowed adaptation to a modernity it kept at a distance, also operated as a political use of the image. In the end, these reflections call for a revision of the notion of "landscape" itself. On several occasions, I have made comparisons with the Hudson River School, showing how that eloquent mid-nineteenth-century landscape painting was vested with an ideological content different from what is discernible in the nocturnes, which formed the negative counterpart, as it were, to that first American landscape painting. The Hudson River School was explicitly engaged in a political discourse that made the projection of an imaginary landscape coincide with specific ambitions. By contrast, the nocturne, whose attitude of detachment was emphasized by its practitioners and critics, evinced not a real political neutrality but an altered relationship to the landscape. At a time when the conquest of the North American continent had come to an end, the country's ambitions had to be transferred to other places and other forms. American imperialism gained a foothold in Cuba and the Philippines, but it developed primarily as a global and more diffuse domination that was less military than economic. In a certain way, the nocturnal landscape also reflected that transition toward an increasingly abstract and invisible domination. Whereas the aim of the landscapes of the Hudson River School was partly to make "manifest" a political project, the conspicuous detachment of the nocturnes may have entailed what Michael Cox calls a "denial" of empire.[1] In reality, the nocturne merely concealed power relations that continued to exist.

That no doubt explains the transient dimension of the vogue for nocturnes. As the United States entered World War I with a certain optimism, the American public's fascination with the nostalgic visions conveyed by the nocturnes seemed to wane. In 1915, for example, a critic reviewing the collections of the Metropolitan Museum for the newspaper *The Forum* included several nocturnes among the works he judged to be without further interest: "There are better artists working now in New York than the great majority of those hung in the Museum. Indeed the greater part of them could be dispensed with to the betterment of the collection, for many of the canvases are not representative of the merits of their authors: they are simply bad examples of more or less competent men's work. For instance, Whistler's *Nocturne in Green and Gold,* Myers's *The Night Mission,* Dabo's *The Cloud,* also Whistler's *Edward G. Kennedy, Lady in Grey* and his *Connie Gilchrist,* Benson's *Portrait of a Lady,* Winslow Homer's *Searchlight* . . . could be put in dark corners, or entirely hidden, and the rooms in which they are now hung would take on a better aspect."[2] Ironically, the critic, in proposing to relegate the nocturnes to the

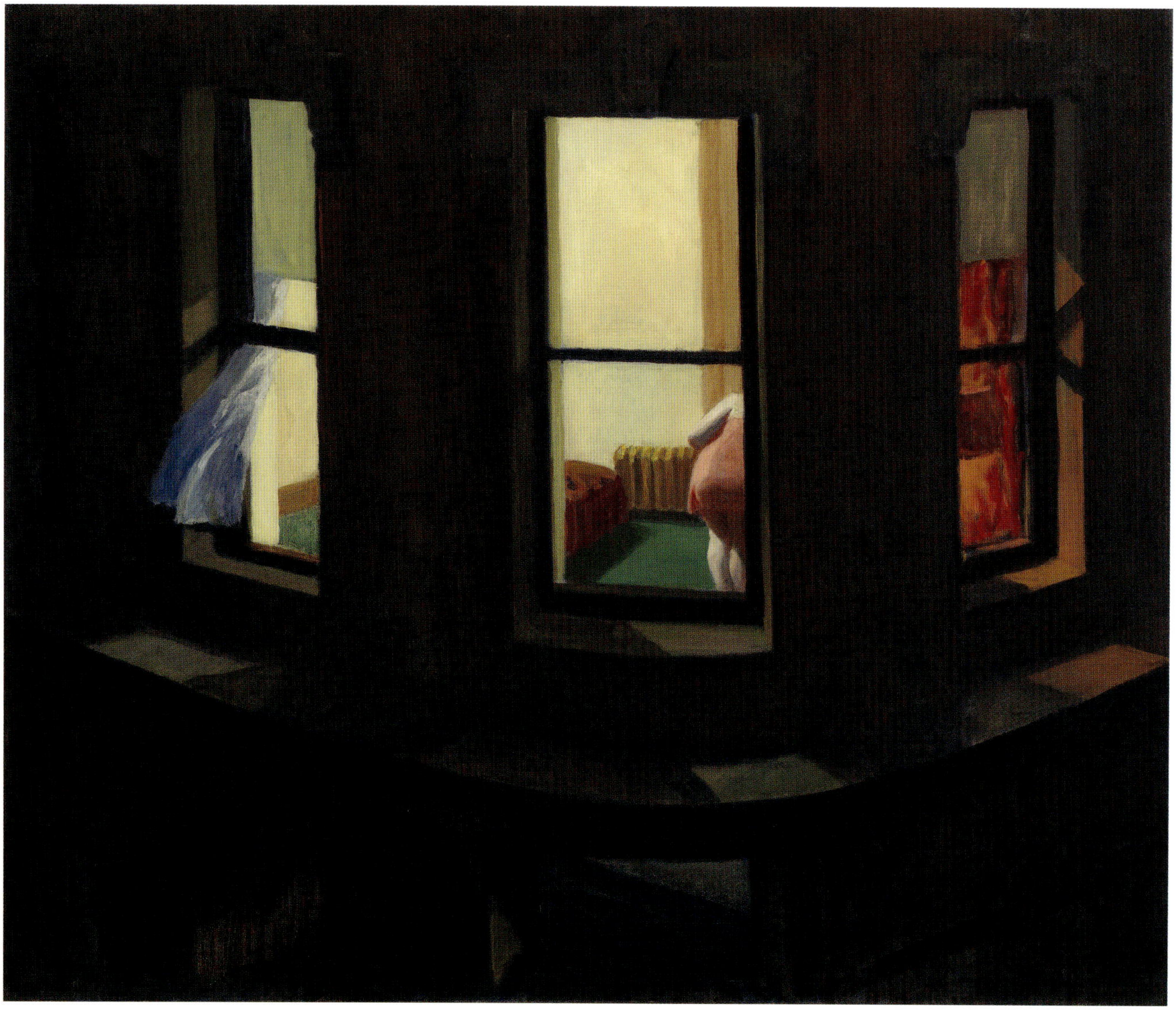

FIG. 151. Edward Hopper, *Night Windows*, 1928. Oil on canvas, 73.7 × 86.4 cm (29 × 34 in.). Museum of Modern Art, Gift of John Hay Whitney.

museum's "dark corners," was ultimately consigning them to the same fate that the *Eruption*, discussed in the introduction to this book, had suffered some twenty years earlier.

In the years surrounding World War I, especially with the self-proclaimed introduction of modernist art at the Armory Show of 1913,[3] a new role for night took shape in art. In Edward Hopper's *Night Windows*, painted in 1928, it is still possible to discern the legacy of the older models, especially that of John Sloan, whose title Hopper directly borrows. But the picture adopts, not without humor, a deliberately modernist point of view, emphasizing the fragmentation of forms and the almost abstract play of light and color (fig. 151). In that scene of the New York night, a furtive view from the dark street of an illuminated interior, the beholder perceives the partially concealed body of an anonymous woman, whose skimpy attire suggests she is preparing for bed. With obvious pleasure, the artist exploits the new potential of vision offered by the nocturnal urban space, multiplying points of view, reducing distances, and isolating zones of light in the darkness to form so many glimpses into the private lives of city dwellers. Like the Marches in *A Hazard of New Fortunes*, Hopper is probably watching the young woman from the elevated subway train, which, for a brief instant, takes him up to her windows. The gaze implicitly staged in *Night Windows* is to be distinguished from that which suffuses many other of Hopper's works, where the painter shows women alone and motionless, sometimes undressed as well, engrossed in their thoughts or in the contemplation of an object invisible to the beholder. Most often in Hopper's paintings, the female figures are looking out the window, symbolically mirroring the beholder's gaze. In *Night Windows,* the artist inverts that *profil perdu* of sorts, and pushes it to the point of the grotesque. The buttocks framed by the central window appear almost to be a gesture of derision, a thumbing of the nose by the painter, and the three illuminated windows form an ironic, ultimately trivial triptych. By contrast, the window, which in other works by Hopper marks the projection outward of a meditative interiority, encourages a centripetal gaze oriented toward an ordinary domestic interior, personified by the woman bent over her task and oblivious to external eyes.

That interior is unique in Hopper's oeuvre for another reason: it is peculiarly decomposed and must be understood as an image in motion. The movement indicated by the curve of the young woman's back, replicated by the curtain being lifted by the breeze (perhaps produced by the passing train) removes the scene from the fixed intensity of a voyeuristic gaze. The billowing curtain also suggests, somewhat naughtily, that the short robe the young woman is wearing could be whipped off just as easily. The three panels of light separate, into distinct moments as it were, the various parts of the room: the darkness that frames them accentuates the differences in luminosity between the left and middle windows, lit by harsh electric light, and a final panel on the right, where a lampshade placed behind a red cloth diffuses a crepuscular light. From one to the other, the beholder feels propelled toward a waning light, as the train's course accompanies the passage of time through the woman's bedroom. Hopper's painting adds to the paradox by fixing that transient vision on canvas: the gaze it casts on the scene is both a passing and a past gaze, which would account for its fragmented, incomplete aspect. The humor Hopper displays in *Night Windows* is thus self-deprecating, and the artist combines a mischievous fondness for the trivial and ephemeral with a certain amusement at his own finite gaze. This is a long way from the nocturne's diffuse and static contemplation. If the painting thematizes absorption, it does so by waxing ironic about its fleetingness. Hopper closes the opening that John Sloan's *Night Windows* had made: by 1928, the night painted by his predecessor already seemed destined for a medium other than painting. That threefold view could indeed begin to move, and the arrangement of the windows along the curving façade might bring to mind the frames of an unspooling film. Coinciding with the transition from silent films to talking pictures, Hopper's painting seems to portend the rich future of the night on America's silver screen.[4] After nocturnes, in fact, American film of the 1940s to 1950s would take hold as the artistic form best able to draw on the symbolic reserves of the night. *Night Windows,* suspended between two visions of the night, marks a major turning point in both the literal and the figurative sense: between the antimodernism of the nocturnes and the exploration of darkness on the big screen by film noir directors such as John Huston and Otto Preminger, a whole society had learned to see the night differently and to exploit all its aesthetic resources, projecting onto it the fears and aspirations of their own time.

Notes

INTRODUCTION

1. "A Chapter in Art," *Puck's Library* 35 (May 1890): 6–7.
2. On Manifest Destiny, see, for example, Thomas Hietala, *Manifest Design: American Exceptionalism and Empire* (Ithaca, NY: Cornell University Press, 2002). For its representation in art, see Albert Boime, *The Magisterial Gaze* (Washington, DC: Smithsonian Institution, 1991); and Angela Miller, *The Empire of the Eye: Landscape Representations and American Cultural Politics, 1825–1875* (Ithaca, NY: Cornell University Press, 1998).
3. Frederic Edwin Church, *Cotopaxi*, 1862, oil on canvas, 122 × 216 cm (48 × 85 in.), Detroit Institute of Arts.
4. Letter from James McNeill Whistler to Frederick Richards Leyland, November 2–9, 1872, Library of Congress manuscripts, Pennel-Whistler coll. PWC 6B/21/3, http://www.whistler.arts.gla.ac.uk/correspondence/people/display/?cid=8794&nameid=Leyland_FR&sr=0&rs=42&surname=Leyland&firstname=Frederick (last consulted in January 2018).
5. Letter from James McNeill Whistler to Walter Greaves, 1871–76, Library of Congress manuscripts, Penn-Whistler coll. PWC 9/639, http://www.whistler.arts.gla.ac.uk/correspondence/exhibit/display/?rs=1&exhibid=LoSFA-1872&sort= (last consulted in January 2018).
6. Sales catalogues formerly held in the archives of the Frick Collection and the Metropolitan Museum of Art in New York.
7. Scott A. Shields, "Evening Meditations: Peters and the Mystery of Monterey," in his *Artists at Continent's End: The Monterey Peninsula Art Colony, 1875–1907* (Berkeley: University of California Press, 2006), 59–83.
8. "Clark Pays $24,000 for Two Paintings," *New York Times*, April 3, 1913. A century later, a photographic print of Edward Steichen's *The Pond—Moonlight* sold for a record $2,928,000, a price that attests to the appeal the nocturne genre continues to exert and also, no doubt, to the artistic aura it confers on photography.
9. "Exhibition by the Fakirs: Weird Canvases Ready for Eleventh Annual Function," *New York Times*, April 29, 1902. The caricature recalls the collection of monochromes published a few years earlier by French humorist Alphonse Allais in *Album primo-avrilesque* (Paris: P. Ollendorff, 1897).
10. James McNeill Whistler, "The Red Rag," *World*, May 22, 1878, repr. in James McNeill Whistler, *The Gentle Art of Making Enemies* (1892; London: Dover, 1976), 126–28.
11. Minutes of the Whistler-Ruskin trial, reproduced in Linda Merrill, *A Pot of Paint: Aesthetics on Trial in Whistler v. Ruskin* (Washington, DC: Smithsonian Institution Press, 1992), 144.
12. Joris Karl Huysmans, *Certains* (Paris: Tresse & Stock, 1889), 67–68.
13. Nikolai Cikovsky and Charles Brock, "Whistler and America," in Richard Dorment and Margaret McDonald, eds., *James McNeill Whistler* (New York: Harry N. Abrams, 1995), 29–38.
14. Henry James, "The Picture Season in London," in *The Painter's Eye: Notes and Essays on the Pictorial Arts by Henry James*, ed. John L. Sweeney (Madison: University of Wisconsin Press, 1956), 143.
15. John Ruskin, *Fors Clavigera: Letters to the Workmen and Labourers of Great Britain* (1871–84; New York: Greenwood, 1968), 73.
16. Linda Merrill, "Whistler in America," in *After Whistler: The Artist and His Influence on American Painting*, ed. Linda Merrill (New Haven, CT: Yale University Press, 2003), 15–16.
17. James McNeill Whistler, *Arrangement in Grey and Black No. 1: Portrait of the Artist's Mother*, 1871, oil on canvas, 144.3 × 162.5 cm (56 3/4 × 63 7/8 in.), Paris, Musée d'Orsay.
18. Ezra Pound, "To Whistler, American," *Poetry: A Magazine in Verse* (October 1912). Whistler's role as a tutelary figure is particularly important here, given that the poem was published in the review's very first issue.
19. "Art and Mr. Whistler," *Art Journal* 46, no. 120 (1894): 358.
20. John Van Dyke, "What Is All This Talk about Whistler?" *Ladies' Home Journal* (March 1904): 10.
21. See, for example, Clara Ruge, "The Tonal School of America," *International Studio* 27, no. 105 (January 1906): 57–68; and, for the adoption of the term by art historians in the twentieth century, Wanda Corn, *The Color of Mood: American Tonalism, 1880–1910* (San Francisco: M. H. De Young Museum, 1972).
22. Wolfgang Schivelbusch, *Disenchanted Night: The Industrialization of Light in the Nineteenth Century*, trans. Angela Davies (Berkeley: University of California Press, 1995); Murray Melbin, *Night as Frontier: Colonizing the World after Dark* (New York: Free Press, 1987).
23. Paul Valéry, *Oeuvres*, 2 vols. (1931; Paris: Gallimard, 1959–60), 2: 919–20; David E. Nye, *Electrifying America: Social Meanings

of a New Technology (Cambridge, MA: MIT Press, 1990).

24. Nye, *Electrifying America*, 29–84.
25. Ibid., 145 and 172. See also David E. Nye, *American Technological Sublime* (Cambridge, MA: MIT Press, 1994).
26. James McNeill Whistler, "Mr. Whistler's 'Ten O'Clock'" (1885), in Whistler, *The Gentle Art of Making Enemies*, 144.
27. Birge Harrison, *Landscape Painting* (New York: Charles Scribner's Sons, 1909), 249–50.
28. Lena M. McCauley, "An Epoch in National Art," *Brush and Pencil* 14, no. 5 (December 1904): 297.
29. T. J. Jackson Lears, *No Place of Grace: Antimodernism and the Transformation of American Culture, 1880–1920* (Chicago: University of Chicago Press, 1981), xv.
30. This tendency is visible, for instance, in the titles given to shows and books on the topic, including Ralph Sessions, *Poetic Vision: American Tonalism* (New York: Spanierman Gallery, 2005) and Harvey L. Jones, *Twilight and Reverie: California Tonalist Painting, 1890–1930* (Oakland: Oakland Museum, 1995).
31. Marc Simpson, ed., *Like Breath on Glass: Whistler, Inness, and the Art of Painting Softly* (New Haven, CT: Yale University Press, 2008).
32. Sarah Burns, "Dirty Pictures," in her *Painting the Dark Side: Art and the Gothic Imagination in Nineteenth-Century America* (Berkeley: University of California Press, 2004), 221–45.
33. Nancy Anderson, ed., *Frederic Remington: The Color of Night* (Washington, DC: National Gallery of Art, 2003). The book's first essay by William C. Sharpe also provides a brief overview of nocturnal landscape painting in American art.
34. Joachim Homann, ed., *Night Visions: Nocturnes in American Art, 1860–1960* (New York: Prestel, 2015)
35. See the exhibition of the artist's works at the Freer Gallery in 2014: *Kiyochika: Master of the Night*, alongside an exhibition of views of the Thames painted by Whistler in the 1870s, http://www.asia.si.edu/exhibitions/current/kiyochika (last consulted in January 2018).
36. Charles C. Eldredge discusses these transatlantic exchanges and draws up a list of formal and thematic parallels between the symbolist movement and comparable trends in the United States. See his *American Imagination and Symbolist Painting* (New York: Grey Art Gallery and Study Center, New York University, 1979).
37. On this subject, see Neil Harris, *The Artist in American Society: The Formative Years* (Chicago: University of Chicago Press, 1982); and Sarah Burns, *Inventing the Modern Artist: Art and Culture in Gilded Age America* (New Haven, CT: Yale University Press, 1996).
38. Marilyn S. Kushner, Kimberly Orcutt, and Casey Nelson Blake, *The Armory Show at 100: Modernism and Revolution* (New York: New-York Historical Society, 2013).

CHAPTER 1. A PARADOXICAL AESTHETICS

1. Leon Battista Alberti, *On Painting*, trans. John R. Spencer, rev. ed. (New Haven, CT: Yale University Press, 1966).
2. André Félibien, *Entretiens sur la vie et les ouvrages de Nicolas Poussin* (Geneva: P. Cailler, 1947), 194.
3. "A Dazzling Picture-Show," *New York Times*, March 3, 1894.
4. *Literary World* (June 1882), excerpts from critical reviews cited by Whistler and published in James McNeill Whistler, *Etchings and Drypoints: Venice, Second Series* (London: Fine Arts Society, 1883), 8.
5. Neil Harris, *The Land of Contrasts: 1880–1901* (New York: George Braziller, 1970), 7.
6. Quoted in Walter Sickert, "The New Life of Whistler," *Fortnightly Review*, December 1, 1908, 1025.
7. "'Airscapes,' by the Brothers Dabo at the Modern Gallery Recently," *New York Times*, February 25, 1906.
8. "Winter Exhibitions," *Saturday Review*, October 28, 1871.
9. On this subject, see Jennifer C. Raab, *Frederic Church: The Art and Science of Detail*, (New Haven, CT: Yale University Press, 2015).
10. Birge Harrison, *Landscape Painting* (New York: Charles Scribner's Sons, 1909), 73–74.
11. Cody Hartley, "The Illusions of Soft Painting," in *Like Breath on Glass: Whistler, Inness, and the Art of Painting Softly*, ed. Marc Simpson (New Haven, CT: Yale University Press, 2008), 77.
12. Maurice Merleau-Ponty, *Phenomenology of Perception*, trans. Donald A. Landes (London: Routledge, 2012), 296.
13. Eli Wildner, *The Gilded Edge: The Art of the Frame* (San Francisco: Chronicle Books, 2000), 60–82.
14. David Park Curry, "Total Control: Whistler at an Exhibition," in *James McNeill Whistler: A Reexamination*, ed. Ruth E. Fine (Washington, DC: National Gallery of Art, 1987), 67–82. Kathleen Pyne links Whistler's aesthetic commitments, which according to her verged on a sacralization of art, to the fascination exerted in the United States by Richard Wagner and his *Gesamtkunstwerk* (total work of art) in the 1890s. See her *Art and the Higher Life: Painting and Evolutionary Thought in Late Nineteenth-Century America* (Austin: University of Texas Press, 1996), 85.
15. Kenneth Myers, *Mr. Whistler's Gallery: Pictures at an 1884 Exhibition* (Washington, DC: Freer Gallery of Art, Smithsonian Institution, 2003).
16. Quoted in Charles Colbert, *Haunted Visions: Spiritualism and American Art* (Philadelphia: University of Pennsylvania Press, 2011), 130.
17. Charles Caffin, *The Story of American Painting: The Evolution of Painting in America from Colonial Times to the Present* (New York: Frederick A. Stokes, 1907), 451.
18. "Dudley Gallery—Cabinet Pictures in Oil," *Times (London)*, November 14, 1871; quoted in *The Paintings of James McNeill Whistler*, ed. Andrew McLaren Young, Margaret MacDonald, Robin Spencer, and Hamish Miles (New Haven, CT: Yale University Press, 1980), 103.
19. Elizabeth Robins Pennell and Joseph Pennell, *The Life of James McNeill Whistler* (Philadelphia: J. B. Lippincott, 1911), 165.
20. Joyce Hill Stoner uses the word "weavism" to describe that practice: see her "Materials for Immateriality," in Simpson, ed., *Like Breath on Glass*, 101.
21. Hartley, "The Illusions of Soft Painting," 84.
22. "Pictures by J. H. Johnson," *New York Times*, February 22, 1894.
23. Quoted in Linda Merrill, *A Pot of Paint: Aesthetics on Trial in Whistler v. Ruskin* (Washington, DC: Smithsonian Institution, 1992), 146.
24. James McNeill Whistler, "The Red Rag," *World*, May 22, 1878, repr. in James McNeill Whistler, *The Gentle Art of Making Enemies* (1892; London: Dover, 1967), 126–28.
25. Letter from James McNeill Whistler to Frederick Leyland, November 2, 1872, Library of Congress, manuscripts, Pennell-Whistler coll., PWC 6B/21/3, http://www.whistler.arts.gla.ac.uk/correspondence/people/display/?cid=8794&nameid=Leyland_FD&sr=0&rs=4&surname=Leyland&firstname=Frederick (last consulted in January 2018).
26. Bernhard Sickert, *Whistler* (London: Duckworth, 1908), 32–33.

27. Stéphane Mallarmé, "Lettre à Henri Cazalis," October 30, 1864, in *Correspondance,* ed. Bertrand Marchal (Paris: Gallimard, 1996), 206. "To name an object is to eliminate three-quarters of the poem's pleasure, which is composed of the happiness of discerning it little by little; to suggest it, such is the dream." Stéphane Mallarmé, "Réponse à Jules Huret [*Enquête sur l'évolution littéraire*]," *L'Écho de Paris,* March 14, 1891, repr. in his *Oeuvres complètes,* ed. Bertrand Marchal, 2 vols. (Paris: Gallimard, 2003), 1: 307.
28. James McNeill Whistler, "Mr. Whistler's 'Ten O'Clock,'" repr. in Whistler, *The Gentle Art of Making Enemies,* 135–59.
29. In that sense, Whistler's art for art's sake is consistent with what Clement Greenberg later described as modern art, which is preoccupied with itself and its own medium rather than engaged in a mimetic relationship with reality. As such, it is interesting to contrast the aesthetic "modernism" of the nocturnes with their politically reactionary and antimodern character. See Clement Greenberg, *Modernist Painting* (Washington, DC: Voice of America, 1959).
30. Pyne, *Art and the Higher Life,* 110.
31. Thomas R. Way, *Memories of James McNeill Whistler, the Artist* (London: John Lane, 1912), 14.
32. Otto Bacher, *With Whistler in Venice* (New York: Century, 1909), 31.
33. Frederic Remington, *Journal,* Ogdensburg, Frederic Remington Art Museum, March 24, 1909.
34. Ibid., March 19, 1908.
35. Birge Harrison, "The 'Mood' in Modern Painting," *Art and Progress* 4, no. 9 (July 1913): 1015–20.

CHAPTER 2. THE IMAGE IN CRISIS

1. On this matter, see Robert Slifkin, "James Whistler as the Invisible Man: Anti-Aestheticism and Artistic Vision," *Oxford Art Journal* 29, no. 1 (March 2006): 53–75.
2. Jonathan Crary, *Techniques of the Observer: On Vision and Modernity in the Nineteenth Century* (Cambridge, MA: MIT Press, 1990).
3. "Looking Into the Unseen," *Sacramento Daily Record-Union,* October 25, 1896.
4. François Brunet, *La Naissance de l'idée de photographie* (Paris: Presses Universitaires de France, 2000).
5. On the various stages leading to the creation of photographic film, see ibid., 229 and 275–76; and Lorraine Daston and Peter Galison, "The Image of Objectivity," *Representations* 40 (Autumn 1992): 81–128, special issue, "Seeing Science."
6. Brunet, *La Naissance de l'idée de photographie,* 278.
7. Headlines conveyed scientists' uncertainty in the face of that discovery: "Nature of the X-Rays; Scientists Trying to Learn What They Really Are. Prof. Roentgen's Cautious Theory. May be Due to the Longitudinal Vibration of Ether—European Experts Studying the New Discovery," *New York Times,* February 16, 1896; "Radioactivity Has Dumbfounded Science," *World,* July 5, 1903; "Photographs Reveal Strange Shadow Shapes," *Washington Post,* March 3, 1907.
8. In her account of 1895 as the year of the "split image," Monique Sicard concludes that a certain notion of scientific progress as linear and uninterrupted had become obsolete: "Paradoxically, the opacity of the world was gaining strength: scholars and scientists were no longer unaware that the universe will always partly escape cognition." *L'Année 1895: L'image écartelée entre voir et savoir* (Le Plessis-Robinson: Synthélabo, 1994), 18.
9. Newspaper clipping, *New York Evening Journal,* December 1, 1903 William J. Hammer papers, Smithsonian National Museum of American History, Washington, D.C.
10. Henry Adams, "The Dynamo and the Virgin," in his *Education of Henry Adams* (Boston: Houghton Mifflin, 1918), 382–83.
11. Ibid.
12. Ibid.
13. The following remarks take up and expand research published in my essay "The *Dynamo and the Virgin*": *Henry* Ossawa Tanner's Religious Nocturnes," in Anna O. Marley, ed., *Henry Ossawa Tanner: Modern Spirit* (Berkeley: University of California Press, 2012), 127–34.
14. See, for example, the portrait he painted of his mother in 1898, which replicates the characteristic pose and sobriety of Whistler's *Arrangement in Black and Grey.*
15. Tanner was invited to present a paper on the role of African Americans in the fine arts at the exposition congress. See Dewey F. Mosby, *Henry O. Tanner* (Philadelphia: Philadelphia Museum of Art, 1991), 91.
16. Joseph Weltzer, "Electric Lamps Fed from Space, and Flames That Do Not Consume," *Harper's Weekly* 35, no. 1803 (July 11, 1891): 524.
17. In his history of spiritualism and the science of the paranormal in the United States, Robert Laurence Moore singles out the example of the telegraph, a technology used to illustrate metaphorically the phenomenon of supernatural communication. See his *In Search of White Crows: Spiritualism, Parapsychology, and American Culture* (Oxford: Oxford University Press, 1977), 22.
18. Clément Cheroux and Andreas Fischer, eds., *Le Troisième Œil: La photographie et l'occulte* (Paris: Gallimard, 2004).
19. "Can Spirits Be Photographed?" *Ogden Standard,* July 17, 1914.
20. Tom Gunning, "Invisible Worlds, Visible Media," in *Brought to Light: Photography and the Invisible, 1840–1900,* ed. Corey Keller (San Francisco: San Francisco Museum of Modern Art, 2008), 51–57.
21. In 1869, during a trial widely followed by the press and the general public, which saw a parade of Mumler's and P. T. Barnum's victims pass through the courtroom, spirit photography was denounced as a dubious medium, at most a source of entertainment. In that case, the circulation of information made possible by photography undermined the scientific value of the spirit photograph. See Michael Leja, "Mumler's Fraudulent Photographs," in *Looking Askance: Skepticism and American Art from Eakins to Duchamp* (Berkeley: University of California Press, 2004), 21–58.
22. David Starr Jordan, "The Sympsychograph: A Study in Impressionist Physics," *Popular Science Monthly* 49 (September 1896): 597–602.
23. David Starr Jordan, "An Almost Too Successful Joke," *Popular Science Monthly* 50 (September 1896): 123–25.
24. Ernest Renan, *Vie de Jésus* (Paris: Michel Lévy Frères, 1863).
25. Tanner, who took Thomas Eakins's classes at the Pennsylvania Academy of the Fine Arts beginning in 1879, was witness to the scandal created by Eakins's hyperrealist *Crucifixion* when it was first exhibited in 1880. See Elizabeth Milroy, "'Consummatum est . . .': A Reassessment of Thomas Eakins's Crucifixion of 1880," *Art Bulletin* 71, no. 2 (June 1989): 269–84.
26. Henry Ossawa Tanner, *And He Vanished Out of Their Sight,* 1897, oil on canvas, 65.4 × 81.3 cm (25 ¾ × 32 in.), private collection.
27. Crary, *Techniques of the Observer,* 98. Crary describes the interest sparked by the phenomenon in Europe and the United States beginning in the 1820s, especially through the invention of optical toys such as the

thaumatrope, the phenakistoscope, and the zootrope. Ibid., 102–7.

28. "Dr. Gabriel's Experiment," *New York Times*, April 13, 1890.
29. "When the Murderer's Photograph Is in His Victim's Eye," *Current Literature* 39, no. 6 (December 1905): 656; "All in the Mind's Eye: That Assassin's Image in the Victim's Retina Is Ascribed to Hypnotism," *Washington Post*, January 27, 1892; L. Ramakers, "Photography of the Interior of the Eye," *Scientific American* 91, no. 25 (December 17, 1904): 435.
30. William James, *Principles of Psychology* (1890; Cambridge, MA: Harvard University Press, 1981), 607.
31. Michel Eugène Chevreul, *De la Loi du contraste simultané des couleurs et de l'assortiment des objets colorés* (Paris: Pitois-Levrault, 1839); Ogden Rood, *Modern Chromatics: With Applications to Art and Industry* (New York: D. Appleton, 1879).
32. Birge Harrison, *Landscape Painting* (New York: Charles Scribner's Sons, 1907), 12.
33. Michael Quick, *George Inness: A Catalogue Raisonné*, 2 vols. (New Brunswick, NJ: Rutgers University Press, 2007); Rachael Z. DeLue, *George Inness and the Science of Landscape* (Chicago: University of Chicago Press, 2005); Adrienne Baxter Bell, *George Inness and the Visionary Landscape* (New York: George Braziller, 2003).
34. Of Inness's students, the painter's son mentioned Carleton Wiggins and Louis C. Tiffany in particular. George Inness Jr., *Life, Art and Letters of George Inness* (New York: Century, 1917), 68.
35. See Bell, *George Inness and the Visionary Landscape*, 151–59.
36. "Art Notes," *Art Review* 1, no. 5 (March 1887): 15.
37. Quick, *George Inness*, 1: 21–22.
38. Ibid., 24. On Inness's affinities with the nocturne aesthetics, see Mark Simpson, ed., *Like Breath on Glass: Whistler, Inness, and the Art of Painting Softly* (New Haven, CT: Yale University Press, 2008).
39. Childe Hassam, letter to Roland Knoedler, March 11, 1917, quoted in Bell, *George Inness and the Visionary Landscape*, 100.
40. George W. Sheldon, "George Inness," *Harper's Weekly* 26 (April 22, 1882): 246.
41. George Inness, quoted in George Calvert, "George Inness: Painter and Personality," *Bulletin of the Art Association of Indianapolis* 13, nos. 5–8 (November 1926): 36.
42. See esp. DeLue, *George Inness and the Science of Landscape*, 59–90 and 171–234.
43. Emanuel Swedenborg, *The Animal Kingdom* (London: West Newberry, 1843).
44. George Inness, "Colors and Their Correspondences," *New Jerusalem Messenger* 13 (November 13, 1867): 78–79, repr. in Sally Promey, "The Ribband of Faith: George Inness, Color Theory, and the Swedenborgian Church," *American Art Journal* 26, nos. 1–2 (1994): 44–65.
45. Promey, "The Ribband of Faith," 47.
46. Inness, "Colors and Their Correspondences," 60.
47. On the construction of Homer as a virile and realistic artist, see Sarah Burns, "Being Big: Winslow Homer and the American Business Spirit," in her *Inventing the Modern Artist: Art and Culture in Gilded Age America* (New Haven, CT: Yale University Press, 1996), 187–220.
48. "Art Notes," *Art Interchange* 26, no. 3 (January 3, 1891): 33.
49. Unidentified press clipping in Nicolai Cikovsky Jr. and Franklin Kelly, *Winslow Homer* (Washington, DC: National Gallery of Art, 1994), 318.
50. William H. Downes, *The Life and Works of Winslow Homer* (Boston: Houghton Mifflin, 1911), 160.
51. Ibid.
52. Web site of the Musée d'Orsay, http://www.musee-orsay.fr/ (last consulted in January 2018).
53. Although that female couple may now seem strange, it was not uncommon at the time to see women—particularly young, unmarried women—dancing together rather than with men. The suspicion of homosexuality may have contributed somewhat to the critics' discomfort but does not explain it altogether.
54. "Some Questions of Art," *New York Sun*, January 25, 1891; quoted in Cikovsky and Kelly, *Winslow Homer*, 318.
55. "The Winslow Homer Pictures," *Art Amateur* 24 (February 1891): 55.
56. "Four Paintings by Homer," *New York Times*, January 16, 1891.
57. "A Boom at Bar Harbor: Real Estate at Maine's Summer Resort," *New York Times*, June 14, 1887; Portland Historical Society, *Mapping Portland, 1690–1900* (Portland, ME: Portland Historical Society, 2000), 3; "Checkley House Hotel," Maine Historical Society, http://www.mainememory.net/artifact/33661/ (last consulted in January 2018).
58. "American-Edison Combination," *New York Times*, August 29, 1885.
59. Winslow Homer, quoted in William Sheldon, "Sketches and Studies," *Art Journal* (April 1880).
60. Downes, *The Life and Works of Winslow Homer*, 173, my emphasis.
61. See, for instance, *Moonlight on the Water*, oil on canvas, 39.85 × 79.8 cm (15 11/16 × 31 7/16 in.), Los Angeles County Museum of Art, Paul Rodman Mabury Collection, and *Summer Night-Dancing by Moonlight*, 1890, oil on canvas, dimensions unknown, private collection, reproduced in Sue Canterbury (ed.), *Noble Dreams & Simple Pleasures: American Masterworks from Minnesota Collections* (Minneapolis: Minneapolis Institute of the Arts, 2009), 6.
62. "Art Notes," *Art Interchange* 26, no. 3 (January 3, 1891): 33.
63. "The Winslow Homer Pictures."
64. W. K. Burton, "Backgrounds and How to Hang Them," *American Journal of Photography* 11 (1890): 358–70.
65. Marta Braun, *Eadweard Muybridge* (London: Reaktion, 2010), 182–237. Michael Leja analyzes the works of the other great realist painter of the period, Thomas Eakins, in their relation to Muybridge's photography. Leja demonstrates that if Eakins's paintings show "disjunctions" introduced by technology and science, Eakins more successfully overcomes the limitations of vision to produce convincing "reality effects." Leja, "Eakins's Reality Effects," in *Looking Askance*, 59-92.
66. See in particular plates 400–404, 406–409 of his 1887 *Animal Locomotion* series. Braun argues that, unlike Étienne-Jules Marey's work, Muybridge's studies responded to both aesthetic and scientific imperatives. The photographer in fact manipulated his results, dwelled on subjects of limited scientific interest merely for aesthetic pleasure, and manifested a desire to model his images on the academic canons of his time. And in *Summer Night*, Homer seems to have shared Muybridge's fondness for the fall of drapery and his fascination with the motion of water. Formally speaking, then, Homer's painting and Muybridge's photos of dancing and water might be a kind of intermediate space, halfway between science and art and expressed in two different media. See Marta Braun, "Muybridge le magnifique," trans. Thierry Gervais and André Gunthert, *Études photographiques* 10 (November 1, 2001), http://etudes photographiques.revues.org/262 (last consulted in January 2018).
67. "It is interesting that in Paris, more than any other city the birthplace of Symbolism, Homer's *A Summer Night* hangs compatibly with Symbolist paintings in

the Musée d'Orsay." Cikovsky and Kelly, *Winslow Homer,* 250–51.

68. On openness as a characteristic of symbolist work, see Dario Gamboni, *Potential Images: Ambiguity and Indeterminacy in Modern Art* (London: Reaktion, 2004).

CHAPTER 3. THE WORK OF ART IN THE AGE OF MECHANICAL REPRODUCTION

1. Reese V. Jenkins, "Technology and the Market: George Eastman and Mass Amateur Photography," *Technology and Culture* 16 (January 1975): 1–19.
2. Tom Gunning, "The Cinema of Attractions: Early Film, Its Spectator and the Avant-Garde," *Wide Angle* 8, nos. 3–4 (Fall 1986): 63–70, reprinted in *Early Cinema: Space, Frame, Narrative,* ed. Thomas Elsaesser (London: British Film Institute, 1990), 56–62.
3. Eileen Bowser, *The Transformation of Cinema, 1907–1915* (Berkeley: University of California Press, 1984), 6.
4. Estelle Jussim, *Visual Communication and the Graphic Arts: Photographic Technologies in the Nineteenth Century* (New York: R. R. Bowker, 1974).
5. Ted Smythe, "The Commercial Press and New Technologies, 1886–1895," in his *Gilded Age Press, 1865–1900* (Westport, CT: Praeger, 2003), 123–49.
6. See, for example, the edition of Frederic Remington's illustrations by Peggy Samuels and Harold Samuels, *Remington: The Complete Prints* (New York: Crown, 1989).
7. Philip Rodney Paulding, "Illustrators and Illustrating," *Munsey's Magazine* 13, no. 2 (May 1895): 151–63; Walt Reed, *The Illustrator in America, 1860–2000* (New York: Harper Collins, 2001). On the relation between the fine arts and illustration, and on the professionalization of illustrators, see also Michelle Bogart, *Artists, Advertising, and the Borders of Art* (Chicago: University of Chicago Press, 1999).
8. Bogart, *Artists, Advertising, and the Borders of Art,* 42.
9. Sidney Fairfield, "The Tyranny of the Pictorial," *Lippincott's Monthly Magazine* (June 1895): 861–64.
10. Charles L. Congdon, "Over-Illustration," *North American Review* 139, no. 336 (November 1884): 480–91.
11. Ibid., 486.
12. Ibid., 483.
13. Samuel D. Warren and Louis D. Brandeis, "The Right to Privacy," *Harvard Law Review* 4, no. 5 (December 15, 1890): 193–220.
14. See, for example, T. J. Jackson Lears, *No Place of Grace: Antimodernism and the Transformation of American Culture, 1880–1920* (Chicago: University of Chicago Press, 1981), 15–16.
15. Walter Benjamin, "A Short History of Photography" (1931), in his *On Photography,* ed.and trans. Esther Leslie (London: Reaktion Books, 2015), n.p.
16. Walter Benjamin, "The Work of Art in the Age of Mechanical Reproduction" (1935), in his *Illuminations,* trans. Harry Zohn (New York: Schocken, 1968), 224 (translation modified).
17. Ibid., 234 (translation modified).
18. Dora M. Morell, "Hermann Dudley Murphy," *Brush and Pencil* 5, no. 2 (November 1899): 55.
19. Letter from Thomas Dewing to Charles Freer, November 16, 1901, archives of the Freer Gallery of Art and Arthur M. Sackler Gallery, Washington, DC.
20. Letter from Dwight Tryon to Charles Freer, June 17, 1895, archives of the Freer Gallery of Art and Arthur M. Sackler Gallery, Washington, DC.
21. I am following here the analyses of Sarah Burns, *Inventing the Modern Artist: Art and Culture in Gilded Age America* (New Haven, CT: Yale University Press, 1996), 296. Burns's book explores in detail the changes in the art market and the rivalries between American painters and illustrators at the turn of the twentieth century.
22. Burns, *Inventing the Modern Artist,* 296.
23. Birge Harrison, *Landscape Painting* (New York: Charles Scribner's Sons, 1909), 207.
24. Kenyon Cox, "William H. Chase, Painter," *Harper's New Monthly* 78 (March 1889): 549–57.
25. Alfred Trumble, "Things of the Time," *Collector* 3, no. 4 (December 15, 1891): 49–50.
26. Ibid.
27. Henry Peter Emerson, *Naturalistic Photography for Students of the Art* (London: Sampson Low, Marston, Searle & Rivington, 1889).
28. Henry Peter Emerson, "Photographing, a Pictorial Art," *Philadelphia Photographer* 23, no. 272 (April 17, 1886): 249–52.
29. Michel Poivert, "Une Photographie dégénérée?" *Études photographiques* 23 (May 15, 2009): 192–206.
30. Emerson, *Naturalistic Photography,* 257.
31. Ibid., 254.
32. Alfred Stieglitz, *Camera Notes* 1, no. 1 (July 1897): 3.
33. Edward Steichen, "Painting and Photography," *Camera Work* 23 (July 1908): 3–5.
34. See also, on the same theme, George Bernard Shaw, "The Unmechanicalness of Photography," *Amateur Photography* 36 (October 9, 1902): 286–89.
35. Edward Steichen, "Ye Fakers," *Camera Work* 1, no. 1 (1903): 48–49.
36. See Jay Bochner, *An American Lens: Scenes from Alfred Stieglitz's New York Secession* (Cambridge, MA: MIT Press, 2005).
37. Alfred Stieglitz, "The Hand Camera: Its Present Importance," *American Annual of Photography* (1897): 18–27.
38. Ibid.
39. Jay Bochner, "The Cost of Aura," in his *American Lens,* 27–31.
40. See Nancy Anderson, ed., *Frederic Remington: The Color of Night* (Washington, DC: National Gallery of Art, 2003). My argument in the following pages owes a lot to the excellent analyses proposed by this exhibition regarding Remington's adaptation to the nocturne and what he borrowed from Whistler.
41. Peggy Samuels and Harold Samuels, *Frederic Remington: A Biography* (New York: Doubleday, 1982), 26–27; Giles Edgerton, "Frederic Remington, Painter and Sculptor: A Pioneer in Distinctive American Art," *Craftsman* 15 (March 1909): 659.
42. Edgerton, "Frederic Remington, Painter and Sculptor," 661.
43. Emerson Hough, "Wild West Faking," *Collier's* 42, no. 13 (December 19, 1908): 18–22. On Remington's construction of his "Western" image, see Alexander Nemerov, "Doing the 'Old America': The Image of the American West, 1880–1920," in William Truettner, ed., *The West as America: Reinterpreting Images of the Frontier, 1820–1920* (Washington, DC: Smithsonian Institution, 1991).
44. "Sketches by Remington," *New York Times,* June 10, 1899.
45. Quoted in Samuels and Samuels, *Remington,* 15.
46. "The Week in Art," *New York Times,* November 11, 1899.
47. Scott A. Shields, "Evening Meditations: Peters and the Mystery of Monterey," in his *Artists at Continent's End: The Monterey Peninsula Art Colony, 1875–1907* (Berkeley: University of California Press, 2006), 65.
48. "Society Views Five Paintings," *San Francisco Call,* December 19, 1902.
49. Alexander Nemerov, *Frederic Remington and Turn-of-the-Century America* (New Haven, CT: Yale University Press, 1995), 44.
50. "A Closed Chapter of Life," *New York Times,* December 23, 1906.
51. "New Remington Paintings," *New York Times,* December 5, 1907.
52. Frederic Remington, *Journal,* Ogdensburg, Frederic Remington Art Museum, December 9, 1909.

53. See, for example, the cover of the *New York Tribune* of July 15, 1920, which consists of a color reproduction of *The Silence of Night*, painted by Johnson in 1919; see also the artist's obituary, published on January 2, 1939, in the *New York Times* ("Frank Tenney Johnson, a Noted Painter").
54. See in particular Nancy Anderson, ed., *Frederic Remington: The Color of Night* (Washington, DC: National Gallery of Art, 2003): 59–71.
55. "Artists in Black and White," *New York Times*, February 7, 1903. See also Estelle Jussim, *Frederic Remington: The Camera and the Old West* (Fort Worth: Amon Carter Museum, 1983), 83.
56. "American Paintings," *New York Times*, April 10, 1890.
57. Remington, *Journal*, March 28, 1908.
58. "Gallery Notes," press clipping inserted into Remington's *Journal*, December 8, 1909.
59. Remington, quoted in Edwin Wildman, "Frederic Remington, the Man," *Outing* 42 (March 1903): 715.
60. See, in particular, the interpretation of *The Eye of the Mind* in Nemerov, *Frederic Remington and Turn-of-the-Century America*, 89.

CHAPTER 4. VISIONS OF THE MIND AND SPIRIT

1. Birge Harrison, *Landscape Painting* (New York: Charles Scribner's Sons, 1909), 171.
2. John Van Dyke, *Art for Art's Sake* (New York: Charles Scribner's Sons, 1893), 34.
3. Sadakichi Hartmann, *The Whistler Book* (Boston: L.C. Page, 1910), 92.
4. Laura Bride Powers, "With Masters of the Brush," *San Francisco Call*, February 12, 1905.
5. Jerome Eddy, *Recollections and Impression of James A. McNeill Whistler* (Philadelphia: Lippincott, 1903), 214.
6. See, for example, David Cleveland, *Intimate Landscapes: Charles Warren Eaton and the Tonalist Movement* (Houston: De Menil Gallery, 2006).
7. Raymond Henniker-Heaton, *An Art Museum: Its Concept and Conduct* (Muskegon: Hackley Art Gallery, 1914), 31.
8. Richard Muther, *The History of Modern Painting* (1896; London: Macmillan, 1907), 13.
9. Frederic Fairchild Sherman, *American Painters of Yesterday and Today* (New York: Priv. Print., 1919), 18.
10. Otto H. Bacher, *With Whistler in Venice* (New York: Century, 1908), 31.
11. Joyce Hill Stoner, "Materials for Immateriality," in *Like Breath on Glass: Whistler, Inness, and the Art of Painting Softly*, ed. Marc Simpson (New Haven, CT: Yale University Press, 2008).
12. Press clipping (*The Echo*), repr. in James McNeill Whistler, *The Gentle Art of Making Enemies* (London: W. Heinemann, 1890), 323.
13. "American Art in Paris and London Exhibitions," *Brush and Pencil* 17, no. 5 (1906): 189.
14. "Art Notes," *Brush and Pencil* 3, no. 5 (February 1899): 314.
15. Birge Harrison, "The 'Mood' in Modern Painting," *Art and Progress* 4, no. 9 (July 1913): 1015.
16. William James, *Principles of Psychology* (1890; Cambridge, MA: Harvard University Press, 1981), 246. On the philosophical role of the notion of the "vague" in James, see William Joseph Gavin, *William James and the Reinstatement of the Vague* (Philadelphia: Temple University Press, 1992).
17. William James, *Principles of Psychology*, 18.
18. In 1902 Frank Podmore published a critical history of modern spiritualism. Half of the first volume was devoted entirely to the American spiritualist movement since the mid-nineteenth century: see his *Modern Spiritualism: A History and Criticism*, 2 vols. (London: Methuen, 1902).
19. James McNeill Whistler, *Nocturne: Blue and Silver—Bognor*, 1872, oil on canvas, 50.17 × 86.04 cm (19.75 × 33.88 in.), Freer Gallery of Art, Washington, DC.
20. Charles Colbert, *Haunted Visions: Spiritualism and American Art* (Philadelphia: University of Pennsylvania Press, 2011), 122. Sarah Burns shows how Whistler himself contributed to that antimaterialistic or spiritualist interpretation of his works: see her "Old Maverick to Old Master: Whistler in the Public Eye in Turn-of-the-Century America," *American Art Journal* 22, no. 1 (Spring 1990): 28–49. See also Kathleen A. Pyne, *Art and the Higher Life: Painting and Evolutionary Thought in Late Nineteenth-Century America* (Austin: University of Texas Press, 1996), 84–134.
21. Charles Caffin, *The Story of American Painting: The Evolution of Painting in America from Colonial Times to the Present* (New York: Frederick A. Stokes, 1907), 296.
22. Christian Brinton, "Whistler from Within," *Munsey's Magazine* 36 (October 1906): 20.
23. On the shift from spiritualism to psychology and the romantic origins of the metaphor, see esp. Terry Castle, *The Female Thermometer: Eighteenth-Century Culture and the Invention of the Uncanny* (Oxford: Oxford University Press, 1995), 174–89.
24. George Beard, *American Nervousness, Its Causes and Consequences: A Supplement to Nervous Exhaustion* (New York: Putnam, 1881); on this subject, see also Tom Lutz, *American Nervousness 1903: An Anecdotal History* (Ithaca, NY: Cornell University Press, 1981).
25. H. Addington Bruce, "Insanity and the Nation," *North American Review* (January 1908): 73.
26. William Dean Howells, *Between the Dark and the Daylight* (New York: Harper and Brothers, 1907).
27. To cite only two examples, there were also popularizing works such as John Bigelow's *The Mystery of Sleep* (New York: Harper's, 1896), which was reissued four times between 1896 and 1905; and Gustavus Hindman Miller's *Ten Thousand Dreams Interpreted: or, What's in a Dream, a Scientific and Practical Exposition* (Chicago: M.A. Donohue, 1901).
28. Henry James, *Portrait of a Lady* (1886; Oxford: Oxford University Press, 2004), 207.
29. William James, *The Varieties of Religious Experience: A Study in Human Nature* (1902; Cambridge, MA: Harvard University Press, 1985), 385.
30. Nathan G. Hale, *Freud and the Americans: The Beginnings of Psychoanalysis in the United States, 1876–1917* (Oxford: Oxford University Press, 1995).
31. J. Mark Baldwin, "Psychology Past and Present," *Princeton Contributions to Psychology* 1 (1896): 6.
32. William James, *Principles of Psychology*, 233.
33. Colbert, who points out the importance of painting in William James's life, calls his psychology a "philosophical tonalism." Colbert, *Haunted Visions*, 150–52.
34. William James, *Principles of Psychology*, 250.
35. Ibid., 220 and 249.
36. Hartmann, *The Whistler Book*, 91.
37. William James, *The Varieties of Religious Experience*, 304.
38. William James, *On Vital Reserves: The Gospel of Relaxation* (New York: H. Holt, 1911), 56–58.
39. On this matter, see Sarah Burns, "Painting as Rest Cure," in her *Inventing the Modern Artist: Art and Culture in Gilded Age America* (New Haven, CT: Yale University Press, 1996), 120–56; Kathleen A. Pyne, "Aesthetic Strategies in the 'Age of Pain': Thomas Dewing and the Art of Life," in her *Art and the Higher Life*, 135–219; Kathleen A. Pyne, "John Twachtman and the Therapeutic

Landscape," in Deborah Chotner, Lisa N. Peters, and Kathleen A. Pyne, *John Twachtman: Connecticut Landscapes* (Washington, DC: National Gallery of Art, 1989), 49–65; and Elizabeth Lee, "Therapeutic Beauty: Abbott Thayer, Antimodernism, and the Fear of Disease," *American Art* 18, no. 3 (Autumn 2004): 32–51.

40. Kenyon Cox, "The Art of Whistler," *Architectural Record* 15 (May 1904): 479, quoted in Burns, "Old Maverick to Old Master," 40.
41. George Moore, *Modern Painting* (1893; London: W. Scott, 1908), 6.
42. Kathleen A. Pyne, "Portrait of a Collector as an Agnostic: Charles Lang Freer and Connoisseurship," *Art Bulletin* 78, no. 1 (March 1996): 75–97.
43. Downes and Robinson, clipping from the *Art Interchange*, mid-1890s quoted in Burns, *Inventing the Modern Artist*, 147.
44. On the "oceanic feeling" elicited by Dewing's landscapes, see Kathleen A. Pyne's *Art and the Higher Life*, 154–57.
45. Christian Brinton, *Modern Artists* (New York: Baker and Taylor, 1908), 111–12.
46. That is the dominant theme, for example, of Charlotte Perkins Gilman's short story "The Yellow Wallpaper," inspired by her own experience of a forced rest cure. The heroine of the story, confined to her bedroom, is ultimately invaded by the yellow of its wallpaper. See Charlotte Perkins Gilman, "The Yellow Wallpaper: A Story" (1892), in her *Yellow Wallpaper and Other Stories* (Mineola, NY: Dover, 1997).
47. Edward A. Ayers, "Color Blindness," *Century Magazine* (April 1907): 885.
48. Van Dyke, *Art for Art's Sake*, 90.
49. Harrison, *Landscape Painting*, 23–24.
50. George Inness, "A Painter on Painting," *Harper's New Monthly Magazine* 56 (February 1878): 458–61.
51. Harrison, "The 'Mood' in Modern Painting," 1020.
52. Pyne, *Art and the Higher Life*. See also Michael Leja's analysis of Helen Abbott Michael's pessimistic interpretation of Claude Monet's art in "Impressionism and Nature's Deceptions" in *Looking Askance: Skepticism and American Art from Eakins to Duchamp* (Berkeley: University of California Press, 2006): 93–123.
53. Alfred Trumble, "Things of the Time," *Collector* 3, no. 4 (December 15, 1891): 70.
54. See, for example, Paul Staiti's interpretation of Winslow Homer's later works: "Winslow Homer and the Drama of Thermodynamics," *American Art* 15, no. 1 (Spring 2001): 10–33.
55. Thomas J. J. See, "The Solar System in the Light of Recent Discoveries," *Atlantic Monthly* 83, no. 498 (April 1899): 464–74.
56. Letter from Herbert Spencer to John Tyndall, in Herbert Spencer and David Duncan, *Life and Letters of Herbert Spencer*, 2 vols. (New York: Appleton, 1908), 2: 104.
57. See also Cynthia Eagle Russett, *The Concept of Equilibrium in American Social Thought* (New Haven, CT: Yale University Press, 1996).
58. Camille Flammarion, "End of the World: Various Ways in Which Our World May Cease to Exist," *New York Tribune*, April 8, 1906.
59. Henry Adams, *A Letter to American Teachers of History* (Baltimore: J. H. Furst, 1910), 203–4; see also Keith R. Burich, "Henry Adams, the Second Law of Thermodynamics, and the Course of History," *Journal of the History of Ideas* 48, no. 3 (September 1987): 467–82.
60. Max Simon Nordau, *Degeneration*, translated from the second German edition (1895; New York: D. Appleton, 2014). On the influence of Nordau's ideas in American culture, see Burns, *Inventing the Modern Artist*, 79–119.
61. Charles Caffin, "The Story of American Painting: French Influence," *American Illustrated Magazine* 41 (March 1906): 590–99.
62. "The Beginning and Growth of Mural Painting in America," *Bookman* 28 (October 1908): 138.
63. Caffin, "The Story of American Painting," 599. On the idea of a feminine sensibility in art and its perceived dangers, see Burns, *Inventing the Modern Artist*, 159–220.
64. Grant Allen, "Woman's Intuition," *Forum* 9 (May 1890): 334, quoted in Burns, *Inventing the Modern Artist*, 170.
65. Allen, "Woman's Intuition," 340.
66. Letter from James McNeill Whistler to Henri Fantin-Latour, September 1867, Library of Congress, manuscripts, Pennell-Whistler collection, PWC 1/33/25, http://www.whistler.arts.gla.ac.uk/correspondence/date/display/?cid=8045&year=1867&month=09&rs=12.
67. Charles Caffin, *American Masters of Painting* (New York: Doubleday, Page, 1909), 47.
68. "Art at Home and Abroad: The Eleventh Exhibition of the Notable 'Ten American Painters,'" *New York Times*, March 29, 1908.
69. Caffin, "The Story of American Painting," 599.
70. Sherman, *American Painters of Yesterday and Today*, 13.
71. Laurence Moore, *In Search of White Crows: Spiritualism, Parapsychology, and American Culture* (Oxford: Oxford University Press, 1977). Moore places the emergence of these figures within the social context of the late nineteenth century, emphasizing especially the level of freedom that the career of medium granted to American women, in a society that otherwise confined them to the roles of wives and mothers subject to the constraints of domestic life.
72. Bailey Van Hook, "'Milk White Angels of Art': Images of Women in Turn-of-the-Century America," *Woman's Art Journal* 11, no. 2 (Autumn 1990): 23–29; Martha Banta, *Imaging American Women: Ideas and Ideals in Cultural History* (New York: Columbia University Press, 1987). On the more explicitly negative aspect of feminine imagery in European art, see Bram Dijkstra, *Idols of Perversity: Fantasies of Feminine Evil in Fin-de-Siècle Culture* (Oxford: Oxford University Press, 1986).
73. Kate Chopin, *The Awakening* (1899; New York: Norton, 1994), 67–68.
74. Cesare Lombroso, *The Man of Genius*, translated from the Italian (London: Walter Scott, 1891), 341.
75. As Sarah Burns has shown, Lombroso's and Nordau's theories on genius and madness had a major impact on American culture and were widely discussed in the mainstream press. See, for example, Aline Gorren, "The New Criticism of Genius," *Atlantic Monthly* 74, no. 446 (December 1894): 794–801; Cesare Lombroso, "Nordau's *Degeneration*, Its Values and Errors," *Century* 50, no. 6 (October 1895): 940–52; Enrico Ferri, "The Delinquent in Art and Literature," *Atlantic Monthly* 80, no. 478 (August 1897): 233–41; "Nordau's *Degeneration*," *New York Times*, March 24, 1895; "Max Nordau's *Degeneration*," *Chicago Daily Tribune*, March 9, 1895; "The Intimate Relation of Genius to Insanity," *New York Times*, March 31, 1907.
76. Sarah Burns, "Dirty Pictures," in her *Painting the Dark Side: Art and the Gothic Imagination in Nineteenth-Century America* (Berkeley: University of California Press, 2004), 221–45.
77. The effect of that technique was to age the paintings in very similar ways, which contributed after the fact to the tendency to compare the two artists. See Abraham A. Davidson, *Ralph Albert Blakelock* (University Park: Pennsylvania State University Press, 1996).
78. I would like to thank Sylvia Yount for our conversation on Blakelock's internment

and concomitant commercial success, and especially for sharing with me her conference paper "Marketing Madness: The Artistic Identity Construction of Albert Blakelock" (1991, College Art Association). See also Abraham A. Davidson, "Art and Insanity, One Case: Blakelock at Middletown," *Smithsonian Studies in American Art* 3, no. 3 (1989): 54–71.

79. Elliott Daingerfield, *Ralph Albert Blakelock* (New York: Priv. Print., 1914), 15.
80. Norman A. Geske, *Beyond Madness: The Art of Ralph Blakelock, 1847–1919* (Lincoln: University of Nebraska Press, 2007).
81. The forgery cases added to the sensational nature of Blakelock's story and were often discussed in the press, including after the artist's death. See, for instance, "Name on Pictures Forged," *New York Times*, December 23, 1903; "Trying to Call Blakelock Back to His Art," *New York Times*, April 2, 1916; "More Bogus Blakelocks," *New York Times*, May 28, 1918; "Bogus Art Not Painted Here," *New York Sun*, June 4, 1918; "Blakelock Paintings, Often Faked, Is Charge," *Evening Star*, August 16, 1923; "Fake Blakelocks Flood Art Market," *New York Times*, January 20, 1928.
82. "$20,000 Is Paid for Blakelock Painting," *New York Times*, February 23, 1916.
83. Harrison, *Landscape Painting*, 167.
84. Ibid., 187.
85. Ibid., 197.
86. Daingerfield, *Ralph Albert Blakelock*, 11.

PART II

1. Harvey L. Jones, *Twilight and Reverie: California Tonalist Painting 1890–1930* (Oakland: Oakland Museum, 1995), 1.
2. For a nuanced view of the ideological commitments of the artists of the Hudson River School, see Angela Miller, *The Empire of the Eye: Landscape Representations and American Cultural Politics, 1825–1875* (Ithaca, NY: Cornell University Press, 1998).
3. On this subject, see Albert Boime, *The Magisterial Gaze* (Washington, DC: Smithsonian Institution, 1991).
4. Rudyard Kipling, "The White Man's Burden: The United States and the Philippine Islands," *McClure's Magazine* 12, no. 4 (February 1899): 290.
5. "Executive Order," proclamation of President McKinley, December 21, 1898, http://www.presidency.ucsb.edu/ws/?pid=69309 (last consulted in January 2018).
6. Snaït B. Gissis analyzes the formation of the concept of race in the eighteenth century and demonstrates that it resulted from the merging of two categories, nature and "society, culture, and civilization." See his "Visualizing 'Race' in the Eighteenth Century," *Historical Studies in the Natural Sciences* 41, no. 1 (Winter 2011): 41–103.
7. Theodore Roosevelt, speech delivered at Oxford University on June 7, 1910, published under the title *Biological Analogies in History* (Oxford: Oxford University Press, 1910), 4.
8. Michael Leja, "Progress and Evolution at the U.S. World's Fairs, 1893–1915," *Nineteenth Century Art Worldwide* 2, no. 2 (Spring 2003), special issue, "The Darwin Effect: Evolution and Nineteenth Century Visual Culture," http://www.19thc-artworldwide.org/spring03/76-spring03/spring03article/221-progress-and-evolution-at-the-us-worlds-fairs-18931915 (last consulted in January 2018).
9. On the ethnic questions at the U.S. world's fairs, see Robert Rydell, *All the World Is a Fair: Visions of Empire at American International Expositions, 1876–1916* (Chicago: University of Chicago Press, 1987).
10. Madison Grant, *The Passing of the Great Race, or, The Racial Basis of European History* (New York: Scribner's 1916).
11. Such is the theme explored in Alan Trachtenberg's *Shades of Hiawatha: Staging Indians, Making Americans, 1880–1930* (New York: Hill and Wang, 2005).
12. Frederick Jackson Turner, "The Significance of the Frontier in American History" (1883), in John Mack Faragher, ed., *Rereading Frederick Jackson Turner: The Significance of the Frontier in American History, and Other Essays* (New Haven, CT: Yale University Press, 1999).
13. Edward S. Curtis, *The North American Indian* (Seattle: E. S. Curtis, 1907–30).
14. Thomas Dixon, *The Clansman* (New York: Doubleday, Page, 1905); D. W. Griffith, *The Birth of a Nation*, Griffith Feature Films, 1915. Alan Trachtenberg compares and contrasts the attitudes of the white American elite toward Indians on one hand and immigrants arriving en masse from southern and eastern Europe on the other, taking care to show how both these groups were ultimately assimilated into American identity, whereas African Americans remained marginalized. Trachtenberg, *Shades of Hiawatha*, xi–xii, 34.

CHAPTER 5. INVERTED LIGHT

1. White studies, developed by historians and literary critics such as Toni Morrison and David Roediger, complements the various disciplines of minority studies by offering an analysis of the dominant (often white and male) point of view. Like these areas of study, white studies is cross-disciplinary, encompassing academic fields from literature to social history to gender studies. Examples of this disciplinary diversity within the field include such works as Grace Elizabeth Hale's *Making Whiteness: The Culture of Segregation in the South, 1890–1940* (New York: Vintage, 1999); Toni Morrison's *Playing in the Dark: Whiteness and the Literary Imagination* (Cambridge, MA: Harvard University Press, 1992; repr. New York: Vintage, 1999); and Martin Berger's *Sight Unseen: Whiteness and American Visual Culture* (Berkeley: University of California Press, 2005).
2. Richard Dyer, *White* (London: Routledge, 1997).
3. The art historian Albert Boime contrasts the formal, even material elements of art to its ideological contents, lamenting that the peculiar blurring of different categories has often been neglected: "There probably never was a time when artists used black without symbolic or ethnic significance." See his *Art of Exclusion: Representing Blacks in the Nineteenth Century* (Washington, DC: Smithsonian Institution Press, 1990), 1–5.
4. Morrison, *Playing in the Dark*. See also Patrick Brantlinger, *Rule of Darkness: British Literature and Imperialism 1830–1914* (Ithaca, NY: Cornell University Press, 1988).
5. On the interactions between image and text, see W. J. T. Mitchell, *Iconology: Image, Text, Ideology* (Chicago: University of Chicago Press, 1986). On the structuring power of metaphor, see George Lakoff and Mark Johnson, *Metaphors We Live By* (Chicago: University of Chicago Press, 1980). For a detailed analysis of the use of metaphor in one instance of imperialist discourse, see Louis A. Perez Jr., *Cuba in the American Imagination: Metaphor and the Imperial Ethos* (Chapel Hill: University of North Carolina Press, 2008).
6. John Van Dyke, *American Painting and Its Tradition* (New York: Charles Scribner's Sons, 1919), 17.
7. John Van Dyke, "Painting at the Fair," *Century Magazine* 48, no. 26 (July 1894): 446.
8. Charles Caffin, *The Story of American Painting: The Evolution of Painting in America from Colonial Times to the Present* (New York: Frederick A. Stokes, 1907), 331–32.
9. Melody Barnett Deusner, "A Network of Associations: Aesthetic Painting and Its

Patrons, 1870–1914" (Ph.D. diss., University of Delaware, 2010).

10. Birge Harrison, "The Future of American Art," *North American Review* 189, no. 638 (January 1909): 26–27.
11. Van Dyke, "Painting at the Fair," 442.
12. Ibid., 446. On the Scandinavian art of the period, see Kirk Varnedoe, *Northern Light: Nordic Art at the Turn of the Century* (New Haven, CT: Yale University Press, 1988).
13. Royal Cortissoz, *Art and Common Sense* (New York: Charles Scribner's Sons, 1913), 71.
14. Birge Harrison, *Landscape Painting* (New York: Charles Scribner's Sons, 1919), 1–3.
15. Ibid., 252–53.
16. See Thomas Cole, "Essay on American Scenery," *American Monthly Magazine* 1 (January 1836), http://thomascole.org/wp-content/uploads/Essay-on-American-Scenery.pdf (last consulted in January 2018).
17. John Muir, *Our National Parks* (Boston: Houghton Mifflin, 1901).
18. "The Color Scheme: Tints of the Pan-American Will Be Symbolical," *Saint Paul Globe,* May 6, 1901; see also C. Y. Turner, "The Color Scheme," in David Gray, ed., *Art Hand-Book: Official Handbook of Architecture and Sculpture and Art Catalogue to the Pan-American Exposition* (Buffalo: David Gray, 1901), 20.
19. Haywood Laudendale, "The Art of Northern Europe," *Brush and Pencil* 14, no. 5 (December 1904): 307–9, 311–15, 317–20.
20. Eunice Tietjens, "Henry O. Tanner," 1914, unpublished, Tanner Papers, Archives of American Art, Washington, DC.
21. On the interrelations between Asian and American art, see Cynthia Mills, Lee Glazer, and Amelia A. Goerlitz, eds., *East-West Interchanges in American Art: A Long and Tumultuous Relationship* (Washington, DC: Smithsonian Institution, 2011).
22. "The Japanese Fine Arts Exhibit at the Columbian Exposition," *Decorator and Furnisher* 24, no. 6 (September 1894): 215.
23. Ernest Fenollosa, *The Masters of Ukioye: A Complete Historical Description of Japanese Paintings and Color Prints of the Genre School* (New York: Knickerbocker, 1896).
24. Frederic J. Haskin, "The 'Yellow Peril' Bogey at Close View," *Salt Lake Herald,* July 30, 1905.
25. On the ambiguous position of Asian artifacts in the eyes of American collectors, see Steven Conn, "Where Is the East?" in his *Do Museums Still Need Objects?* (Philadelphia: University of Pennsylvania Press, 2010), 86–137.
26. Van Dyke, *American Painting and Its Tradition,* 163.
27. Sadakichi Hartmann, *A History of American Art* (Boston: L. C. Page, 1901), 167.
28. Ibid., 158.
29. John Van Dyke, *A Textbook of the History of Painting* (London: Longmans, Green, 1894), 276.
30. Ernest Fenollosa, *East and West* (New York: T. Y. Crowell, 1893), v–vi.
31. Van Dyke, *American Painting and Its Tradition,* 16.
32. David E. Nye, *American Technological Sublime* (Cambridge, MA: MIT Press, 1994), 148.
33. David Conaby, *China under Searchlight* (London: T. Fisher Unwin, 1901); David Newton E. Campbell, *Searchlight on the Panama Canal, or America's Greatest Enterprise* (Baltimore: Baltimore Book, 1909).
34. Rudyard Kipling, "The White Man's Burden: The United States and the Philippine Islands," *McClure's Magazine* 12, no. 4 (February 1899).
35. *Official Catalogue and Guide Book to the Pan-American Exposition* (Buffalo: Charles Ahrhart, 1901): 40–41; Robert Rydell, *All the World Is a Fair: Visions of Empire at American International Expositions, 1876–1916* (Chicago: University of Chicago Press, 1987), 126–53.
36. Randolph Wellford Smith, *Benighted Mexico* (New York: John Lane, 1916): 5.
37. Kenyon Cox, *Winslow Homer* (New York: Priv. Print., 1914), 32.
38. Van Dyke, *American Painting and Its Tradition,* 106.
39. Cox, *Winslow Homer,* 32.
40. "Spanish Awed by Searchlight," *New York Times,* June 15, 1898. See also Admiral Sampson's account of the battle: William T. Sampson, "The Atlantic Fleet in the Spanish War," *Century Magazine* 57, no. 6 (April 1898): 866–913.
41. Randall C. Griffin, *Winslow Homer: An American Vision* (New York: Phaidon, 2006), 187, 205.
42. Nicolai Cikovsky Jr. and Franklin Kelly, *Winslow Homer* (Washington, DC: National Gallery of Art, 1994), 379. On that "modernist" reading of Homer, see the review of Nicolai Cikovsky Jr. and Franklin Kelly's exhibition *Winslow Homer:* Sarah Burns, "Modernizing Winslow Homer," *American Quarterly* 49, no. 3 (September 1997): 615–39.
43. Edwin S. Porter, *Sampson-Schley Controversy* (N.p: Edison Manufacturing, 1901), http://www.loc.gov/item/00694297 (last consulted in January 2018).
44. Significantly, the expression "yellow journalism" refers to another image: that of the "Yellow Kid," a street urchin and hero of one of the first American comic strips, which appeared in the series *Hogan's Alley,* published in the *New York World* between 1894 and 1896.
45. On the historical sources of the anecdote, see J. Campbell, "Not Likely Sent: The Remington-Hearst 'Telegrams,'" *Journalism and Mass Communication Quarterly* 77, no. 2 (June 2000): 405–22.
46. Peter H. Wood, *Weathering the Storm: Inside Winslow Homer's Gulf Stream* (Athens: University of Georgia Press, 2004), 44–47.
47. Amy Kaplan, "Black and Blue on San Juan Hill," in Amy Kaplan and Donald E. Pease, eds., *Cultures of United States Imperialism* (Durham, NC: Duke University Press, 1993), 219–37.
48. Theodore Roosevelt, *The Rough Riders* (New York: Scribner, 1899), 143.
49. Ibid., 81.
50. Ibid., 21.
51. "The Colored Man in Cuba," *New York Times,* January 26, 1899.
52. On this topic, see in particular Kaplan's discussion of race in the movies narrating the Spanish-American War in Cuba as well as in the Philippines to American audiences. Amy Kaplan, "The Birth of an Empire," *PMLA* 114, no. 5 (October 1999): 1068–79.
53. On the racist rhetoric of soap advertising, see Anne McClintock, "Soft-Soaping Empire: Commodity Racism and Imperial Advertising," in *Imperial Leather: Race, Gender and Sexuality on the Colonial Contest* (New York: Routledge, 1995); and Juliann Sivulka, *Stronger than Dirt: A Cultural History of Advertising Personal Hygiene in America, 1875–1940* (Amherst, NY: Humanity, 2001).
54. Dietrich Neumann and Kermit Champa, eds., *Architecture of the Night: The Illuminated Building* (New York: Prestel, 2002), 12.
55. Kipling, "The White Man's Burden."
56. Kenyon Cox, "Searchlight," *Burlington Magazine* 12 (November 1907): 122.
57. Thomas Fleming, *Around the Pan with Uncle Hank: His Trip through the Pan-American Exposition* (New York: Nutshell, 1901).
58. See Carolyn Thomas de la Peña, "'Bleaching the Ethiopian': Desegregating Race and Technology through Early X-Ray Experiments," *Technology and Culture* 47, no. 1 (January 2006): 27–55.

59. Richard J. Powell, introduction to Peter H. Wood and Karen C. Dalton, eds., *Winslow Homer's Images of Blacks: The Civil War and Reconstruction Years* (Austin: University of Texas Press, 1988), 9.
60. John Singleton Copley, *Watson and the Shark*, 1778, oil on canvas, 182.1 × 229.7 cm (71 3/4 × 90 1/2 in.), National Gallery of Art, Washington, DC.
61. Letter from Winslow Homer to Roland Knoedler, February 17, 1902, Archives of American Art, Washington, DC.
62. That is how the American ambassador John Hay described the Cuban conflict in a letter sent to Theodore Roosevelt from London on July 27, 1898. William Roscoe Thayer, *John Hay* (Boston: Houghton Mifflin, 1915), 2:337.
63. Charles Byer, "Pacifying the Moros: American Military Government in the Southern Philippines, 1899–1913," *Military Review* 85, no. 3 (June 2005): 41–45.
64. "Our Flag in the Sulus," *New York Sun*, May 28, 1899.
65. Frank Carpenter, "Human Sacrifice in Mindanao," *St. Louis Republic*, July 8, 1900.
66. "Horrors of Slavery in the Philippines," Washington *Evening Times*, March 8, 1899.
67. Henry O. Dwight, "Uncle Sam's Legacy of Slaves," *Forum* 29 (May 1900): 284.
68. Ibid., 287.
69. Ibid.
70. An article in the *Los Angeles Herald*, for example, described the Spaniards in unflattering terms: "Spaniards . . . shirking their duty like cowards, bunglers, and a perjured, priest-ridden, inferior race" (G. A. Burgess, "Spain's Darkest Hour," *Los Angeles Herald*, July 31, 1898).
71. JoAnne Mancini, "Destructive Creation: The U.S.-Philippine Relationship in American Art," in Mills, Glazer, and Goerlitz, eds., *East-West Exchanges in American Art*, 36–49.
72. Phelps Whitmarsh, "The Sulu Archipelago," *Outlook* 66, no. 10 (November 1900): 578.
73. Hubert Howe Bancroft, *The Book of the Fair* (San Francisco: Bancroft, 1893), 58.
74. "They Do Not Like Royalty," *Herald*, June 25, 1893.
75. Mancini, "Destructive Creation."
76. William Jennings Bryan, "Imperialism" (1900), in *Under Other Flags: Travels, Lectures, Speeches* (Lincoln: Woodruff-Collins, 1904), 305–39.
77. Mark Twain, "To the Person Sitting in Darkness," *North American Review* 531 (February 1901). The expression is a reference to Matthew 4:16: "The people who sat in darkness have seen a great light, And upon those who sat in the region and shadow of death Light has dawned" (NKJV).
78. Twain, "To the Person Sitting in Darkness."
79. Ibid.
80. Thomas Cole, *The Course of Empire: Desolation*, 1836, oil on canvas, 160.7 × 100 cm (63 1/4 × 39 3/8 in.), New-York Historical Society.

CHAPTER 6. VANISHING INDIANS

1. Mathilde Arrivé, "'Utterly Lost'? L'Indien et la photographie à l'épreuve de l'(anti-) modernité dans *The North-American Indian* d'Edward S. Curtis" (Ph.D. thesis, Université Michel de Montaigne-Bordeaux III, 2009).
2. Patrick Brantlinger, *Dark Vanishings: Discourse on the Extinction of Primitive Races, 1800–1930* (Ithaca, NY: Cornell University Press, 2003); on the myth of the vanishing Indian in American culture from the late eighteenth to the nineteenth century, see, in particular, chap. 3, "Vanishing Americans," 44–67. See also Brian W. Dippie, *The Vanishing American: White Attitudes and U.S. Indian Policy* (Middletown, CT: Wesleyan University Press, 1982).
3. Alan Trachtenberg, *Shades of Hiawatha: Staging Indians, Making Americans, 1880–1930* (New York: Hill and Wang, 2005), 193.
4. Ibid., 170–71.
5. On mythology and tradition as factors of national identity for Americans since the nineteenth century, see Michael Kammen, *Mystic Chords of Memory: The Transformation of Tradition in American Culture* (New York: Knopf, 1991).
6. In 1898 Peters found artistic inspiration in the conflict, as Homer would a few years later. The California artist painted the warship *Oregon* meeting up with Sampson's fleet in Key West and chose a nocturnal atmosphere for his rendering. See "Recent Work of the Artists," *San Francisco Call*, September 8, 1898.
7. Joseph K. Dixon, *The Vanishing Race: The Last Great Indian Council* (New York: Doubleday, Page, 1914).
8. Philip Freneau, "The Indian Burying Ground" (1787), quoted in Dippie, *The Vanishing American*, 3.
9. Speech by Chief Seattle, delivered in 1854 and published by Henry A. Smith in the *Seattle Sunday Star* on October 29, 1887. Serious doubt has been cast on the authenticity of the speech, and it is now believed that Smith may have been its author. See Jerry L. Clark, "Thus Spoke Chief Seattle: The Story of an Undocumented Speech," *Prologue Magazine* 18, no. 1 (Spring 1985), http://www.archives.gov/publications/prologue/1985/spring/chief-seattle.html (last consulted in January 2018).
10. On the massacre of Wounded Knee and the Indian extermination policy, see the now-classic work by Dee Brown, *Bury My Heart at Wounded Knee* (New York: Holt, Rinehart, and Winston, 1970); Richard E. Jensen, R. Eli Paul, and John Carter, eds., *Eyewitness at Wounded Knee* (Lincoln: University of Nebraska Press, 1991); and Élise Marienstras, *Wounded Knee ou l'Amérique fin de siècle* (Paris: Complexe, 1992).
11. Marienstras, *Wounded Knee*, 225.
12. *Report on Indians Taxed and Indians Not Taxed in the United States* (Washington, DC: Department of the Interior, 1894), 5.
13. *Collier's* published James Fenimore Cooper's complete works in an illustrated series of 1891, reissued by Putnam in 1896. Scribner's brought out a version illustrated by the illustrator N. C. Wyeth in 1919.
14. Ella Higginson, *The Vanishing Race and Other Poems* (Bellingham, WA: C. M. Sherman, 1911).
15. Edward S. Curtis, "Vanishing Indian Types: The Tribes of the Southwest," *Scribner's Magazine* 39, no. 5 (May 1906): 513–29; Edward S. Curtis, "Vanishing Indian Types: The Tribes of the Northwest Plains," *Scribner's Magazine* 39, no. 6 (June 1906): 657–72; on this subject, see John M. Coward, *The Newspaper Indian: Native American Identity in the Press, 1820–90* (Urbana: University of Illinois Press, 1999).
16. Higginson, *The Vanishing Race*, 5.
17. Edward S. Curtis, *The North American Indian* (Seattle: E. S. Curtis, 1907–1930), vol. 1, pl. 1.
18. Arrivé, "'Utterly Lost'?" 598.
19. The topos even appears in the œuvre of the realist artist Thomas Eakins, who in 1874 painted a *Hiawatha* depicting the hero, shown only in silhouette, bent over his own shadow against the background of a setting sun. Thomas Eakins, *Hiawatha*, about 1874, oil on canvas mounted on a wood panel, 35.7 × 44.6 cm (14 1/8 × 17 5/8 in.), Hirshhorn Museum and Sculpture Garden, Washington, DC.
20. Dixon, *The Vanishing Race, 219.*
21. Dixon, *The Vanishing Race*, 220, 223, 225.
22. Royal Cortissoz, "Frederic Remington: A Painter of American Life," *Scribner's Magazine* 47, no. 22 (February 1910): 181–95.
23. Anonymous critic, press clipping inserted into Frederic Remington's journal,

Ogdensburg, Frederic Remington Art Museum, 1909, December 11, 1909.

24. William Hornaday, *Our Vanishing Wild Life, Its Extermination and Preservation* (New York: Charles Scribner's Sons, 1913), 8.
25. Ibid., 88.
26. Remington's article focuses on feats of "bravery" by the U.S. Army and flippantly mentions his failed visit to the site of the massacre with the burial party, on account of his need for a good breakfast. Despite the partiality of his narrative, Remington must at least have heard striking descriptions of the battlefield from the burial party in question. Frederic Remington, "The Sioux Outbreak in South Dakota," *Harper's Weekly* 35, no. 24 (January 1891): 57–61.
27. Brantlinger, *Dark Vanishings*, 62.
28. Scott A. Shields, *Artists at Continent's End: The Monterey Peninsula Art Colony, 1875–1907* (Berkeley: University of California Press, 2006).
29. Benjamin Madley, *An American Genocide: The United States and the Californian Indian Catastrophe* (New Haven, CT: Yale University Press, 2016).
30. Eloise J. Roorbach, "The Indigenous Art of California: Its Pioneer Spirit and Vigorous Growth," *Craftsman*, August 22, 1912, 490; quoted in Shields, *Artists at Continent's End*, 114.
31. Dolores Estrada, "The Passing of the Spanish in California," *Overland Monthly* 50, no. 2 (July 1907): 28, quoted in Shields, *Artists at Continent's End*, 119.
32. See, for example, Paul Elder, *The Old Spanish Missions of California: An Historical and Descriptive Sketch* (San Francisco: Paul Elder, 1913), http://memory.loc.gov/service/gdc/scd0001/2007/20070807003ol/20070807003ol.pdf (last consulted in January 2018).
33. Lenore Kothe, "Artistic Homes of San Francisco," *San Francisco Call*, January 1, 1911.
34. "The Evolution of the Mud House," *San Francisco Call*, June 25, 1899.
35. On this subject, see Dippie, *The Vanishing American*, 284–90.
36. On the California tonalists' pronounced taste for adobe structures, see also Scott A. Shields, "An Atmosphere of Nostalgia: McCormick and the 'Adobe Painters,'" in his *Artists at Continent's End*, 111–29.
37. "The Evolution of the Mud House."
38. Theodore Roosevelt, *The Winning of the West*, 4 vols. (New York: Putnam, 1889), 3: 309.
39. Ibid., 1:13.
40. Hornaday, *Our Vanishing Wild Life*, 88.
41. Ibid., 234.
42. J. M. Guinn, "The Passing of the Old Pueblo," *Annual Publication of the Historical Society of Southern California and Pioneer Register, Los Angeles* 5, no. 2 (1901): 113–20.
43. Letter from Frederic Remington to his wife, 1900, quoted in Peggy Samuels and Harold Samuels, *Frederic Remington: A Biography* (New York: Doubleday, 1982), 307.
44. "A Few Words from Mr. Remington," *Collier's Weekly* 34, March 18, 1905, 16.
45. Scott A. Shields, *Artists at Continent's End, 114-119*. On that decorative arts movement, which originated in Great Britain, and especially on its antimodern tendencies, aslo see T. J. Jackson Lears, "The Figure of the Artisan: Arts and Crafts Ideology," in his *No Place of Grace: Antimodernism and the Transformation of American Culture, 1880–1920* (Chicago: University of Chicago Press, 1981), 59–96.
46. Hannah Astrup Larsen, "Carmel by the Sea Plans to Hold an Art Exhibition," *San Francisco Call*, April 29, 1907, quoted in Shields, *Artists at Continent's End*, 115.
47. On rural postal delivery, see the online exhibition of the National Postal Museum of the Smithsonian Institution (with a special page devoted to mailboxes), called "Reaching Rural America," http://postalmuseum.si.edu/exhibits/current/customers-and-communities/reaching-rural-america/index.html (last consulted in January 2018).
48. "Odd Photographs," *San Francisco Sunday Call*, November 24, 1907.
49. Louis J. Stellman, *The Vanished Ruin Era: San Francisco's Classic Artistry of Ruin Depicted in Picture and Song* (San Francisco: Paul Elder, 1910), 16–19.
50. Charles Rollo Peters, *Portals of the Past*, 1906. Oil on canvas, 30 × 40 1/4 in. (76.2 × 102.24 cm), private collection, reproduced in Shields, *Artists at Continent's End*, 79.
51. Kathleen Pyne, *Art and the Higher Life: Painting and Evolutionary Thought in Late Nineteenth-Century America* (Austin: University of Texas Press, 1996), chap. 1, "The American Response to Darwinism."
52. Michael Leja analyzes the ideological contradictions underlying the visual depictions of progress at the world's fairs in the United States, particularly through their architecture and carved decorations: "Progress and Evolution at the U.S. World's Fairs, 1893–1915," *Nineteenth Century Art Worldwide* 2, no. 2, special issue, "The Darwin Effect: Evolution and Nineteenth Century Visual Culture" (Spring 2003), http://www.19thc-artworldwide.org/spring03/76-spring03/spring03article/221-progress-and-evolution-at-the-us-worlds-fairs-18931915 (last consulted in January 2018).
53. John Van Dyke, *Nature for Its Own Sake: First Studies in Natural Appearances* (New York: Charles Scribner's Sons, 1898), 210–11.
54. Henry A. Smith, "Chief Seattle's Speech of 1854," *Seattle Sunday Star*, October 29, 1887.
55. Trachtenberg, *Shades of Hiawatha*, 22.
56. For another view on the problematic responses white Americans found to the perceived threats to their identity, see Alexander Nemerov, "Vanishing Americans: Abbott Thayer, Theodore Roosevelt, and the Attraction of Camouflage," *American Art* 11, no. 2 (Summer 1997): 50–81.
57. Lears, *No Place of Grace*, 188. Michael Kammen analyzes the multiple forms taken by that interest in genealogy among Americans at the turn of the twentieth century, he too underscoring the racist and classist dimension of the movement: see his *Mystic Chords of Memory*, 215–28.
58. Trachtenberg, *Shades of Hiawatha*, 256–66.
59. *National American Indian Memorial Groundbreaking Ceremonies Program* (Philadelphia: Wanamaker, 1914), 4.
60. See, for example, the analyses of the figure of prehistoric man in Remington's works, in Alexander Nemerov, "Stirring and Crawling," in his *Frederic Remington and Turn-of-the-Century America* (New Haven, CT: Yale University Press, 1995), 7–52.
61. Jeremiah Curtin, *Creation Myths of Primitive America* (Boston: Little, Brown, 1898).
62. Curtis, *The North American Indian*, xv.
63. On this subject, see William Sharpe, "What's Out There?" in *Frederic Remington*, ed. Nancy Anderson (Washington, DC: National Gallery of Art, 2003), 18–51.
64. Ibid., 68. Frederic Remington, *Shotgun Hospitality*, 1908, oil on canvas, 68.6 × 101.6 cm (27 × 40 in.), Hood Museum of Art, Dartmouth College, Hanover, NH.
65. Frederic Remington, *Against the Sunset*, 1906, oil on canvas, 55.9 × 76.2 cm (22 × 30 in.), private collection.
66. Renée L. Bergland, *The National Uncanny: Indian Ghosts and American Subjects* (Hanover, NH: University Press of New England, 2000).
67. Ibid., 5.
68. Ibid., 161.
69. *Sioux Ghost Dance*, Thomas A. Edison Company, 1894, http://loc.gov/item/00694139 (last consulted in January 2018).

70. James Mooney, *The Ghost Dance Religion and the Sioux Outbreak of 1890* (Washington, DC: Bureau of Ethnology, 1896).
71. Smith, "Chief Seattle's Speech of 1854."
72. James Mooney, "Parallels with Other Systems," in his *Ghost Dance Religion*, 928–48.
73. Frederic W. Morton, "Work of Ralph A. Blakelock," *Brush and Pencil* 9, no. 5 (February 1902): 257–69.
74. Elliott Daingerfield, *Ralph Albert Blakelock* (New York: Priv. Print., 1914), 24.
75. "Dance of the Ghost," *Pittsburg Dispatch*, November 2, 1890.
76. J. A. Mitchell, "Types and People at the Fair," in Francis Davis Millet et al., *Some Artists at the Fair* (New York: Charles Scribner's Sons, 1893), 43–44.
77. H. H. Van Meter, *The Vanishing Fair* (Chicago: Literary Art Company, 1894).
78. Frederick Douglass, introduction to Ida B. Wells et al., *The Reason Why the Colored American Is Not in the World's Columbian Exposition*, ed. Robert W. Rydell (1893; Urbana: University of Illinois Press, 1999).
79. Remington, *Journal*, March 26, 1908.

CHAPTER 7. A BLUEBLOOD LANDSCAPE

1. Amy Kaplan, "Black and Blue on San Juan Hill," in *Cultures of United States Imperialism*, ed. Amy Kaplan and Donald E. Pease (Durham, NC: Duke University Press, 1993).
2. The specialist on the subject was Edward Kemble, who provided the illustrations for *Uncle Remus* and *Uncle Tom's Cabin*, but also published explicitly racist collections: *Kemble's Coons* (New York: R. H. Russell and Son, 1897), and *Comical Coons* (New York: R. H. Russell and Son, 1898).
3. "Black Americans in Congress," U.S. Congress Web site, http://history.house.gov/Exhibitions-and-Publications/BAIC/Black-Americans-in-Congress/ (last consulted in January 2018).
4. *Thirty Years of Lynching in the United States, 1889–1919* (New York: National Association for the Advancement of Colored People, 1919).
5. W. E. B. Du Bois, *The Souls of Black Folks* (Chicago: McClurg, 1903), vii.
6. Toni Morrison, "Unspeakable Things Unspoken: The Afro-American Presence in American Literature," *Michigan Quarterly Review* 28, no. 1 (Winter 1989): 1–34.
7. Henry O. Tanner, quoted in William R. Lester, "Henry Ossawa Tanner, Exile for Art's Sake," *Alexander's Magazine* 7, no. 2 (September 15, 1980): 73.
8. Letter from Henry O. Tanner to Eunice Tietjens, May 25, 1914, Henry O. Tanner Papers, Archives of American Art, Washington, DC. See also Albert Boime, "Henry O. Tanner's Subversion of Genre," *Art Bulletin* 75, no. 3 (September 1993): 415–42; Will South, "A Missing Question Mark: The Unknown Henry O. Tanner," *Nineteenth Century Art Worldwide* 8, no. 2 (Autumn 2009), http://www.19thc-artworldwide.org/autumn09/a-missing-question-mark (last consulted in January 2018); Naurice France Woods and George Dimock, "Affirming Blackness: A Rebuttal of Will South's 'A Missing Question Mark: The Unknown Henry O. Tanner,'" *Nineteenth Century Art Worldwide* 8, no. 2 (Autumn 2009), http://www.19thc-artworldwide.org/autumn10/a-rebuttal-to-will-souths-qa-missing-question-mark-the-unknown-henry-ossawa-tannerq (last consulted in January 2018).
9. F. James Davis, *Who Is Black? A Nation's Definition* (University Park: Pennsylvania State University Press, 1991).
10. Lester, "Henry Ossawa Tanner," 70.
11. "Miss Meta V. Warick and Henry O. Tanner," Henry O. Tanner Papers, Archives of American Art, Washington, DC.
12. Alan Braddock, "Painting the World's Christ: Tanner, Hybridity, and the Blood of the Holy Land," *Nineteenth Century Art Worldwide* 6, no. 1 (2007), http://www.19thc-artworldwide.org/spring07/67-autumn04/autumn04article/298-painting-the-worlds-christ-tanner-hybridity-and-the-blood-of-the-holy-land (last consulted in January 2018).
13. Letter from Tanner to Tietjens.
14. On the practice of passing, see Alison Hobbs, *A Chosen Exile: A History of Racial Passing in American Life* (Cambridge, MA: Harvard University Press, 2014).
15. George M. Cohan, *The Man in the Moon Is a Coon* (New York: Howley, Haviland, 1897).
16. *The Moon, the Coon, and the Little Octoroon* (New York: Shapiro, Bernstein, 1903); Mississippi State University, Charles H. Templeton Digital Sheet Music Collection, http://digital.library.msstate.edu/cdm/ref/collections/SheetMusic/id/26087 (last consulted in January 2018).
17. Kate Chopin, "Désirée's Baby" (1893), in her *Complete Novels and Stories* (New York: Literary Classics of the United States, 2002), 242–48.
18. See, for example, Sir Harry H. Johnson, "The Pygmies of the Great Congo Forest," *McClure's Magazine* 18, no. 4 (February 1902): 349–53.
19. "The Color of the Human Skin," *Literary Digest* 18, no. 8 (February 25, 1899): 222.
20. "How to Make Colored People White," *Literary Digest* 18, no. 24 (June 17, 1899): 699–700.
21. Dewey F. Mosby, *Henry O. Tanner* (Philadelphia: Philadelphia Museum of Art, 1991), 168–69 and 136.
22. Braddock, "Painting the World's Christ."
23. Henry O. Tanner, quoted in Lester, "Henry Ossawa Tanner," 73.
24. "Didn't My Lord Deliver Daniel?" in James Weldon Johnson and J. Rosamond Johnson, *The Books of American Negro Spirituals* (1925; New York: DaCapo, 2002), 148.
25. W. T. Lhamon Jr., *Raising Cain: Blackface Performance from Jim Crow to Hip Hop* (Cambridge, MA: Harvard University Press, 1998), 75–76.
26. On photographs of lynching, see James Allen and Hilton Als, eds., *Without Sanctuary: Lynching Photography in America* (Santa Fe: Twin Palms, 2000); Dora Apel, *Imagery of Lynching: Black Men, White Women, and the Mob* (New Brunswick, NJ: Rutgers University Press, 2004); Dora Apel and Shawn Michelle Smith, *Lynching Photographs* (Berkeley: University of California Press, 2008); and Amy Louise Wood, *Lynching and Spectacle: Witnessing Racial Violence in America, 1890–1940* (Chapel Hill: University of North Carolina Press, 2009), esp. chap. 6, 71–112.
27. Jacqueline Goldsby, *A Spectacular Secret: Lynching in American Life and Literature* (Chicago: University of Chicago Press, 2006).
28. Stephen Crane, "The Monster," *Harper's Magazine* 97, no. 579 (August 1898): 343–76.
29. Ibid., 350.
30. See, for example, S. E. F. Rose, *The Ku Klux Klan or Invisible Empire* (New Orleans: L. Graham, 1914).
31. Stewart E. Tolnay and E. M. Beck, *A Festival of Violence: An Analysis of Southern Lynchings, 1882–1930* (Urbana: University of Illinois Press, 1995), 271.
32. Morrison, *Playing in the Dark*, 33.
33. For his *Lynching in the West: 1850–1935* (Durham: Duke University Press, 2006), the contemporary artist Ken Gonzales-Day visited the sites of lynching and photographed the trees from which the victims were hanged, which he considers the last visible monuments preserving the memory of these crimes.
34. Joseph Pennell, *Adventures of an Illustrator Mostly in Following His Authors in America and Europe* (Boston: Little, Brown, 1925), 54.
35. Paul Laurence Dunbar, "The Haunted

Oak," in his *Lyrics of Love and Laughter* (New York: Dodd and Mead, 1903), 153.

36. Abraham Lincoln, "Gettysburg Address" (1863), http://www.loc.gov/exhibits/gettysburg-address/ (last consulted in January 2018).

PART III

1. Upton Sinclair, *The Jungle* (New York: Doubleday, Page, 1906). The cover of the novel's first edition juxtaposes the word "jungle" with an urban panorama composed of tall buildings and industrial smokestacks, similar to the landscape Whistler transformed in his nocturnes.
2. William H. Tolman, *Municipal Reform Movements in the United States* (New York: Fleming H. Revell, 1895), 35. For a detailed statistical study of urban development in the United States during the nineteenth century, see Adna F. Weber, *The Growth of Cities in the Nineteenth Century* (New York: Macmillan, 1899).
3. Lyman Abbott, introduction to *Darkness and Daylight: or, Lights and Shadows of New York Life: A Woman's Pictorial Record of Gospel, Temperance, Mission, and Rescue Work "in His Name,"* ed. Helen Campbell, Thomas Wallace Knox, and Thomas Byrnes (Hartford: A. D. Worthington, 1900), 40, 42.
4. Edward Bellamy, *Looking Backward, 2000 to 1887* (Boston: Houghton Mifflin, 1887).
5. James Gilbert, *Perfect Cities: Chicago's Utopias of 1893* (Chicago: University of Chicago Press, 1993).
6. This, of course, is not exclusively true of American art. T. J. Clark shows that French painting of the Second Empire, though it reflects the influence of Haussmannization on the city, primarily reveals the new relationship that Parisians maintained with their physical and social environment, a relationship he says was dominated by the image: see the chapter "The View from Notre-Dame," in his *Painting of Modern Life: Paris in the Art of Manet and His Followers* (Princeton: Princeton University Press, 1984), 23–78.
7. On nighttime in the major European capitals, see Joachim Schlör, *Nights in the Big Cities: Paris, Berlin, London 1840–1930* (1991), trans. Pierre Gottried Imhoff and Dafyd Rees Roberts (Chicago: University of Chicago Press, 1998); Simone Delattre, *Les Douze Heures noires* (Paris: Albin Michel, 2000); Christopher Otter, *The Victorian Eye: A Political History of Light and Vision in Britain, 1800–1910* (Chicago: University of Chicago Press, 2008).
8. John M. Gillette, *Constructive Rural Sociology* (New York: Sturgis and Walton, 1913), 97, 86.
9. James McNeill Whistler, *Mr. Whistler's Ten O'Clock* (London: Chatto and Windus, 1888), 15.
10. Nathalie Cochoy, *Passante à New York* (Bordeaux: Presses Universitaires de France, 2010), 12.
11. See, in particular, Thomas Bender, *Toward an Urban Vision: Ideas and Institutions in Nineteenth-Century America* (Baltimore: Johns Hopkins University Press, 1982); and Liam Kennedy and Maria Balshaw, eds., *Urban Space and Representation* (London: Pluto, 2000).
12. David Peters Corbett, comparing Sloan's scenes of urban life with the deserted modernist landscapes of the painter Charles Sheeler, attempts to show the unity of the two visions, detecting a certain distance in Sloan and, conversely, a humanization of the urban landscape in Sheeler. See David Peters Corbett, "Ashcan Perspectives," *American Art* 25, no. 1 (Spring 2011): 13–15.
13. In the introduction to her book on the Ashcan School, Rebecca Zurier explains that the school's name was acquired only belatedly and was never accepted by those it was supposed to designate, namely, John Sloan, George Bellows, George Luks, Everett Shinn, and William Glackens, all students of Robert Henri. Nevertheless, because the term reflects these artists' ideological position, I will use it here in preference to the more neutral term for the group, "the Eight," which includes artists less clearly committed to these positions, such as Ernest Lawson. See Rebecca Zurier, *Picturing the City: Urban Vision and the Ashcan School* (Berkeley: University of California Press, 2006); "Eight Independent Painters," *New York Sun*, May 15, 1907.

CHAPTER 8. CONTRAST, CONFRONTATION, AND SPECTACLE

1. Theodore Dreiser, *Sister Carrie* (New York: Doubleday, Page, 1900), 9.
2. Lyman Abbott, introduction to *Darkness and Daylight, Or, Lights and Shadows of New York Life: A Woman's Pictorial Record of Gospel, Temperance, Mission, and Rescue Work "in His Name,"* ed. Helen Campbell, Thomas Wallace Knox, and Thomas Byrnes (Hartford: A. D. Worthington, 1900), 42.
3. On the electrification of American cities, see Wolfgang Schivelbusch, *Disenchanted Night: The Industrialization of Light in the Nineteenth Century*, trans. Angela Davies (Berkeley: University of California Press, 1995); Andreas Bluhm and Louise Lippincott, *Light! The Industrial Age, 1750–1900: Art and Science, Technology and Society* (London: Thames and Hudson, 1999); David E. Nye, *Electrifying America: Social Meanings of a New Technology* (Cambridge, MA: MIT Press, 1990); John A. Jakle, *City Lights: Illuminating the American Night* (Baltimore: Johns Hopkins University Press, 2001).
4. Joachim Schlör, "Digression: In a New Light," in his *Nights in the Big City: Paris, Berlin, London, 1840–1930* (1991), trans. Pierre Gottfried Imhoff and Dafyd Rees Roberts (Chicago: University of Chicago Press, 1998), 57–71.
5. James Fullarton Muirhead, *The Land of Contrasts: A Briton's View of His American Kin* (Leipzig: Baedeker, 1893), 207.
6. Eugène Sue, *Les Mystères de Paris* (1842–43; Paris: Gallimard, 2009).
7. George G. Foster, *New York by Gaslight and Other Urban Sketches* (1850; Berkeley: University of California Press, 1990); Matthew Hale Smith, *Sunshine and Shadow in New York* (Hartford: J. B. Burr, 1868); James Dabney McCabe, *The Secrets of the Great City* (Philadelphia: Jones Brothers, 1868); Edward Crapsey, *The Nether Side of New York, or, The Vice, Crime and Poverty of the Great Metropolis* (New York: Sheldon, 1872); Charles Loring Brace, *The Dangerous Classes of New York , and Twenty Years' Work among Them* (New York: Wynkopp and Hallenbeck, 1872); Edward Savage, *Police Recollections or Boston by Daylight and Gaslight* (Boston: John P. Dale, 1873); James D. McCabe, *New York by Sunlight and Gaslight* (Philadelphia: Hubbard Brothers, 1881); J. W. Buel, *Metropolitan Life Unveiled: The Mysteries and Miseries of America's Great Cities, Embracing New York, Washington City, San Francisco, Salt Lake City, and New Orleans* (San Francisco: A. L. Bancroft, 1882). An online exhibition of the Library Company of Philadelphia gives a detailed presentation of several of these books: "Capitalism by Gaslight: The Shadow Economies of 19th-Century America," http://librarycompany.org/shadoweconomy/index.htm (last consulted in January 2018).
8. The vogue continued after 1890, alternating between a moralistic view marked through and through by religious references (Thomas Dewitt Talmage, *Night Scenes of City Life* [New York: Donohue, Henneberry, 1891]) and a discourse addressed to tourists, particularly those

visiting the big cities that played host to the world's fairs, these texts being the most generously illustrated (*Mysteries and Miseries of Chicago by Day and by Night* [Chicago: Garden City, 1893]). Jack London also produced works in that genre, though he chose London as his field of investigation: see his *People of the Abyss* (New York: Macmillan, 1903).

9. Christopher Otter's interpretations in *The Victorian Eye: A Political History of Light and Vision in Britain, 1800–1910* (Chicago: University of Chicago Press, 2008), take the opposite approach from those inspired by Michel Foucault and Guy Debord, which reduce artificial lighting to surveillance or spectacle. Otter defends the idea that the introduction of artificial lighting generated progressive social and cultural practices. Although surveillance and spectacle provide effective models for understanding certain aspects of representations of the nocturnal city, I shall also draw on the nuances introduced by Otter, in order to avoid too systematic an interpretation.
10. On the social transformations allowed by urban night, see Jacques Rancière's study of popular education in the French working class in the 1830s. Jacques Rancière, *Proletarian Nights: The Workers' Dream in Nineteenth-Century France*, trans. John Dury (London: Verso, 2012).
11. Maxim Gorky, "Boredom," *Independent*, August 8, 1907.
12. Thorstein Veblen, *The Theory of the Leisure Class: An Economic Study of Institutions* (1899; New York: Penguin, 1994).
13. Daniel Burnham, the architect of the World's Columbian Exposition in Chicago, was thus in charge of revising the master plans for Chicago and Washington, D.C., at the turn of the century. Burnham was one of the most important figures in the City Beautiful movement, which championed an architecture inspired by the neoclassical style and the fine arts, as well as a rational and harmonious organization of the city. See William H. Wilson, *The City Beautiful Movement* (Baltimore: Johns Hopkins University Press, 1989).
14. "Editor's Table," *New England Magazine* 16, no. 3 (May 1894): 388.
15. David E. Nye, *American Technological Sublime* (Cambridge, MA: MIT Press, 1994), 147. Whereas the Exposition Universelle de Paris, which Chicago sought to emulate, could project only the equivalent of 1 million candelas, the illumination of Jackson Park exceeded 11.4 million candelas. On electric lighting at the World's Columbian Exposition in Chicago, see Murat Halstead, "Electricity at the Fair," *Cosmopolitan* 15, no. 5 (September 1893): 577–83; "Under the Electric Glare: The First Grand Illumination of the Exposition Grounds," *New York Times*, May 9, 1893; John Patrick Barrett, *Electricity at the Columbian Exposition* (Chicago: Donnelley and Sons, 1894).
16. Halstead, "Electricity at the Fair," 578.
17. On electric lighting during the U.S. world's fairs between 1876 and 1915 see Nye, *Electrifying America*, 37–47.
18. John Kasson, "Reading the City: The Semiotics of Everyday Life," in his *Rudeness and Civility: Manners in Nineteenth-Century Urban America* (New York: Hill and Wang, 1990), 66.
19. Rem Koolhaas, *Delirious New York: A Retroactive Manifesto for Manhattan* (New York: Oxford University Press, 1978), 23.
20. The problem was such that the Tenement Commission of New York City ordered a study of emergency exits and fire escapes in 1900: see Hugh Bonner and Laurence Veiller, *Tenement House Fire Escapes in New York and Brooklyn* (New York: Evening Post Job Printing House, 1900).
21. See Nye, "The Great White Way," in *Electrifying America*, 29–84.
22. Rupert Hughes, *The Real New York* (New York: Smart Set, 1904), 91.
23. Dreiser, *Sister Carrie*, 27.
24. Stephen Crane, *Maggie, a Girl of the Streets* (1893; New York: Norton, 1979), 76–77.
25. William Z. Ripley, "Races in the United States," *Atlantic Monthly* 102, no. 6 (December 1908): 745–59.
26. Thomas Bender, *American Abyss: Savagery and Civilization in the Age of Industry* (Ithaca, NY: Cornell University Press, 2009), 72–73.
27. Jacob Riis, *How the Other Half Lives: Studies among the Tenements of New York*, ed. Hasia R. Diner (1890; New York: Norton, 2010). See also, by the same author, *The Children of the Poor* (New York: Scribner's, 1892) and *The Battle with the Slum* (New York: Macmillan, 1902).
28. Paul Underwood Kellogg, *The Pittsburgh Survey* (New York: Charity Organization Society of the City of New York, 1914). Didier Aubert points out that Lewis Hine signed only slightly more than 80 prints of the 350 that illustrate the book, though Kellogg gives them a preeminent place in its promotion: see Didier Aubert, "Lewis Hine et les images anonymes du Pittsburgh Survey," *Études photographiques* 17 (November 2005): 112–35.
29. On American documentary photography, see Maren Stange, *Symbols of Ideal Life: Social Documentary Photography in America 1890–1950* (Cambridge: Cambridge University Press, 1989).
30. Jane Addams, *Twenty Years at Hull House* (New York: Macmillan, 1910); Louise W. Knight, *Jane Addams: Spirit in Action* (New York: Norton, 2010).
31. On American progressive reformism, see Richard Hofstadter, *The Age of Reform* (New York: Vintage, 1955); Lewis L. Gould, *America in the Progressive Era, 1890–1914* (New York: Longman, 2001); Michael McGheer, *A Fierce Discontent: The Rise and Fall of the Progressive Movement in America, 1870–1920* (Oxford: Oxford University Press, 2005).
32. Jacob Riis, *The Making of an American* (London: Macmillan, 1901), 267.
33. Peter B. Hales, *Silver Cities: Photographing American Urbanization, 1839–1939* (1984; Philadelphia: Temple University Press, 2006), 194.
34. See esp. the two central chapters of Schlör, *Nights in the Big City:* "Night and Security" (71–163) and "Night and Morality" (164–274).
35. Riis, *The Making of an American*, 267.
36. Ibid., 265.
37. In addition to Maren Stange, *Symbols of Ideal Life: Social Documentary Photography in America 1890–1950* (New York: Cambridge University Press, 1989), see Sandra S. Phillips, Simon Baker, Philip Brookman, Marta Gili, Carol Squiers, and Richard B. Woodward, *Exposed: Voyeurism, Surveillance and the Camera* (New Haven, CT: Yale University Press, 2010). The introduction of urban lighting stemmed in large part from these reflections on the control of the city's visible space. On the political investment in light in the nocturnal city, see Schivelbusch, *Disenchanted Night*, 80–114.
38. Otter, *The Victorian Eye*, 54.
39. Rebecca Zurier, *Art for the Masses: A Radical Magazine and Its Graphics, 1911–1917* (Philadelphia: Temple University Press, 1988).
40. For a general survey of the reception given these picturesque spectacles, see, for example, Frank H. Smith, *Art, History, Midway Plaisance and World's Columbian Exposition* (Chicago: Foster Press, 1893); Richard H. Barry, *Snapshots on the Midway at the Pan-American Exposition* (Buffalo: Robert Allen Reid, 1901).
41. For a detailed analysis of women's presence at the 1893 fair, see Meg Armstrong,

"'A Jumble of Foreignness': The Sublime Musayums of Nineteenth-Century Fairs and Expositions," *Cultural Critique* 23 (Winter 1992–93): 199–250.

42. William Z. Ripley examined the question of mixed marriages between different groups of immigrants and between immigrants and native-born Americans, concluding there was an "Anglo-Saxon's burden" "to nourish, uplift, and inspire all these immigrant peoples of Europe [so] that, in due course of time, even if the Anglo-Saxon stock be physically inundated by the engulfing flood, the torch of its civilization and ideals may still continue to illuminate the way." Ripley, "Races in the United States."
43. That was also how Jacob Riis divided up *How the Other Half Lives,* with chapters devoted to "Chinatown" (49–55), "Jew-town" (92–101), and "The Italian in New York" (102–19).
44. *Brentano's Views of the City of Chicago* (New York: Brentano's, 1892, 40.
45. Riis, *How the Other Half Lives,* 67.
46. Henry James, *The American Scene* (New York: Harper's, 1907), 83.
47. Ibid., 201.
48. Postcards of this type were called "hold to light" postcards. http://www.chicagopostcardmuseum.org/glossary_of_postcard_terms.html#H (last consulted January 2018). See also Martin Willoughby, *A History of Postcards: A Pictorial Record from the Turn of the Century to the Present Day* (London: Bracken, 1992), 101–2.
49. Robert Louis Stevenson, *New Arabian Nights* (London: Chatto and Windus, 1882). James Joyce's short story "Araby" (1914) was published at the end of the period studied here. In it, Dublin is seen through the prism of the exotic imagery of the *Thousand and One Nights* (in James Joyce, *Dubliners* [New York: Norton, 2006], 29–37). See Richard van Leeuwen and Ulrich Marzolph, *The Arabian Nights Encyclopedia,* 2 vols. (Santa Barbara: ABC Clio, 2004), 2: 612–13, 710–11.
50. O. Henry, "A Madison Square Arabian Night," in his *Trimmed Lamp, and Other Stories of the Four Million* (New York: Doubleday, Page, 1907), 22–32.
51. Ibid., 25–26.
52. "Street Arabs," in Riis, *How the Other Half Lives,* 196–209.
53. Hasia R. Diner, Jeffrey Shandler, and Beth S. Wenger, eds., *Remembering the Lower East Side: American Jewish Reflections* (Bloomington: Indiana University Press, 2000). Jacob Riis also notes that, among the various communities scattered among New York neighborhoods, the Arabs were clustered on Washington Street (*How the Other Half Lives,* 22).
54. Ernest Ingersoll, "A Ramble at Night," in *Handy Guide to New York City, Brooklyn, Staten Island, and Other Districts* (Chicago: Rand, McNally, 1907), 109–18.
55. In her analysis of the urban picturesque genre in American literature, Carrie Tirado Bramen shows how it functioned as a factor of assimilation, which transformed ethnic and economic divisions within the metropolis into an aesthetic spectacle: "The Urban Picturesque and the Spectacle of Americanization," *American Quarterly* 52, no. 3 (September 2000): 444–77.
56. Edward Said, *Orientalism* (New York: Vintage, 1979), 5–6.
57. On the formation of the urban space under the influence of capitalism, see David Harvey, "Money, Time, Space and the City," in his *Consciousness and the Urban Experience: Studies in the History and Theory of Capitalist Urbanization* (Baltimore: Johns Hopkins University Press, 1985), 1–35.
58. Bender, *American Abyss,* 71.
59. Ibid., 84–90; Alan Trachtenberg, *Shades of Hiawatha: Staging Indians, Making Americans, 1880–1930* (New York: Hill and Wang, 2005), 34.
60. For example, the organizers of the exhibition planned to hand out free watermelons to all African American visitors on that day. On the (non)participation of African Americans at the World's Columbian Exposition in Chicago, see Ida B. Wells, ed., *The Reason Why the Colored American Is Not in the World's Columbian Exposition* (1893; Urbana: University of Illinois Press, 1999), and Christopher R. Reed, *All the World Is Here! Black Presence at White City* (Bloomington: Indiana University Press, 2002).
61. A few exceptions can be noted, such as George Bellows's *Both Members of This Club* (1909, National Gallery of Art, Washington, D.C.), which depicts a boxing match between a white man and the black boxer Joe Gans; and Robert Henri's portrait of the young Willie Gee (1904, Newark Museum).

CHAPTER 9. SHADOW PRESENCES

1. On the visual sociology of cities, see Jerome Krase, "Visualisation du changement urbain," trans. Arjan Kok and Fabio La Rocca, *Sociétés* 95, no. 1 (2007): 65–87, http://www.cairn.info/revue-societes-2007-1-page-65.htm (last consulted in January 2018).
2. Georg Simmel, "Sociology of the Senses" (1903), translated from the German, in Robert E. Park and Ernest W. Burgess, *Introduction to the Science of Sociology* (Chicago: University of Chicago Press, 1921), 656–51.
3. Thorstein Veblen, *The Theory of the Leisure Class: An Economic Study of Institutions* (1899; New York: Penguin, 1994), 87.
4. See esp. Rebecca Zurier, "The Cartoonist's Vision: William Glackens and the Legible City," in her *Picturing the City: Urban Vision and the Ashcan School* (Berkeley: University of California Press, 2006), 181–212.
5. Kevin Lynch, *The Image of the City* (Cambridge, MA: MIT Press, 1960).
6. John Kasson, "Reading the City: The Semiotics of Everyday Life," in his *Rudeness and Civility: Manners in Nineteenth-Century Urban America* (New York: Hill and Wang, 1990).
7. William Dean Howells, *A Hazard of New Fortunes* (1890; New York: New American Library, 1983), 66.
8. Richard Sennett, "The Turmoil of Public Life in the 19th Century," in his *The Fall of Public Man* (Cambridge: Cambridge University Press, 1974), 125–255.
9. Ibid., 20 and 153.
10. Lawrence Frank, *Victorian Detective Fiction and the Nature of Evidence: The Scientific Investigations of Poe, Dickens, and Doyle* (New York: Macmillan, 2003).
11. Sigmund Krausz, *Street Types of Chicago: Character Studies* (Chicago: M. Stern, 1892).
12. On police photography, see Thomas Byrnes, *Professional Criminals of America* (New York: Cassell, 1886).
13. Helen Campbell, Thomas Wallace Knox, and Thomas Byrnes, eds., *Darkness and Daylight, Or, Lights and Shadows of New York Life: A Woman's Pictorial Record of Gospel, Temperance, Mission, and Rescue Work "in His Name"* (Hartford: A. D. Worthington, 1900), x.
14. Zurier notes that, at the turn of the century, crowds and mobs were sufficient in and of themselves to merit an item in the newspaper in her *Picturing the City,* 193.
15. Gerald Stanley Lee, *Crowds, a Moving Picture of Democracy* (Garden City: Doubleday, Page, 1913).
16. "The psychological crowd is a provisional being formed of heterogeneous elements, which for a moment are combined, exactly as the cells which constitute a living body form by their reunion a new being which displays characteristics very different from those possessed by each of the cells

singly." Gustave Le Bon, *The Crowd: A Study of the Popular Mind,* translated from the French (1896; Kitchener, Ont.: Batoche, 2001), 15.

17. Ibid., 40.
18. Mrs. Schuyler Van Rensselaer, "People in New York," *Century Magazine* 49, no. 4 (February 1895): 535–36. On the visual uniformity resulting from the neutralizing effect of dress codes, see Sennett, *The Fall of Public Man,* 161–65.
19. H. G. Wells, *The Future in America: A Search for Realities* (New York: Harper and Brothers, 1906), 38–39, quoted in Zurier, *Picturing the City,* 197.
20. "Control of Crowds an Engineering Problem," *Literary Digest* 40, no. 9 (February 26, 1910): 393.
21. The term "carnivalesque," borrowed from Mikhail Bakhtin, can also be applied to the political context of the scene Sloan describes, since, as in the carnival analyzed by Bakhtin, what is at stake is the celebration of a "dethronement" and a "coronation," in their modern and democratic versions. See Mikhail Bakhtin, "Popular-Festive Forms and Images in Rabelais," in his *Rabelais and His World,* trans. Helene Iswolsky (Bloomington: Indiana University Press, 1984), 196–277.
22. Diary of John Sloan, November 5, 1907, quoted in Zurier, *Picturing the City,* 260.
23. Many articles in the popular press examined the subject. See, for example, Charles Johnston, "Nihilism and Anarchy," *North American Review* 171, no. 5 (September 1900): 302–13; Francis H. Nichols, "The Anarchists in America," *Outlook* 8, no. 28 (August 10, 1901): 859–63; Ray Stannard Baker, "The Reign of Lawlessness," *McClure's Magazine* 23, no. 1 (May 1904): 43–56; Joseph E. Gary, "The Chicago Anarchists of 1886," *Century Magazine* 45 (April 1893): 803–37. See also Ross Barrett, "Painting and Violence at Century's End," in his *Rendering Violence: Riots, Strikes and Upheaval in Nineteenth-Century American Art* (Berkeley: University of California Press, 2014), 127–54.
24. Frederick Winslow Taylor, *The Principles of Scientific Management* (New York: Harper's, 1911).
25. "When the City Amuses Itself," *Harper's Magazine* 118, no. 708 (May 1909): 879.
26. Everett Shinn, *Fleischmann's Bread Line,* 1900, pastel and watercolor on paper, 21.6 × 34.3 cm (8 1/2 × 13 1/2 in.), private collection.
27. In his novel *The Bread Line* (New York: Century, 1900), Albert Bigelow Paine depicts an artist painting a similar scene. On New Year's Eve, when the streets are filled with reveling crowds, the artist finds himself forced to join the line himself.
28. On the silhouette in the Western pictorial tradition, see Victor Stoichita, *Brève histoire de l'ombre* (Geneva: Droz, 2000); William C. Sharpe, *Grasping Shadows: The Dark Side of Literature, Painting, Photography and Film* (Oxford: Oxford University Press, 2017); on occurrences of the silhouette in late nineteenth-century French art, see Nancy Forgione, "'The Shadow Only': Shadow and Silhouette in Late Nineteenth-Century Paris," *Art Bulletin* 1, no. 3 (September 1999): 490–512. Gwendolyn DuBois Shaw questioned silhouettes in relation to racial identity with her work on the recently rediscovered silhouette art of Moses Williams, a slave of the Peale family in the early nineteenth century. Gwendolyn DuBois Shaw, "Moses Williams, Cutter of Profiles: Silhouettes and African American Identity in the Early Republic," *Proceedings of the American Philosophical Society* 149, no. 1 (March 2005): 22–39.
29. Charles Caffin, *Photography as a Fine Art* (New York: Doubleday, Page, 1901), 37.
30. "Hackmen and Their Ways," in *Chicago by Day and Night: The Pleasure Seeker's Guide to the Paris of America* (Chicago: Thompson and Zimmerman, 1892), 134–38.
31. George J. Kneeland, *Commercialized Prostitution in New York* (New York: Century, 1913), 13.
32. Stephen Crane, *Maggie, a Girl of the Streets* (1893; New York: Norton, 1979).
33. Timothy Gilfoyle, introduction to *Journal of the History of Sexuality* 18, no. 3 (September 2009): 359–66. See also Timothy Gilfoyle, *City of Eros: New York City, Prostitution and the Commercialization of Sex, 1790–1920* (New York: Norton, 1992); Elizabeth Alice Clement, *Love for Sale: Courting, Treating, and Prostitution in New York City, 1900–1945* (Chapel Hill: University of North Carolina Press, 2006); Kathy Peiss, *Cheap Amusements: Working Women and Leisure in Turn-of-the-Century New York* (Philadelphia: Temple University Press, 1986); and, for a comparison with France, S. Hollis Clayson, *Painted Love: Prostitution in French Art of the Impressionist Era* (Los Angeles: Getty Research Institute, 2003).
34. J. W. Buel, *Metropolitan Life Unveiled: The Mysteries and Miseries of America's Great Cities, Embracing New York, Washington City, San Francisco, Salt Lake City, and New Orleans* (San Francisco: A. L. Bancroft, 1882), 61–62.
35. Rupert Hughes, *The Real New York* (New York: Smart Set, 1904), 92.
36. Everett Shinn, *Girl on Stage,* 1906, oil on canvas, 25.4 × 30.4 cm (10 × 12 in.), private collection.
37. Kneeland, *Commercialized Prostitution in New York,* 164.
38. Ernest A. Bell, *Fighting the Traffic in Young Girls: War on the White Slave Trade* (Chicago: G. S. Ball, 1910); Jane Addams, "An Analogy," in her *A New Conscience and an Ancient Evil* (New York: Macmillan, 1912), 3–13.
39. Clayson, *Painted Love.*
40. S. Hollis Clayson, "Outsiders: American Painters and Cosmopolitanism in the City of Light, 1870–1914," in *La France dans le regard des États-Unis,* ed. Frédéric Monneyron and Martine Xiberras (Perpignan: Presses Universitaires de Perpignan, 2006), 57–71.
41. John Barrett Kerfoot, "Black Art," *Camera Work* 8 (October 1904), repr. in *Camera Work: A Critical Anthology,* ed. Jonathan Green (New York: Aperture, 1973), 47–49.
42. The exhibition "The Darker Side of Light" held at the National Gallery in Washington, D.C., in 2010 analyzes the culture of privacy in the second half of the nineteenth century through a collection of engravings, relating intimacy to the private space of darkness, but also to the medium of engraving itself. Peter Parshall, ed. *The Darker Side of Light: Arts of Privacy, 1850–1900* (Washington, DC: National Gallery of Art, 2010).

CHAPTER 10. THE URBAN NOCTURNE AND THE REDEFINITION OF THE AMERICAN LANDSCAPE

1. Thomas Bender, *Toward an Urban Vision: Ideas and Institutions in Nineteenth-Century America* (Baltimore: Johns Hopkins University Press, 1982).
2. Ibid., 161–87.
3. Lewis Mumford, *The Brown Decades: A Study of the Arts in America, 1865–1895* (1955; New York: Dover, 1971), 88.
4. Sadakichi Hartmann, "Plea for the Picturesqueness of New York," *Camera Notes* 4 (October 1900): 91–97.
5. William Sharpe, "New York, Night and Cultural Mythmaking: The Nocturne in Photography, 1900–1925," *Smithsonian Studies in American Art* 2, no. 3 (Autumn 1988): 2–21.

6. James B. Carrington, "New York at Night," *Scribner's Magazine* 27, no. 3 (March 1900); 326–36. Carrington published a second series of nocturnal prints of New York in the same magazine in 1918: "Some Night Views of New York," *Scribner's Magazine* 5, no. 3 (March 1918): 293–300.
7. "The Picturesqueness of New York Streets: Illustrated in the Paintings of Birge Harrison," *Craftsman* 13, no. 4 (January 1908): 397–99.
8. Didier Aubert, "Photographie et utopie industrielle: Pittsburgh au début du XXe siècle," *Revue Française d'Études Américaines* 3 (2001): 35.
9. Quoted in Richard Haw, *War of the Brooklyn Bridge: A Visual History* (New York: Routledge, 2008), 77.
10. Didier Aubert, "Photographie et progressisme: *The Pittsburgh Survey*, 1907–1914" (Ph.D. thesis, Université de Lyon 2, 2000), 76.
11. Alan Trachtenberg, *The Incorporation of America: Culture and Society in the Gilded Age* (New York: Hill and Wang, 1982), 115.
12. David E. Nye, *American Technological Sublime* (Cambridge, MA: MIT Press, 1994).
13. Nye makes the taste for the sublime an essential factor, at least as significant as economic and technological factors, in the development of skyscrapers. See ibid., 89.
14. William Dean Howells, *A Hazard of New Fortunes* (1890; New York: New American Library, 1983), 66–67.
15. William Sharpe, *New York Nocturne: The City after Dark in Literature, Painting, and Photography, 1850–1950* (Princeton: Princeton University Press, 2008), 123.
16. Henry James, *The American Scene* (New York: Harper's, 1907), 83.
17. Carrington, "New York at Night," 334.
18. Meir Wigoder, "The 'Solar Eye' of Vision: Emergence of the Skyscraper-Viewer in the Discourse on Heights in New York City, 1890–1920," *Journal of the Society of Architectural Historians* 61, no. 2 (June 2002): 152–69.
19. James, *The American Scene,* 89.
20. "Churches Smothered by Skyscrapers," *New York Tribune,* November 4, 1906.
21. On the regulations established in New York in 1916, see the New York City website: http://www.nyc.gov/html/dcp/html/subcats/zoning.shtml (last consulted in January 2018).
22. "The Church Spire to Be a Thing of the Past," *Los Angeles Herald,* April 29, 1909.
23. Carrington, "New York at Night," 327.
24. Ibid., 326.
25. Sylvester Baxter, "Civic Improvement and Architecture," *Century Magazine* 64, no. 6 (October 1902): 912–21; Hartmann, "A Plea for the Picturesqueness of New York," 97.
26. Hartmann, "A Plea for the Picturesqueness of New York," 95.
27. Charles G. D. Roberts, *New York Nocturnes* (Boston: Lamson, Wolffe, 1898).
28. Alan Trachtenberg, *Brooklyn Bridge, Fact and Symbol* (Chicago: University of Chicago Press, 1967).
29. Montgomery Schuyler, "The Skyscraper Problem," *Scribner's Magazine* 34, no. 2 (August 1903): 256.
30. Edgar Saltus, "The Colossal City," *Munsey's Magazine* 32, no. 6 (March 1905): 789.
31. David E. Nye, *Electrifying America: Social Meanings of a New Technology* (Cambridge, MA: MIT Press, 1990), 60. See particularly Nye's discussion of what he calls the "unintended" electrical sublime in the urban context in his *American Technological Sublime,* 173–98.
32. "The Lighted Wonder of the World," *Saint Paul Globe,* January 3, 1904.
33. Ibid.
34. Ezra Pound, "Patria Mia," *New Age* 11, no. 21 (September 19, 1912): 492.
35. "The Lighted Wonder of the World."
36. The reference to Karl Marx and Friedrich Engels's *Communist Manifesto* is taken from Marshall Berman, *All That Is Solid Melts into Air: The Experience of Modernity* (New York: Penguin, 1982).
37. Trachtenberg, *The Incorporation of America,* 112–21.
38. Ibid., 119.
39. Nye, *American Technological Sublime,* 195–96. In its early days in the 1880s, the Edison Pearl Street power station was the hub of a dense network of electric cables, but they gradually vanished from city dwellers' sight: those of the White City, which served as a testing ground in that domain, were systematically buried. See John Patrick Barrett, *Electricity after the Columbian Exposition* (Chicago: Donnelley and Sons, 1894), 192–205.
40. John W. Breyfogle, "291," *Camera Work* 47 (January 1915), repr. in Green, *Camera Work*, 292.
41. Arthur G. Dove, "291," *Camera Work* 47 (January 1915), repr. in Green, *Camera Work, 292.*
42. For a detailed analysis of the painting, see Marianne Doezema, "The Excavation" in her *George Bellows and Urban America* (New Haven, CT: Yale University Press, 1992), 9–66.
43. Joseph A. Schumpeter, "The Process of Creative Destruction," in his *Capitalism, Socialism and Democracy* (1942; New York: Routledge, 2008), 81–87.
44. Mme Léon Grandin, *A Parisienne in Chicago: Impressions of the World's Columbian Exposition* (1894), trans. Mary Beth Raycraft (Urbana: University of Illinois Press, 2010), xi.
45. James, *The American Scene,* 133.
46. Michael Leja, *Looking Askance: Skepticism and American Art from Eakins to Duchamp* (Berkeley: University of California Press, 2007), 169–71; John F. Kasson, *Amusing the Million: Coney Island at the Turn of the Century* (New York: Hill and Wang, 1978), 71–72; Max Page, *The Creative Destruction of Manhattan, 1900–1940* (Chicago: University of Chicago Press, 1999).
47. H. H. Van Meter, *The Vanishing Fair* (Chicago: Literary Art Company, 1894), 13; Grandin, *A Parisienne in Chicago,* 67–68.

CONCLUSION

1. Cox's reflections concern the historiography of the United States in particular: Michael Cox, "Empire by Denial: The Strange Case of the United States," *International Affairs* 81, no. 1 (January 1, 2005): 15–30.
2. Willard Huntington Wright, "The Paintings of the Metropolitan Museum," *Forum* 54 (November 1915): 529.
3. On the construction of the Armory Show as a key moment in the transition toward modernism, see JoAnne Mancini, *Pre-Modernism: Art-World Change and American Culture from the Civil War to the Armory Show* (Princeton: Princeton University Press, 2005).
4. On this subject, see Erika Doss, "Edward Hopper, *Nighthawks* and Film Noir," *Post-Script: Essays in Film and the Humanities* 2, no. 2 (Winter 1986): 14–36.

Bibliography

PRIMARY SOURCES

Adams, Henry. *A Letter to American Teachers of History.* Baltimore: J. H. Furst, 1910.

——. *The Education of Henry Adams.* Boston: Houghton Mifflin, 1918.

Addams, Jane. *Twenty Years at Hull House.* New York: Macmillan, 1910.

Bacher, Otto H. *With Whistler in Venice.* New York: Century, 1908.

Bancroft, Hubert Howe. *The Book of the Fair.* San Francisco: Bancroft, 1893.

Barrett, John Patrick. *Electricity at the Columbian Exposition.* Chicago: Donnelley and Sons, 1894.

Barry, Richard H. *Snapshots on the Midway at the Pan-American Exposition.* Buffalo: Robert Allen Reid, 1901.

Beard, George. *American Nervousness: Its Causes and Consequences: A Supplement to Nervous Exhaustion.* New York: Putnam, 1881.

Bellamy, Edward. *Looking Backward, 2000 to 1887.* Boston: Houghton Mifflin, 1887.

Bonner, Hugh, and Lawrence Veiller. *Tenement House Fire Escapes in New York and Brooklyn.* New York: Evening Post Job Printing House, 1900.

Brinton, Christian. "Whistler from Within." *Munsey's Magazine* 36 (October 1906): 3–20.

——. *Modern Artists.* New York: Baker and Taylor, 1908.

Bruce, H. Addington. "Insanity and the Nation." *North American Review* (January 1908): 70–79.

Bryan, William Jennings. "Imperialism." 1900. In his *Under Other Flags: Travels, Lectures, Speeches,* 305–39. Lincoln: Woodruff-Collins Printing, 1904.

Caffin, Charles. *Photography as a Fine Art.* New York: Doubleday, Page, 1901.

——. *The Story of American Painting: The Evolution of Painting in America from Colonial Times to the Present.* New York: Frederick A. Stokes, 1907.

——. *American Masters of Painting.* New York: Doubleday, Page, 1909.

Calvert, George. "George Inness: Painter and Personality." *Bulletin of the Art Association of Indianapolis* 13, nos. 5–8 (November 1926): 35–57.

Campbell, Helen, Thomas Wallace Knox, and Thomas Byrnes. *Darkness and Daylight, Or, Lights and Shadows of New York Life.* Hartford: A. D. Worthington, 1900.

Carrington, James B. "New York at Night." *Scribner's Magazine* 27, no. 3 (March 1900): 326–36.

Chopin, Kate. "Désirée's Baby." 1893. In her *Complete Novels and Stories.* New York: Literary Classics of the United States, 2002.

——. *The Awakening.* 1899. New York: Norton, 1994.

Cole, Thomas. "Essay on American Scenery." *American Monthly Magazine* 1 (January 1836), http://www.tc.umn.edu/~danp/rhet8520/winter99/cole.html (last consulted in September 2015).

Congdon, Charles L. "Over-Illustration." *North American Review* 139, no. 336 (November 1884): 480–91.

Cortissoz, Royal. "Frederic Remington: A Painter of American Life." *Scribner's Magazine* 47, no. 22 (February 1910): 181–95.

——. *Art and Common Sense.* New York: Charles Scribner's Sons, 1913.

Cox, Kenyon. "William M. Chase, Painter." *Harper's New Monthly* 78 (March 1889): 549–57.

——. *Winslow Homer.* New York: Priv. Print., 1914.

Crane, Stephen. *Maggie, a Girl of the Streets.* 1893. New York: Norton, 1979.

——. "The Monster." *Harper's Magazine* 97, no. 579 (August 1898): 343–76.

Curtin, Jeremiah. *Creation Myths of Primitive America.* Boston: Little, Brown, 1898.

Curtis, Edward S. "Vanishing Indian Types: The Tribes of the Southwest." *Scribner's Magazine* 39, no. 5 (May 1906): 513–29.

——. *The North American Indian.* 20 vols. Seattle: E. S. Curtis, 1907–30.

Daingerfield, Elliott. *Ralph Albert Blakelock.* New York: Priv. Print., 1914.

Dixon, Joseph K. *The Vanishing Race: The Last Great Indian Council.* New York: Doubleday, Page, 1914.

Dixon, Thomas. *The Clansman.* New York: Doubleday, Page, 1905.

Downes, William H. *The Life and Works of Winslow Homer.* Boston: Houghton Mifflin, 1911.

Dreiser, Theodore. *Sister Carrie.* New York: Doubleday, Page, 1900.

Du Bois, W. E. B. *The Souls of Black Folks.* Chicago: McClurg, 1903.

Dunbar, Paul Laurence. "The Haunted Oak." In *Lyrics of Love and Laughter.* New York: Dodd and Mead, 1903, 152–56.

Eddy, Jerome. *Recollections and Impressions of James A. McNeill Whistler.* Philadelphia: Lippincott, 1903.

Emerson, Henry Peter. "Photographing, a Pictorial Art." *Philadelphia Photographer* 23, no. 272 (April 17, 1886): 249–52.

——. *Naturalistic Photography for Students of the Art.* London: Sampson Low, Marston, Searle and Rivington, 1889.

Fairfield, Sidney. "The Tyranny of the Pictorial." *Lippincott's Monthly Magazine* (June 1895): 861–64.

Fenollosa, Ernest. *East and West.* New York: T. Y. Crowell, 1893.

——. *The Masters of Ukioye: A Complete Historical Description of Japanese Paintings and Color Prints of the Genre School.* New York: Knickerbocker, 1896.

Gilman, Charlotte Perkins. *Yellow Wallpaper and Other Stories.* 1892. Mineola, NY: Dover, 1997.

Grandin, Mme Léon. *A Parisienne in Chicago: Impressions of the World's Columbian Exposition.* 1894. Translated by Mary Beth Raycraft. Urbana: University of Illinois Press, 2010.

Grant, Madison. *The Passing of The Great Race; or, The Racial Basis of European History.* New York: Scribner's, 1916.

Gray, David, ed. *Art Hand-Book: Official Handbook of Architecture and Sculpture and Art Catalogue to the Pan-American Exposition.* Buffalo: David Gray, 1901.

Griffith, D. W. *The Birth of a Nation.* Griffith Feature Films, 1915.

Halstead, Murat. "Electricity at the Fair." *Cosmopolitan* 15, no. 5 (September 1893): 577–83.

Harrison, Birge. *Landscape Painting.* New York: Charles Scribner's Sons, 1909.

——. "The Future of American Art." *North American Review* 189, no. 638 (January 1909): 26–27.

——. "The 'Mood' in Modern Painting." *Art and Progress* 4, no. 9 (July 1913): 1015–1020.

Hartmann, Sadakichi. "A Plea for the Picturesqueness of New York." *Camera Notes* 4 (October 1900): 91–97.

——. *A History of American Art.* Boston: L. C. Page, 1901.

——. *The Whistler Book.* Boston: L. C. Page, 1910.

Henniker-Heaton, Raymond. *An Art Museum: Its Concept and Conduct.* Muskegon: Hackley Art Gallery, 1914.

Henry, O. "A Madison Square Arabian Night." In his *The Trimmed Lamp, and Other Stories of the Four Million*, 22–32. New York: Doubleday, Page, 1907.

Higginson, Ella. *The Vanishing Race and Other Poems.* Bellingham, WA: C.M. Sherman, 1911.

Hornaday, William. *Our Vanishing Wild Life, Its Extermination and Preservation.* New York: Charles Scribner's Sons, 1913.

Hough, Emerson. "Wild West Faking." *Collier's Magazine* 42, no. 13 (December 19, 1908): 18–22.

Howells, William Dean. *A Hazard of New Fortunes.* 1890. New York: New American Library, 1983.

——. *Between the Dark and the Daylight.* New York: Harper and Brothers, 1907.

Hughes, Rupert. *The Real New York.* New York: Smart Set, 1904.

Huysmans, Joris-Karl. *Certains.* Paris: Tresse et Stock, 1889.

Inness, George. "A Painter on Painting." *Harper's New Monthly Magazine* 56 (February 1878): 458–61.

Inness, George Jr. *Life, Art and Letters of George Inness.* New York: Century, 1917.

James, Henry. *Portrait of a Lady.* 1886. Oxford: Oxford University Press, 2004.

——. *The American Scene.* New York: Harper's, 1907.

——. *The Painter's Eye: Notes and Essays on the Pictorial Arts by Henry James.* Edited by John L. Sweeney. Madison: University of Wisconsin Press, 1956.

James, William. *Principles of Psychology.* 1890. Cambridge, MA: Harvard University Press, 1981.

——. *The Varieties of Religious Experience: A Study in Human Nature.* 1902. Cambridge, MA: Harvard University Press, 1985.

——. *On Vital Reserves: The Gospel of Relaxation.* New York: H. Holt, 1911.

Kellogg, Paul Underwood. *The Pittsburgh Survey.* New York: Charity Organization Society of the City of New York, 1914.

Kerfoot, John Barrett. "Black Art." *Camera Work* 8 (October 1904). Reprinted in *Camera Work: A Critical Anthology*, edited by Jonathan Black. New York: Aperture, 1973, 47–49.

Kipling, Rudyard. "The White Man's Burden: The United States and the Philippine Islands." *McClure's Magazine* 12, no. 4 (February 1899): 290–91.

Kneeland, George J. *Commercialized Prostitution in New York.* New York: Century, 1913.

Krausz, Sigmund. *Street Types of Chicago: Character Studies.* Chicago: M. Stern, 1892.

Laudendale, Haywood. "The Art of Northern Europe." *Brush and Pencil* 14, no. 5 (December 1904): 307–9, 311–15, 317–20.

Le Bon, Gustave. *The Crowd: A Study of the Popular Mind.* Translated from the French. 1896. Kitchener, Ont.: Batoche, 2001.

Lee, Gerald Stanley. *Crowds, a Moving Picture of Democracy.* Garden City: Doubleday, Page, 1913.

Lombroso, Cesare. *The Man of Genius.* Translated from the Italian. 1889. New York: Scribner's, 1891.

Mooney, James. *The Ghost Dance Religion and Sioux Outbreak of 1890.* Washington, DC: Bureau of Ethnology, 1896.

Moore, George. *Modern Painting.* 1893. London: W. Scott, 1908.

Morell, Dora M. "Hermann Dudley Murphy." *Brush and Pencil* 5, no. 2 (November 1899): 55.

Morton, Frederic W. "Work of Ralph A. Blakelock." *Brush and Pencil* 9, no. 5 (February 1902): 257–69.

Muir, John. *Our National Parks.* Boston: Houghton Mifflin, 1901.

Muirhead, James Fullarton. *The Land of Contrasts: A Briton's View of His American Kin.* Leipzig: Baedeker, 1893.

Muther, Richard. *The History of Modern Painting.* 1896. London: Macmillan, 1907.

Nordau, Max. *Degeneration.* Translated by George L. Mosse. 1892. New York: H. Fertig, 1968.

Paine, Albert Bigelow. *The Bread Line.* New York: Century, 1900.

Paulding, Philip Rodney. "Illustrators and Illustrating." *Munsey's Magazine* 13, no. 2 (May 1895): 151–63.

Pennell, Elizabeth Robins, and Joseph Pennell. *The Life of James McNeill Whistler.* Philadelphia: J. B. Lippincott, 1911.

Pound, Ezra. "To Whistler, American." *Poetry: A Magazine in Verse* (October 1912): 7.

Remington, Frederic. *Journal.* Ogdensburg, NY, Frederic Remington Art Museum, 1907–1909.

——. "The Sioux Outbreak in South Dakota." *Harper's Weekly* 35, no. 24 (January 1891): 57, 60–61.

Riis, Jacob. *How the Other Half Lives: Studies among the Tenements of New York.* 1890. Edited by Hasia R. Diner. New York: Norton, 2010.

——. *The Making of an American.* London: Macmillan, 1901.

Roberts, Charles G. D. *New York Nocturnes.* Boston: Lamson, Wolffe, 1898.

Roosevelt, Theodore. *The Winning of the West.* New York: Putnam, 1889.

——. *The Rough Riders.* New York: Scribner, 1899.

Ruge, Clara. "The Tonal School of America." *International Studio* 27, no. 105 (January 27, 1906): 57–68.

Ruskin, John. *Fors Clavigera: Letters to the Workmen and Labourers of Great Britain.* 1871–1884. New York: Greenwood, 1968.
Schuyler, Montgomery. "The Skyscraper Problem." *Scribner's Magazine* 34, no. 2 (August 1903): 253–56.
Shaw, George Bernard. "The Unmechanicalness of Photography." *Amateur Photographer* 36, no. 9 (October 1902): 286–89.
Sheldon, George W. "George Inness." *Harper's Weekly* 26 (April 22, 1882): 244–46.
——. "Sketches and Studies." *Art Journal* 6 (April 1880): 105–9.
Sherman, Frederic Fairchild. *American Painters of Yesterday and Today.* New York: Priv. Print., 1919.
Sickert, Bernhard. *Whistler.* London: Duckworth, 1908.
Sickert, Walter. "The New Life of Whistler." *Fortnightly Review* 90 (December 1, 1908): 1017–1028.
Simmel, Georg. "Sociology of the Senses: Visual Interaction." Translated from the German. In *Introduction to the Science of Sociology,* edited by R. E. Park and Edward E.W. Burgess, 356–61. Chicago: University of Chicago Press, 1921.
Sinclair, Upton. *The Jungle.* New York: Doubleday, Page, 1906.
Smith, Henry A. "Chief Seattle's Speech of 1854." *Seattle Sunday Star,* October 29, 1887.
Starr Jordan, David. "The Sympsychograph: A Study in Impressionist Physics." *Popular Science Monthly* 49 (September 1896): 597–602.
——. "An Almost Too Successful Joke." *Popular Science Monthly* 50 (September 1896): 123–25.
Steichen, Edward. "Ye Fakers." *Camera Work* 1 (1903): 48–49.
——. "Painting and Photography." *Camera Work* 23 (July 1908): 3–5.
Stellman, Louis J. *The Vanished Ruin Era: San Francisco's Classic Artistry of Ruin Depicted in Picture and Song.* San Francisco: Paul Elder, 1910.
Stevenson, Robert Louis. *New Arabian Nights.* London: Chatto and Windus, 1882.
Stieglitz, Alfred. "The Hand Camera: Its Present Importance." *American Annual of Photography* (1897): 18–27.
Swedenborg, Emanuel. *The Animal Kingdom.* London: West Newbery, 1843.
Taylor, Frederick Winslow. *The Principles of Scientific Management.* New York: Harper's, 1911.
Thirty Years of Lynching in the United States, 1889–1918. New York: National Association for the Advancement of Colored People, 1919.
Trumble, Alfred. "Things of the Time." *Collector* 3, no. 15 (December 1891): 49–50.
Turner, Frederick Jackson. "The Significance of the Frontier in American History." 1893. In *Rereading Frederick Jackson Turner: The Significance of the Frontier in American History, and Other Essays,* edited by John Mack Faragher. New Haven: Yale University Press, 1999.
Twain, Mark. "To the Person Sitting in Darkness." *North American Review* 531 (February 1901): 161–76.
Van Dyke, John. *Art for Art's Sake.* New York: Charles Scribner's Sons, 1893.
——. *A Textbook of the History of Painting.* London: Longmans, Green, 1894.
——. "Painting at the Fair." *Century Magazine* 48, no. 26 (July 1894): 439-47.
——. *Nature for Its Own Sake: First Studies in Natural Appearances.* New York: Charles Scribner's Sons, 1898.
——. "What Is All This Talk about Whistler?" *Ladies' Home Journal* 21 (March 1904): 10.
——. *American Painting and Its Tradition.* New York: Charles Scribner's Sons, 1919.
Van Meter, H. H. *The Vanishing Fair.* Chicago: Literary Art, 1894.
Veblen, Thorstein. *The Theory of the Leisure Class: An Economic Study of Institutions.* 1899. New York: Penguin, 1994.
Warren, Samuel D., and Louis D. Brandeis. "The Right to Privacy." *Harvard Law Review* 4, no. 5 (December 15, 1890): 193–220.
Way, Thomas R. *Memories of James McNeill Whistler, the Artist.* London: John Lane, 1912.
Wells, H. G. *The Future in America: A Search for Realities.* New York: Harper and Brothers, 1906.
Wells, Ida B., ed. *The Reason Why the Colored American Is Not in the World's Columbian Exposition.* 1893. Urbana: University of Illinois Press, 1999.
Weltzer, Joseph. "Electric Lamps Fed from Space, and Flames That Do Not Consume." *Harper's Weekly* 35, no. 1803 (July 11, 1891): 524.
Whistler, James McNeill. *Etchings and Drypoints: Venice, Second Series.* London: Fine Arts Society, 1883.
——. *Mr. Whistler's Ten O'Clock.* London: Chatto and Windus, 1888.
——. *The Gentle Art of Making Enemies.* 1892. London: Dover, 1967.
Wildman, Edwin. "Frederic Remington, the Man." *Outing Magazine* 42 (March 1903): 715–16.

SECONDARY SOURCES

Allen, James, and Hilton Als, eds. *Without Sanctuary: Lynching Photography in America.* Santa Fe: Twin Palms, 2000.
Anderson, Nancy, ed. *Frederic Remington: The Color of Night.* Washington, DC: National Gallery of Art, 2003.
Apel, Dora. *Imagery of Lynching: Black Men, White Women and the Mob.* New Brunswick, NJ: Rutgers University Press, 2004.
Apel, Dora, and Shawn Michelle Smith. *Lynching Photographs.* Berkeley: University of California Press, 2008.
Armstrong, Meg. "'A Jumble of Foreignness': The Sublime Musayums of Nineteenth-Century Fairs and Expositions." *Cultural Critique* 23 (Winter 1992–1993): 199–250.
Arrivé, Mathilde. "'Utterly Lost'? L'Indien et la photographie à l'épreuve de l'(anti-)modernité dans *The North-American Indian* d'Edward S. Curtis." Ph.D. thesis, Université Michel de Montaigne–Bordeaux III, 2009.
Aubert, Didier. "Photographie et progressive: *The Pittsburgh Survey,* 1907–1914." Ph.D. thesis, Université de Lyon 2, 2000.
——. "Lewis Hine et les images anonymes du Pittsburgh Survey." *Études Photographiques* 17 (November 2005): 112–35.
Banta, Martha. *Imaging American Women: Ideas and Ideals in Cultural History.* New York: Columbia University Press, 1987.
Barrett, Ross. "Painting and Violence at Century's End." In his *Rendering Violence: Riots, Strikes and Upheaval in Nineteenth-Century American Art.* Berkeley: University of California Press, 2014, 127–54.
Baxter Bell, Adrienne. *George Inness and the Visionary Landscape.* New York: George Braziller, 2007.
——, ed. *George Inness: Writings and Reflections on Art and Philosophy.* New York: George Braziller, 2006.
Bender, Thomas. *Toward an Urban Vision: Ideas and Institutions in Nineteenth-Century America.* Baltimore: Johns Hopkins University Press, 1982.
——. *American Abyss: Savagery and Civilization in the Age of Industry.* Ithaca, NY: Cornell University Press, 2009.

Benjamin, Walter. "The Work of Art in the Age of Mechanical Reproduction." 1935. In his *Illuminations,* translated by Harry Zohn. New York: Schocken, 1968.

———. "A Short History of Photography." 1931. In his *On Photography,* edited and translated by Esther Leslie. London: Reaktion, 2015.

Berger, Martin. *Sight Unseen: Whiteness and American Visual Culture.* Berkeley: University of California Press, 2005.

Bergland, Renée L. *The National Uncanny: Indian Ghosts and American Subjects.* Hanover, NH: University Press of New England, 2000.

Bluhm, Andreas, and Louise Lippincott. *Light! The Industrial Age, 1750–1900: Art and Science, Technology and Society.* London: Thames and Hudson, 1999.

Bochner, Jay. *An American Lens: Scenes from Alfred Stieglitz's New York Secession.* Cambridge, MA: MIT Press, 2005.

Bogart, Michelle. *Artists, Advertising, and the Borders of Art.* Chicago: University of Chicago Press, 1999.

Boime, Albert. *The Art of Exclusion: Representing Blacks in the Nineteenth Century.* Washington, DC: Smithsonian Institution Press, 1990.

———. *The Magisterial Gaze.* Washington, DC: Smithsonian Institution Press, 1991.

———. "Henry O. Tanner's Subversion of Genre." *Art Bulletin* 75, no. 3 (September 1993): 415–42.

Bowser, Eileen. *The Transformation of Cinema, 1907–1915.* Berkeley: University of California Press, 1984.

Braddock, Alan. "Painting the World's Christ: Tanner, Hybridity, and the Blood of the Holy Land." *Nineteenth Century Art Worldwide* 3, no. 2 (Summer 2004), http://www.19thc-artworldwide.org/index.php/autumn04/298-painting-the-worlds-christ-tanner-hybridity-and-the-blood-of-the-holy-land.

Bramen, Carrie Tirado. "The Urban Picturesque and the Spectacle of Americanization." *American Quarterly* 52, no. 3 (September 2000): 444–77.

Brantlinger, Patrick. *Dark Vanishings: Discourse on the Extinction of Primitive Races, 1800–1930.* Ithaca, NY: Cornell University Press, 2003.

Braun, Marta. "Muybridge le magnifique." Translated by Thierry Gervais and André Gunthert. *Études photographiques* 10 (November 2001), http://etudesphotographiques. revues.org/262

———. *Eadweard Muybridge.* London: Reaktion, 2010.

Brown, Dee. *Bury My Heart at Wounded Knee.* New York: Holt, Rinehart and Winston, 1970.

Brunet, François. *La Naissance de l'idée de photographie.* Paris: Presses Universitaires de France, 2000.

Burich, Keith R. "Henry Adams, the Second Law of Thermodynamics, and the Course of History." *Journal of the History of Ideas* 48, no. 3 (September 1987): 467–82.

Burns, Sarah. "Old Maverick to Old Master: Whistler in the Public Eye in Turn-of-the-Century America." *American Art Journal* 22, no. 1 (Spring 1990): 28–49.

———. *Inventing the Modern Artist: Art and Culture in Gilded Age America.* New Haven: Yale University Press, 1996.

———. "Modernizing Winslow Homer." *American Quarterly* 49, no. 3 (September 1997): 615–39.

———. *Painting the Dark Side: Art and the Gothic Imagination in Nineteenth-Century America.* Berkeley: University of California Press, 2004.

Canterbury, Sue, ed. *Noble Dreams and Simple Pleasures: American Masterworks from Minnesota Collections.* Minneapolis: Minneapolis Institute of the Arts, 2009.

Castle, Terry. *The Female Thermometer: Eighteenth-Century Culture and the Invention of the Uncanny.* Oxford: Oxford University Press, 1995.

Chéroux, Clément, and Andreas Fischer, eds. *Le Troisième Oeil: La photographie et l'occulte.* Paris: Gallimard, 2004.

Chotner, Deborah, Lisa N. Peters, and Kathleen A. Pyne. *John Twachtman: Connecticut Landscapes.* Washington, DC: National Gallery of Art, 1989.

Cikovsky, Nikolai Jr., and Franklin Kelly. *Winslow Homer.* Washington, DC: National Gallery of Art, 1994.

Clayson, S. Hollis. *Painted Love: Prostitution in French Art of the Impressionist Era.* Los Angeles: Getty Research Institute, 2003.

Clement, Elizabeth Alice. *Love for Sale: Courting, Treating, and Prostitution in New York City, 1900–1945.* Chapel Hill: University of North Carolina Press, 2006.

Cleveland, David. *Intimate Landscapes: Charles Warren Eaton and the Tonalist Movement.* Houston: De Menil Gallery, 2006.

Cochoy, Nathalie. *Passante à New York.* Bordeaux: Presses Universitaires de Bordeaux, 2010.

Colbert, Charles. *Haunted Visions: Spiritualism and American Art.* Philadelphia: University of Pennsylvania Press, 2011.

Conn, Steven. *Do Museums Still Need Objects?* Philadelphia: University of Pennsylvania Press, 2010.

Corbett, David Peters. "Ashcan Perspectives." *American Art* 25, no. 1 (Spring 2011): 13–15.

Corn, Wanda. *The Color of Mood: American Tonalism, 1880–1910.* San Francisco: M. H. De Young Museum, 1972.

Crary, Jonathan. *Techniques of the Observer: On Vision and Modernity in the Nineteenth Century.* Cambridge, MA: MIT Press, 1990.

Daston, Lorraine, and Peter Galison. "The Image of Objectivity." *Representations* 40 (Autumn 1992): 81–128. Special issue, "Seeing Science."

Davidson, Abraham A. "Art and Insanity, One Case: Blakelock at Middletown." *Smithsonian Studies in American Art* 3, no. 3 (1989): 54–71.

———. *Ralph Albert Blakelock.* University Park: Pennsylvania State University Press, 1996.

Davis, F. James. *Who Is Black? A Nation's Definition.* University Park: Pennsylvania State University Press, 1991.

Delattre, Simone. *Les Douze Heures noires.* Paris: Albin Michel, 2000.

DeLue, Rachael Z. *George Inness and the Science of Landscape.* Chicago: University of Chicago Press, 2005.

Deusner, Melody Barnett. "A Network of Associations: Aesthetic Painting and Its Patrons, 1870–1914." Ph.D. thesis, University of Delaware, 2010.

Dijkstra, Bram. *Idols of Perversity: Fantasies of Feminine Evil in Fin-de-siècle Culture.* Oxford: Oxford University Press, 1986.

Diner, Hasia R., Jeffrey Shandler, and Beth S. Wenger, eds. *Remembering the Lower East Side: American Jewish Reflections.* Bloomington: Indiana University Press, 2000.

Dippie, Brian W. *The Vanishing American: White Attitudes and U.S. Indian Policy.* Middletown: Wesleyan University Press, 1982.

Doezema, Marianne. *George Bellows and Urban America.* New Haven: Yale University Press, 1992.

Dorment, Richard, and Margaret McDonald, eds. *James McNeill Whistler.* New York: Harry N. Abrams, 1995.

Doss, Erika. "Edward Hopper, *Nighthawks* and Film Noir." *Post-Script: Essays in Film and the Humanities* 2, no. 2 (Winter 1986): 14–36.

DuBois Shaw, Gwendolyn. "'Moses Williams, Cutter of Profiles': Silhouettes and African American Identity in the Early Republic." *Proceedings of the American Philosophical Society* 149, no. 1 (March 2005): 22–39.

Dyer, Richard. *White*. London: Routledge, 1997.

Elcott, Noam M. *Artificial Darkness: An Obscure History of Modern Art and Media*. Chicago: University of Chicago Press, 2016.

Eldredge, Charles C. *American Imagination and Symbolist Painting*. New York: Grey Art Gallery and Study Center, New York University, 1979.

Forgione, Nancy. "'The Shadow Only': Shadow and Silhouette in Late Nineteenth-Century Paris." *Art Bulletin* 81, no. 3 (September 1999): 490–512.

Fine, Ruth E., ed. *James McNeill Whistler: A Reexamination*. Washington, DC: National Gallery of Art, 1987.

Gamboni, Dario. *Potential Images: Ambiguity and Indeterminacy in Modern Art*. London: Reaktion, 2004.

Gavin, William Joseph. *William James and the Reinstatement of the Vague*. Philadelphia: Temple University Press, 1992.

Geske, Norman A. *Beyond Madness: The Art of Ralph Blakelock, 1847–1919*. Lincoln: University of Nebraska Press, 2007.

Gilbert, James. *Perfect Cities: Chicago's Utopias of 1893*. Chicago: University of Chicago Press, 1993.

Gilfoyle, Timothy J. *City of Eros: New York City, Prostitution, and the Commercialization of Sex, 1790–1920*. New York: Norton, 1992.

Goldsby, Jacqueline. *A Spectacular Secret: Lynching in American Life and Literature*. Chicago: University of Chicago Press, 2006.

Griffin, Randall C. *Winslow Homer: An American Vision*. New York: Phaidon, 2006.

Gunning, Tom. "The Cinema of Attractions: Early Film, Its Spectator, and the Avant-Garde." *Wide Angle* 8, no. 3 and 4 (Fall 1986): 63–70. Reprinted in *Early Cinema: Space, Frame, Narrative*, ed. Thomas Elsaesser. London: British Film Institute, 1990.

Hale, Nathan G. *Freud and the Americans: The Beginnings of Psychoanalysis in the United States, 1876–1917*. Oxford: Oxford University Press, 1995.

Hales, Peter B. *Silver Cities: Photographing American Urbanization, 1839–1939*. 1984. Philadelphia, Temple University Press, 2006.

Harris, Neil. *The Land of Contrasts: 1880–1901*. New York: George Braziller, 1970.

——. *The Artist in American Society: The Formative Years*. Chicago: University of Chicago Press, 1982.

Hietala, Thomas. *Manifest Design: American Exceptionalism and Empire*. Ithaca, NY: Cornell University Press, 2002.

Hobbs, Alison. *A Chosen Exile: A History of Racial Passing in American Life*. Cambridge, MA: Harvard University Press, 2014.

Jakle, John A. *City Lights: Illuminating the American Night*. Baltimore: Johns Hopkins University Press, 2001.

Jenkins, Reese V. "Technology and the Market: George Eastman and Mass Amateur Photography." *Technology and Culture* 16 (January 1975): 1–19.

Jones, Harvey L. *Twilight and Reverie: California Tonalist Painting 1890–1930*. Oakland: Oakland Museum, 1995.

Jussim, Estelle. *Visual Communication and the Graphic Arts: Photographic Technologies in the Nineteenth Century*. New York: R. R. Bowker, 1974.

——. *Frederic Remington: The Camera and the Old West*. Fort Worth: Amon Carter Museum, 1983.

Kammen, Michael. *Mystic Chords of Memory: The Transformation of Tradition in American Culture*. New York: Knopf, 1991.

Kaplan, Amy. "The Birth of an Empire." *Publications of the Modern Language Association of America* 114, no. 5 (October 1999): 1068–1079.

Kaplan, Amy, and Donald E. Pease, eds. *Cultures of United States Imperialism*. Durham: Duke University Press, 1993.

Kasson, John F. *Amusing the Million: Coney Island at the Turn of the Century*. New York: Hill and Wang, 1978.

——. *Rudeness and Civility: Manners in Nineteenth-Century Urban America*. New York: Hill and Wang, 1990.

Keller, Corey, ed. *Brought to Light: Photography and the Invisible, 1840–1900*. San Francisco: San Francisco Museum of Modern Art, 2008.

Kennedy, Liam, and Maria Balshaw, eds. *Urban Space and Representation*. London: Pluto, 2000.

Koolhaas, Rem. *Delirious New York: A Retroactive Manifesto for Manhattan*. New York: Oxford University Press, 1978.

Kushner, Marilyn S., Kimberly Orcutt, and Casey Nelson Blake. *The Armory Show at 100: Modernism and Revolution*. New York: New-York Historical Society, 2013.

Lears, T. J. Jackson. *No Place of Grace: Antimodernism and the Transformation of American Culture, 1880–1920*. Chicago: University of Chicago Press, 1981.

Lee, Elizabeth. "Therapeutic Beauty: Abbott Thayer, Antimodernism, and the Fear of Disease." *American Art* 18, no. 3 (Autumn 2004): 32–51.

Leja, Michael. "Progress and Evolution at the U.S. World's Fairs, 1893–1915." *Nineteenth Century Art Worldwide* 2, no. 2 (Spring 2003), http://www.19thc-artworldwide. org/spring03/221-progress-and-evolution-at-the-us-worlds- fairs-18931915.

——. *Looking Askance: Skepticism and American Art from Eakins to Duchamp*. Berkeley: University of California Press, 2004.

Lhamon, W. T. Jr. *Raising Cain: Blackface Performance from Jim Crow to Hip Hop*. Cambridge, MA: Harvard University Press, 1998.

Lutz, Tom. *American Nervousness 1903: An Anecdotal History*. Ithaca, NY: Cornell University Press, 1981.

Madley, Benjamin. *An American Genocide: The United States and the Californian Indian Catastrophe*. New Haven: Yale University Press, 2016.

Mancini, JoAnne. *Pre-Modernism: Art-World Change and American Culture from the Civil War to the Armory Show*. Princeton: Princeton University Press, 2005.

Marienstras, Élise. *Wounded Knee ou l'Amérique fin de siècle*. Paris: Complexe, 1992.

McClintock, Anne. *Imperial Leather: Race, Gender and Sexuality in the Colonial Contest*. New York: Routledge, 1995.

Melbin, Murray. *Night as Frontier: Colonizing the World after Dark*. New York: Free Press, 1987.

Merrill, Linda. *A Pot of Paint: Aesthetics on Trial in Whistler v. Ruskin*. Washington, DC: Smithsonian Institution Press, 1992.

——. ed. *After Whistler: The Artist and His Influence on American Painting*. New Haven: Yale University Press, 2003.

Miller, Angela. *The Empire of the Eye: Landscape Representations and American Cultural Politics, 1825–1875*. Ithaca, NY: Cornell University Press, 1998.

Mills, Cynthia, Lee Glazer, and Amelia A. Goerlitz. *East-West*

Interchanges in American Art: A Long and Tumultuous Relationship. Washington, DC: Smithsonian Institution, 2011.

Mitchell, W. J. T. *Iconology: Image, Text, Ideology.* Chicago: University of Chicago Press, 1986.

Moore, Robert Laurence. *In Search of White Crows: Spiritualism, Parapsychology, and American Culture.* Oxford: Oxford University Press, 1977.

Morrison, Toni. "Unspeakable Things Unspoken: The Afro-American Presence in American Literature." *Michigan Quarterly Review* 28, no. 1 (Winter 1989): 1–34.

——. *Playing in the Dark.* New York: Vintage, 1993.

Mosby, Dewey F. *Henry O. Tanner.* Philadelphia: Philadelphia Museum of Art, 1991.

Mumford, Lewis. *The Brown Decades: A Study of the Arts in America, 1865–1895.* 1955. New York: Dover, 1971.

Myers, Kenneth. *The Artists in American Society: The Formative Years.* Chicago: University of Chicago Press, 1982.

——. *Mr. Whistler's Gallery: Pictures at an 1884 Exhibition.* Washington, DC: Freer Gallery of Art, Smithsonian Institution, 2003.

Nemerov, Alexander. *Frederic Remington and Turn-of-the-Century America.* New Haven: Yale University Press, 1995.

——. "Vanishing Americans: Abbott Thayer, Theodore Roosevelt, and the Attraction of Camouflage." *American Art* 11, no. 2 (Summer 1997): 50–81.

Neumann, Dietrich, and Kermit Champa, eds. *Architecture of the Night: The Illuminated Building.* New York: Prestel, 2002.

Nye, David E. *Electrifying America: Social Meanings of a New Technology.* Cambridge, MA: MIT Press, 1990.

——. *American Technological Sublime.* Cambridge, MA: MIT Press, 1994.

Otter, Christopher. *The Victorian Eye: A Political History of Light and Vision in Britain, 1800–1910.* Chicago: University of Chicago Press, 2008.

Page, Max. *The Creative Destruction of Manhattan, 1900–1940.* Chicago: University of Chicago Press, 1999.

Parshall, Peter, ed. *The Darker Side of Light: Arts of Privacy, 1850–1900.* Washington, D.C.: National Gallery of Art, 2010.

Peiss, Kathy. *Cheap Amusements: Working Women and Leisure in Turn-of-the-Century New York.* Philadelphia: Temple University Press, 1986.

Poivert, Michel. "Une photographie dégénérée?" *Études Photographiques* 23 (May 15, 2009): 192–206.

Promey, Sally. "The Ribband of Faith: George Inness, Color Theory, and the Swedenborgian Church." *American Art Journal* 26, nos. 1–2 (1994): 44–65.

Pyne, Kathleen A. *Art and the Higher Life: Painting and Evolutionary Thought in Late Nineteenth-Century America.* Austin: University of Texas Press, 1996.

——. "Portrait of a Collector as an Agnostic: Charles Lang Freer and Connoisseurship." *Art Bulletin* 78, no. 1 (March 1996): 75–97.

Quick, Michael. *George Inness: A Catalogue Raisonné.* New Brunswick, NJ: Rutgers University Press, 2007.

Raab, Jennifer C. *Frederic Church: The Art and Science of Detail.* New Haven: Yale University Press, 2015.

Rancière, Jacques. *Proletarian Nights: The Workers' Dream in Nineteenth-Century France.* Translated by John Drury. London: Verso, 2012.

Reed, Christopher R. *All the World Is Here! Black Presence at White City.* Bloomington: Indiana University Press, 2002.

Reed, Walt. *The Illustrator in America, 1860–2000.* New York: HarperCollins, 2001.

Rydell, Robert. *All the World Is a Fair: Visions of Empire at American International Expositions, 1876–1916.* Chicago: University of Chicago Press, 1987.

Said, Edward. *Orientalism.* New York: Vintage, 1979.

Samuels, Peggy, and Harold Samuels. *Frederic Remington: A Biography.* New York: Doubleday, 1982.

——. *Remington: The Complete Prints.* New York: Crown, 1989.

Schivelbusch, Wolfgang. *Disenchanted Night: The Industrialization of Light in the Nineteenth Century.* Translated by Angela Davies. Berkeley: University of California Press, 1995.

Schlör, Joachim. *Nights in the Big City: Paris, Berlin, London, 1840–1930.* 1991. Translated by Pierre Gottfried Imhoff and Dafyd Rees Roberts. Chicago: University of Chicago Press, 1998.

Schumpeter, Joseph A. *Capitalism, Socialism and Democracy.* 1942. New York: Routledge, 2006.

Sennett, Richard. *The Fall of Public Man.* Cambridge: Cambridge University Press, 1974.

Sessions, Ralph. *Poetic Vision: American Tonalism.* New York: Spanierman Gallery, 2005.

Sharpe, William. "New York, Night and Cultural Mythmaking: The Nocturne in Photography, 1900–1925." *Smithsonian Studies in American Art* 2, no. 3 (Autumn 1988): 2–21.

——. *New York Nocturne: The City after Dark in Literature, Painting, and Photography, 1850–1950.* Princeton: Princeton University Press, 2008.

——. *Grasping Shadows: The Dark Side of Literature, Painting, Photography, and Film.* Oxford: Oxford University Press, 2017.

Shields, Scott A. *Artists at Continent's End: The Monterey Peninsula Art Colony, 1875–1907.* Berkeley: University of California Press, 2006.

Sicard, Monique. *L'Année 1895: L'image écartelée entre voir et savoir.* Paris: Synthélabo, 1994.

Simpson, Marc, ed. *Like Breath on Glass: Whistler, Inness, and the Art of Painting Softly.* New Haven: Yale University Press, 2008.

Sivulka, Juliann. *Stronger than Dirt: A Cultural History of Advertising Personal Hygiene in America, 1875–1940.* Amherst, NY: Humanity, 2001.

Slifkin, Robert. "James Whistler as the Invisible Man: Anti-Aestheticism and Artistic Vision." *Oxford Art Journal* 29, no. 1 (March 2006): 53–75.

Smythe, Ted C. *The Gilded Age Press, 1865–1900.* Westport, CT: Praeger, 2003.

Staiti, Paul. "Winslow Homer and the Drama of Thermodynamics." *American Art* 15, no. 1 (Spring 2001): 10–33.

Stoichita, Victor. *Brève histoire de l'ombre.* Geneva: Droz, 2000.

Tolman, William H. *Municipal Reform Movements in the United States.* New York: Fleming H. Revell, 1895.

Tolnay, Stewart E., and E. M. Beck. *A Festival of Violence: An Analysis of Southern Lynchings, 1882–1930.* Urbana: University of Illinois Press, 1995.

Trachtenberg, Alan. *Brooklyn Bridge, Fact and Symbol.* Chicago: University of Chicago Press, 1967.

——. *The Incorporation of America: Culture and Society in the Gilded Age.* New York: Hill and Wang, 1982.

——. *Shades of Hiawatha: Staging Indians, Making Americans, 1880–1930.* New York: Hill and Wang, 2005.

Truettner, William, ed. *The West as America: Reinterpreting Images*

of the Frontier, 1820–1920. Washington, DC: Smithsonian Institution, 1991.
Van Hook, Bailey. "'Milk White Angels of Art': Images of Women in Turn-of-the-Century America." *Woman's Art Journal* 11, no. 2 (Autumn 1990): 23–29.
Willoughby, Martin. *A History of Postcards: A Pictorial Record from the Turn of the Century to the Present Day.* London: Bracken, 1992.
Wilner, Eli. *The Gilded Edge: The Art of the Frame.* San Francisco: Chronicle, 2000.
Wood, Amy Louise. *Lynching and Spectacle: Witnessing Racial Violence in America, 1890–1940.* Chapel Hill: University of North Carolina Press, 2009.
Wood, Peter H. *Weathering the Storm: Inside Winslow Homer's Gulf Stream.* Athens: University of Georgia Press, 2004.
Wood, Peter H., and Karen C. Dalton, eds. *Winslow Homer's Images of Blacks: The Civil War and Reconstruction Years.* Austin: University of Texas Press, 1988.
Young, Andrew McLaren, Margaret MacDonald, Robin Spencer, and Hamish Miles. *The Paintings of James McNeill Whistler.* New Haven: Yale University Press, 1980.
Zurier, Rebecca. *Art for the Masses: A Radical Magazine and Its Graphics, 1911–1917.* Philadelphia: Temple University Press, 1988.
——. *Picturing the City: Urban Vision and the Ashcan School.* Berkeley: University of California Press, 2006.

Index

Page numbers in *italics* indicate illustrations.

Illustration Credits

The photographers and the sources of visual material other than the owners indicated in the captions are as follows. Every effort has been made to supply complete and correct credits; if there are errors or omissions, please contact Yale University Press so that corrections can be made in any subsequent edition.

Fig. 3. Copyright © Isabella Stewart Gardner Museum, Boston, MA, USA/Bridgeman Images

Figs. 5, 9. Photo: Erich Lessing/Art Resource, NY

Figs. 7, 125. Photograph copyright © Museum of Fine Arts, Boston

Fig. 10. Bridgeman Images

Fig. 11. Photo: Museo Thyssen-Bornemisza/Scala/Art Resource, NY

Fig. 15. Photo: Hervé Lewandowski. Copyright © RMN-Grand Palais/Art Resource, NY

Fig. 17. Tom Veilleux Gallery, Portland, Maine

Fig. 22. Rich Sanders, Des Moines, Iowa

Figs. 23, 52, 90. Image copyright © Sterling and Francine Clark Art Institute, Williamstown, Massachusetts (photo by Michael Agee)

Figs. 24, 53, 93, 113. Photo copyright © Christie's Images/Bridgeman Images

Figs. 25, 138. Yale University Art Gallery

Fig. 26. Detroit Museum of Art Purchase/Picture Fund/Bridgeman Images

Figs. 36, 91. Photography copyright © Art Institute of Chicago

Figs. 38, 63, 65, 71, 89, 148. Image copyright © Metropolitan Museum of Art. Image source: Art Resource, NY

Fig. 45. Yale University Art Gallery. © 2017 The Estate of Edward Steichen/Artists Rights Society (ARS), New York

Figs. 46, 108, 139, 151. Digital image copyright © Museum of Modern Art/Licensed by SCALA/Art Resource, NY

Fig. 47. Photo: René-Gabriel Ojéda. Copyright © RMN-Grand Palais/Art Resource, NY

Figs. 48, 149: Courtesy George Eastman Museum

Figs. 56, 58, 59, 145. © 2017 The Estate of Edward Steichen/Artists Rights Society (ARS), New York

Figs. 60, 126. Image copyright © Metropolitan Museum of Art. Image source: Art Resource, NY. © 2017 The Estate of Edward Steichen/Artists Rights Society (ARS), New York

Fig. 64. Photo: Addison Gallery of American Art, Phillips Academy, Andover, MA/Art Resource, NY

Fig. 85. Photo: Minneapolis Institute of Art

Figs. 111, 120, 121, 123, 132, 141. © 2017 Delaware Art Museum/Artists Rights Society (ARS), New York

Fig. 128. Copyright © Cleveland Museum of Art

Fig. 131. Photo: SSPL/National Media Museum/Art Resource, NY

Fig. 145. © 2017 The Estate of Edward Steichen/Artists Rights Society (ARS), New York